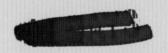

# The New York Times

## BOOK OF

# Medicine

# The New York Times

# BOOK OF

# Medicine

MORE THAN 150 YEARS OF REPORTING
ON THE EVOLUTION OF MEDICINE

*Edited by*
## GINA KOLATA

*Foreword by*
## ABRAHAM VERGHESE

STERLING
New York

STERLING
New York

An Imprint of Sterling Publishing
1166 Avenue of the Americas
New York, NY 10036

ISBN 978-1-4549-0205-8

Distributed in Canada by Sterling Publishing
c/o Canadian Manda Group, 664 Annette Street
Toronto, Ontario, Canada M6S 2C8
Distributed in the United Kingdom by GMC Distribution Services
Castle Place, 166 High Street, Lewes, East Sussex, England BN7 1XU
Distributed in Australia by Capricorn Link (Australia) Pty. Ltd.
P.O. Box 704, Windsor, NSW 2756, Australia

For information about custom editions, special sales,
and premium and corporate purchases, please contact Sterling Special Sales
at 800-805-5489 or specialsales@sterlingpublishing.com.

Manufactured in the United States of America

2 4 6 8 10 9 7 5 3 1

www.sterlingpublishing.com

# CONTENTS

**CHAPTER 18**

# Reproductive Medicine

**CHAPTER 19**

# Surgery

**CHAPTER 20**

# Transplants

**CHAPTER 21**

# Ulcers

**CHAPTER 22:**

# Vaccines

# FOREWORD

I like to remind my interns that what we seem most sure of today, the "evidence-based medicine" we espouse (which by implication suggests that everything before was witchcraft) will in fifty years be viewed as primitive and absurd. An attitude of humility is therefore prudent. But perhaps one has to be humbled first to arrive at this stance.

When I was an intern in America in 1980, there was a palpable sense that medicine had pretty much sorted out all the major puzzles. Many cancers were treatable and even curable, a dizzying array of new antibiotics was coming out, surgeons were doing heroic things through tiny incisions, and transplantation of organs was an industry. The word to describe our attitude in those days was conceit. It was the conceit of *cure*: the sense that there was nothing we couldn't fix. And if we couldn't, it was only because the patient had come too late or the protoplasm was too weak.

Of course that was before AIDS.

I recall *The New York Times* article by Lawrence Altman in July of 1981: "Rare Cancer Seen in 41 Homosexuals." It paralleled reports in the medical journals; these were all harbingers of the epidemic. By that time I'd already decided to pursue a fellowship in infectious diseases in Boston. I had no notion that this one disease—as yet unnamed—would encompass most of what I would do as an infectious disease specialist. I imagined it would be something like Legionnaire's disease or Lyme: a mysterious syndrome at first, but one whose cause would soon be discovered. Then treatment would emerge, and *voila*—it would be a nuisance at best. We could not have imagined AIDS, its magnitude, its scope, and the way it had arrived seemingly from nowhere.

Traveling with the virus was the metaphor it carried, a metaphor of shame and secrecy that was almost as devastating as the disease itself. The metaphor was rooted in those first patients being gay men and intravenous drug users.

The AIDS epidemic changed my career and my life. Among the many things I learned was that when one could not cure, one could *heal*. By that I mean that even in this fatal illness, one could help the patient and the family come to terms with the disease, one could relieve pain and suffering; I learned that healing occurred by one's presence, by caring, by being there for the patient through thick and thin. It was something the horse-and-buggy doctor of a century before understood; even in those pre-antibiotic and pre-vaccine days when scarlet fever and typhoid and tuberculosis were untreatable scourges, the doctor still had much to offer.

It is fitting that this collection of medical reporting and essays from *The New York Times* should begin with AIDS. One sees here the very first report, the first blip of the epidemic's arrival. The reports that follow are the milestones (each unforgettable—I can remember the season and what songs were hot on that new channel, MTV): the finding of the causative virus; the first (much heralded and ultimately disappointing) drug, AZT . . . The last chapter in the AIDS saga is unwritten: a vaccine that prevents the infection, or a treatment that eradicates the virus rather than just keeping it in check. (And lest we think this idea is far-fetched, we have just arrived at that moment with hepatitis C, a terrible scourge for which new drugs offer a complete eradication after a finite course of treatment.)

The art of chronicling the march of medical history, discovery, and the changing landscape of illness is a genre in itself, one that has been a regular feature of *The New York Times* from its inception. Arguably *The Times* defined the genre. We've come to rely on familiar names such as Altman, Kolata, Grady, and others to tell us the story. Their voices, their writing form the fabric of our personal memories of each era. And as this genre of writing has evolved, so has a healthy skepticism, a rigor that makes it unlikely that headlines the equivalent of these two from 1913 could appear: "Cause of Cancer Found at Last by Boston Scientist" or "Diabetes Cure Confirmed by Treatment of 176 Cases." But perhaps we are being unfair to that era; with the extant knowledge and the peer-review process of 1913, those claims might have seemed plausible.

We are now entering the personalized 'omics era where as routinely as we measure our cholesterol, we will soon be mapping out our genome, the proteome, the transcriptome, the metabolome, the phenome, and much more—all this during one office visit. The magnitude of electronic data that we will need to store on any *one* patient will eclipse what is presently in the entire Library of Congress. But what will this mean for public policy, for the individual? And as we harness the power of shared databases, who will "own" our individual data and what are the implications for privacy? Clearly, the progress of science and the shifting landscape of disease (such as the arrival of Ebola on U.S. shores as I write) will require the best of medical reporting. The responsibility of the Fourth Estate to lay out for public debate not just the facts but the ethical and social issues will be huge. It's an important responsibility, one that requires objectivity, skill, research, immersion, and an appreciation of history.

In Camus's *The Plague*, Raymond Rambert, a journalist from Paris, finds himself inadvertently stuck in Oran when the town is quarantined because of the outbreak. When the moment finally comes after many days when he can in fact leave, Rambert decides to stay. He says, "Until now I always felt a stranger in this town . . . But now that I've seen what I have seen, I know that I belong here whether I want it or not. This business is everybody's business."

The business of medicine is truly everybody's business. It is writing of the sort that is in these pages that makes it so.

*Abraham Verghese*
Vice Chair of the Department of Medicine at Stanford University
and author of *Cutting for Stone*

# INTRODUCTION

*T*he *New York Times* was first published on September 18, 1851, with a bold proclamation: "We publish today the first issue of the New-York Daily Times, and we intend to issue it every morning (Sundays excepted) for an indefinite number of years to come."

Life was very different then, and so were human beings. People ate locally grown organic food and exercised more. They did not have the stress of long commutes and, of course, there were no distractions like endless streams of e-mails and texts and Twitter feeds.

But health was another issue. A landmark study of Civil War veterans provided some data. Men of that era were significantly smaller than men today. An average man was five feet seven inches tall and weighed 147 pounds. Today, the average man is 2½ inches taller and weighs 44 pounds more.

People also were sickly. By middle age, most had the sort of chronic debilitating ailments that we now associate with the elderly. Forty-four percent of men aged 50 to 64 had difficulty bending, as compared to less than 8 percent now. Twenty-nine percent had trouble walking, triple that of today.

The transformation from the Civil War era today is so great, in fact, that the late Robert Fogel, a Nobel Prize–winning economist who studied the health of Civil War veterans, said humans in the industrialized world "have undergone a form of evolution that is unique not only to humankind, but unique among the 7,000 or so generations of humans who have ever inhabited the earth."

People are bigger and healthier throughout life. Childhood illnesses like scarlet fever that could leave people with injured hearts for life are gone. Smallpox has disappeared. As people age, they get serious chronic ailments much later in life, if they get them at all. And at every age people are less likely to die. The age-adjusted risk of dying dropped 60 percent from 1935 to 2010. For heart disease and stroke in particular, the change has been stunning. Since 1950, the number of deaths per year from heart disease has fallen by 72 percent and the number of deaths from stroke fell by 77.5 percent.

The evolution in humankind, though, did not involve major genetic changes. Instead, it was the result of enormous advances in medicine, a transformation so profound that it is almost hard to imagine what the world was like when *The Times* was first published. The articles of *The Times*, which form a living history, are revelatory, showing how so much of what we now take for granted in medicine came to be. Treatments for depression, for blood pressure and heart disease, for ulcers and diabetes, were products of the later years of the 20th century. Even antibiotics were unknown until the middle of the century. Viruses were unheard of and no one knew that DNA carried blueprints for life. Every disease, every medical discovery, has a story that unfolds with drama and false turns and blind alleys, and, more often than not, ends in triumph as a mystery is solved.

Cancer, for example, obsessed people in the early 20th century who puzzled over what it was and how to treat it. In 1907, *The Times* published an article saying that the cause of cancer was discovered and a cure was possible. It was caused by spirochaetes, the article reported, a type of bacteria. In 1912, *The Times* reported that cancer was caused by an amoeba and that a vaccine to prevent it was possible. A French doctor, Gaston Odin, announced, "I succeeded in cultivating the microbe in conformity with the most rigorous Pasteur methods, and I have in my tubes of cultures formal proof of my claim. The cancer microbe is a parasite blood amoeba."

There were claims that radium cured cancer, and then the cure was surgery, often radical. Diagnostics lagged. It was not until 1965 that scientists reported finding breast cancer with X-rays—a mammogram. Colonoscopies were first reported in 1974.

The leading killer of Americans today—heart disease—only became preventable and treatable late in the 20th century. Bypass surgery was first done in 1969. Stents came about in 1988. The first successful drug for lowering blood pressure was reported in 1951. Before that, Times articles described a variety of methods like one the one in 1908 that used electric currents. "A senescent patient with arterio-sclerosis may be placed in a solenoid and connected with the high frequency apparatus, or he may be placed in a condenser couch or chair . . . In from twenty to thirty minutes his blood pressure will be reduced from ten to fifteen millimeters."

Later in the century, a popular remedy for high blood pressure was to go on a totally salt-free diet, with many traveling to Duke University for a so-called "rice diet," consisting of rice, fruit and vegetables. Yet, all too often, blood pressure remained high.

Statins, which made lowering cholesterol feasible for almost everyone, first came on the market in 1987.

But although it took most of the past century for effective medical treatments to be discovered, there were huge improvements in health much earlier. Public health campaigns were the reason—requirements for quarantining the sick and repeated instructions in hygiene, including advice not to give babies beer or "swill milk" described as "that bluish white compound of true milk, pus and dirty water."

There were also exhortations to avoid unpasteurized milk. A 1905 article in *The Times* quoted an expert (what kind of expert?) of the era, Nathan Strauss, saying that unpasteurized milk was "worse than a plague." He provided formulas for pasteurizing it. "Milk is the one article of food in which disease and death can lurk without giving any suspicion from its taste, smell, or appearance," he said. He called for pasteurization to "prevent helpless infants [from] developing from puny, sickly childhood into diseased, weakened, and helpless manhood and womanhood."

As the 20th century progressed, various other plagues struck—yellow fever, the terrible 1918 flu, and, more recently, AIDS. With the flu, the articles tell not just of the devastation—the panic and suffering—that the virus caused; they also tell of a remarkable discovery more than half a century later, when researchers found shards of the virus in preserved tissue and reconstructed it.

But not every medical discovery was a happy one. Articles reported as well on disturbing ethical lapses. They describe scandals involving experiments with mentally ill people and prisoners, among others. Codes of ethics were formulated and a new discipline and a new role, the ethicist, came into being. That set the scene for debates over discoveries like cloning and in vitro fertilization and organ transplants that raised ethical questions while offering promises of new treatments.

Some conditions seemed ever-present and ever-perplexing—obesity, for example. An article in 1897 told how many calories and nutrients a man, a woman and children of different ages reported on the stunning intake of some young men who went on a camping trip and that of a well-known strongman. The men were consuming 3,235 calories a day, the strongman 4,462.

In 1959, an article on an insurance company study of 5 million Americans concluded that excess weight is tied to mortality, that those with the lowest weights live longest, and that women were thinner than in decades past while men were fatter.

A few decades later, in 2005, a large study using federal data concluded that the lowest death rate is among people deemed slightly overweight—those of normal weight and those below normal weights did not live as long.

The articles tell of unfolding insights into Alzheimer's, cancer, ulcers and diabetes. They report on the struggles to treat mental illness and the enormous success of vaccines. Every disease, every condition, has a tale that is best appreciated by seeing discoveries and claims triumphed and challenged and accepted. But perhaps the most fascinating aspect of these dramas is the cumulative story of how far medicine has come since those days when people were small and weak and sickly, and how much can now be done for conditions that once seemed just part of humankind.

In assembling this book, I was reminded of a quote by an admissions officer at Harvard University who said he had to turn down so many stellar applicants that he could easily have created a second, parallel class of freshmen just as talented and qualified as the ones he admitted. Because we could only choose a limited number of articles, *Times* researcher Susan Beachy and I felt the same way. We could have compiled another book or maybe even two books with different articles describing discoveries that were just as important and giving insights into life in previous years that were just as evocative. We hope readers will understand that omissions were inevitable given the length constraints.

CHAPTER 1

# AIDS

# Rare Cancer Seen in 41 Homosexuals

By LAWRENCE K. ALTMAN, M.D.

Doctors in New York and California have diagnosed among homosexual men 41 cases of a rare and often rapidly fatal form of cancer. Eight of the victims died less than 24 months after the diagnosis was made.

The cause of the outbreak is unknown, and there is as yet no evidence of contagion. But the doctors who have made the diagnoses, mostly in New York City and the San Francisco Bay area, are alerting other physicians who treat large numbers of homosexual men to the problem in an effort to help identify more cases and to reduce the delay in offering chemotherapy treatment.

The sudden appearance of the cancer, called Kaposi's Sarcoma, has prompted a medical investigation that experts say could have as much scientific as public health importance because of what it may teach about determining the causes of more common types of cancer.

## First Appears in Spots

Doctors have been taught in the past that the cancer usually appeared first in spots on the legs and that the disease took a slow course of up to 10 years. But these recent cases have shown that it appears in one or more violet-colored spots anywhere on the body. The spots generally do not itch or cause other symptoms, often can be mistaken for bruises, sometimes appear as lumps and can turn brown after a period of time. The cancer often causes swollen lymph glands, and then kills by spreading throughout the body.

Doctors investigating the outbreak believe that many cases have gone undetected because of the rarity of the condition and the difficulty even dermatologists may have in diagnosing it.

In a letter alerting other physicians to the problem, Dr. Alvin E. Friedman-Kien of New York University Medical Center, one of the investigators, described the appearance of the outbreak as "rather devastating."

Dr. Friedman-Kien said in an interview yesterday that he knew of 41 cases collated in the last five weeks, with the cases themselves dating to the past 30 months. The Federal Centers for Disease Control in Atlanta is expected to publish the first description of the outbreak in its weekly report today, according to a spokesman,

2

Dr. James Curran. The report notes 26 of the cases—20 in New York and six in California.

There is no national registry of cancer victims, but the nationwide incidence of Kaposi's Sarcoma in the past had been estimated by the Centers for Disease Control to be less than six-one-hundredths of a case per 100,000 people annually, or about two cases in every three million people. However, the disease accounts for up to 9 percent of all cancers in a belt across equatorial Africa, where it commonly affects children and young adults.

In the United States, it has primarily affected men older than 50 years. But in the recent cases, doctors at nine medical centers in New York and seven hospitals in California have been diagnosing the condition among younger men, all of whom said in the course of standard diagnostic interviews that they were homosexual. Although the ages of the patients have ranged from 26 to 51 years, many have been under 40, with the mean at 39.

Nine of the 41 cases known to Dr. Friedman-Kien were diagnosed in California, and several of those victims reported that they had been in New York in the period preceding the diagnosis. Dr. Friedman-Kien said that his colleagues were checking on reports of two victims diagnosed in Copenhagen, one of whom had visited New York.

## Viral Infections Indicated

No one medical investigator has yet interviewed all the victims, Dr. Curran said. According to Dr. Friedman-Kien, the reporting doctors said that most cases had involved homosexual men who have had multiple and frequent sexual encounters with different partners, as many as 10 sexual encounters each night up to four times a week.

Many of the patients have also been treated for viral infections such as herpes, cytomegalovirus and hepatitis B as well as parasitic infections such as amebiasis and giardiasis. Many patients also reported that they had used drugs such as amyl nitrite and LSD to heighten sexual pleasure.

Cancer is not believed to be contagious, but conditions that might precipitate it, such as particular viruses or environmental factors, might account for an outbreak among a single group.

The medical investigators say some indirect evidence actually points away from contagion as a cause. None of the patients knew each other, although the theoretical

3

possibility that some may have had sexual contact with a person with Kaposi's Sarcoma at some point in the past could not be excluded, Dr. Friedman-Kien said.

Dr. Curran said there was no apparent danger to nonhomosexuals from contagion. "The best evidence against contagion," he said, "is that no cases have been reported to date outside the homosexual community or in women."

Dr. Friedman-Kien said he had tested nine of the victims and found severe defects in their immunological systems. The patients had serious malfunctions of two types of cells called T and B cell lymphocytes, which have important roles in fighting infections and cancer.

But Dr. Friedman-Kien emphasized that the researchers did not know whether the immunological defects were the underlying problem or had developed secondarily to the infections or drug use.

The research team is testing various hypotheses, one of which is a possible link between past infection with cytomegalovirus and development of Kaposi's Sarcoma.

*July 3, 1981*

# New U.S. Report Names
# Virus That May Cause AIDS

By LAWRENCE K. ALTMAN, M.D.

Federal researchers announced today that they had found a virus that they believe is the cause of acquired immune deficiency syndrome, or AIDS.

They called it HTLV-3 and said they had developed a process to mass-produce it for the purpose of developing the tools needed to finally conquer the mysterious disease that has afflicted more than 4,000 Americans.

The announcement follows the attention recently given to the discovery of a virus called LAV by researchers at the Pasteur Institute in Paris. The head of the Centers for Disease Control in Atlanta said over the weekend that he believed LAV was the cause of AIDS.

Margaret M. Heckler, Secretary of Health and Human Services, said today that she thought the two viruses "will prove to be the same."

With the new process, the Federal researchers said they had developed a test that could reliably detect the virus that causes AIDS in blood that is donated for a wide variety of uses, including the treatment of hemophilia. They said they applied for a patent on the process today and that they expected the test to be widely available within six months.

The optimism surrounding the American and French research appears to reflect a high point in what has been one of the most challenging international scientific efforts to battle any modern disease.

Finding the cause of AIDS will not necessarily lead to any treatment of the disease soon, nor will it necessarily result in a method of prevention. But the finding led the American researchers to express the hope that a vaccine would be developed and ready for testing "in about two years."

Even as the French and American researchers' confidence has grown steadily in recent weeks, a degree of uncertainty still clings to the findings, and the tension of the exhaustive search was apparent in interviews and visits to the research facilities. There was a sense of quiet triumph in the halls of the Atlanta centers last week, but the euphoria that might have been expected was tempered by the knowledge that months of research are still required to firmly ascertain whether LAV and HTLV-3 are the same, and whether the virus is the cause of AIDS. Dr. Robert C. Gallo of the National Cancer Institute, who headed the team that is reporting its

5

findings in four papers in the journal *Science*, said that if the two viruses "turn out to be the same I will say so."

Dr. Gallo said he had isolated the virus from more than 50 patients and had detected evidence of antibodies that are a kind of record of the existence of the virus in the blood in about 85 percent of patients with AIDS and in about 80 percent of patients with a condition he called pre-AIDS.

After the first cases of AIDS were recognized in New York and California in 1981, Federal researchers quickly identified homosexual and bisexual males as the primary group affected. Epidemiologists also identified intravenous drug users, people of Haitian descent and hemophiliacs as other groups at risk of AIDS.

Early in the course of the investigation, Federal epidemiologists at the Centers for Disease Control in Atlanta determined that a transmissible agent was the only plausible factor that could satisfactorily explain the cause of AIDS in such widely different risk groups. The researchers said they strongly suspected that the transmissible agent was a micro-organism and they presumed it was a virus.

After initial tests failed to identify any known virus—or any other micro-organism—as the cause, researchers turned their attention to a new group called retroviruses. Retroviruses are so named because they contain an enzyme called reverse transcriptase that can copy the RNA of the virus into the DNA form, thus reversing the usual direction of the flow of genetic information.

By May 1983, researchers from the National Cancer Institute, the Harvard University School of Public Health, the Centers for Disease Control, the Kimron Veterinary Institute of Israel, New York University, the New York Veterans Administration Hospital, Litton Bionetics Inc. of Maryland and the Raymond Poincare Hospital in France published several reports in *Science* about a retrovirus called HTLV-1, which was put forward as the leading candidate as the cause of AIDS. HTLV-1, initially reported in 1981, had been found to cause a rare type of leukemia in southern Japan and the Caribbean islands. HTLV originally stood for human T-cell leukemia virus, but now the initials are used for human T-lymphotropic retroviruses to broaden the name.

In the same issue of *Science* last May, a team from the Pasteur Institute in Paris reported the discovery of LAV. LAV stands for lymphadenopathy-associated virus. The French researchers had isolated LAV from one of the many swollen lymph nodes in the body of a French man who said he had more than 50 homosexual partners each year and who had traveled to many European countries, North Africa, India and the United States. His last trip to New York was in 1979.

At the time of the first LAV report, Federal and other researchers said they were not excited by the prospects of that retrovirus as the cause of AIDS.

The significance of LAV began to become apparent for two reasons. One was that researchers could not detect HTLV-1 in all AIDS cases and because AIDS was rare in Japan. The other reason was the progress made by the French researchers who were expanding their studies on LAV.

The turning point came at a meeting in Park City, Utah, last January, according to one of the participants in the meeting. "We all got very excited" at the French presentation, the scientist said. Until then, some researchers believed that the LAV was not a retrovirus but a member of an entirely different family.

Dr. Luc Montagnier said his Pasteur Institute team has isolated "about a dozen" viruses that are either identical to or similar to LAV according to electron microscope and immunologic studies.

The viruses have been isolated from patients with AIDS or from members of the high-risk groups who have swollen lymph glands throughout their body. The condition is called lymphadenopathy, and many doctors suspect that it is a form of AIDS that cannot be now diagnosed as such because of the lack of a diagnostic test.

The patients have included French men as well as people from Haiti and Zaire, two countries where large numbers of AIDS cases are being diagnosed.

One of the many challenges facing AIDS researchers is to determine why the tests for the LAV or HTLV-3 were negative in some cases of patients presumed to have AIDS.

One thesis advanced by Dr. Montagnier is that the tests themselves may not be able to detect LAV at a certain stage of the disease. Another is that the technology of LAV testing is still too crude to detect all cases.

It remains remotely possible that the viruses observed by French and American researchers are not the cause of AIDS, but part of it. They could be just a newly recognized opportunistic infection of the type that afflict AIDS victims. Opportunistic infections are those that are caused by micro-organisms that usually do not make ill those people whose immune systems are working properly.

Dr. Montagnier said that his team considered that possibility "unlikely" because LAV was isolated from a patient whose immune system was not depressed and because similar isolates have come from people who had no evidence of a reversal of the so-called T4-T8 lymphocytes that seems to develop in patients with AIDS and suspected of having it.

After the Pasteur Institute team reported its findings with LAV, it began sending samples of the virus to any other scientific team that asked for it. As of today, Dr. Montagnier said the number of laboratories was "about 10" and they were located throughout the United States and Europe.

Cooperation between labs was further indicated today by Dr. Gallo, who recalled that one of the French researchers had trained in his laboratory in Bethesda, Md.

The French virus was sent to Dr. Gallo at the National Cancer Institute last July, Dr. Montagnier said, "but he told me this isolate did not work, so we sent it again in September."

It is customary for researchers to send specimens of new organisms to other laboratories interested in the problem. But in the words of Dr. Donald Francis, who heads the Centers for Disease Control team of virologists investigating AIDS: "Not many people are calling the French every week asking for that virus. You have to be cautious about working with what you think is the cause of AIDS."

Because the disease at present is so insidious and incurable, it generates some fear among the public and considerable concern even among the scientists working with it.

One of the classic ways to determine if a micro-organism causes disease is to inject it into animals. Thus, researchers at the Atlanta centers, the Pasteur Institute and elsewhere have injected the AIDS-linked viruses into animals but, as of today, none have shown any evidence of AIDS.

If the suspect viruses become indisputably linked to AIDS and a test to detect the virus in blood for transfusion is successfully developed, it would be applied an estimated 23 million times a year for the 3 million blood transfusions given in the United States each year, the researchers said today.

The risk probably was not great in any case. Reassuring data already comes from tests the French researchers have made on blood donated for transfusions in France. Dr. Montagnier said that the team could find evidence of LAV in "only one out of more than 100" units of blood tested.

Researchers are hoping that the LAV and HTLV-3 are the same. Dr. James Curran, who heads the Atlanta centers' AIDS investigating team, said that if tests show the viruses to be different in major ways, "then something is wrong because one virus causes AIDS."

Dr. Curran said that there may be several other so-called co-factors involved in explaining why some who are exposed to the virus that causes AIDS get it and others do not. "Not everyone who smokes gets lung cancer," Dr. Curran said.

It is possible that genetic factors or certain infections could act to increase the vulnerability of an individual to the virus.

Research growing out of the new work may help explain why AIDS has such a long incubation period—a period that can range apparently from nine months to more than five years.

*April 24, 1984*

# AIDS Drugs Offer Hope but Cure Remains Distant

## By HAROLD M. SCHMECK JR.

This year the AIDS epidemic is being transformed from an utterly hopeless situation to one in which many, perhaps most American victims of the disease will have access to drug treatments that may give precious extra months of life.

One anti-AIDS drug appears to be nearing Federal approval, and trials of potential new drugs are being set up or expanded at a fast pace. But like every other aspect of the deadly epidemic, the drug outlook is marked by controversy and anguish.

The pace of progress seems agonizingly slow to patients who know they only have 6 to 18 months more to live.

### "They Are Desperate"

"Many of them are much better informed about AIDS than the average physician, and they are desperate," said Dr. Michael Lange, of St. Luke's–Roosevelt Hospital Center in New York.

At present only a handful of drugs look promising enough for trial in patients. Most are in short supply and many patients have to be told they must wait, even for a spot in an experiment.

"I would like to try something even if it doesn't work," one patient told Dr. Lange. "Just to sit there and think and do nothing about it is very, very difficult."

### Push for Treatments

On the other side is the huge effort medical scientists are making to cope with the growing menace of acquired immune deficiency syndrome. The virus that causes AIDS was discovered less than five years ago. Today, knowing its identity and having already discovered a wealth of detail about it, scientists are trying to exploit every weak point the virus offers.

Medical scientists are mounting what is probably the greatest concentrated effort ever made to find therapies for a single virus disease. And, in an unusual approach that they hope will quicken the pace of progress, Federal officials are sponsoring new research consortiums involving Government, university and industry scientists.

10

The drug most widely tried against the AIDS virus is azidothymidine, AZT. Nearly 5,000 patients have used it and the numbers are growing rapidly. The Food and Drug Administration is expected to approve the drug within weeks.

The evidence indicates that AZT has prolonged many lives. But so far the success is measured in months only, and the drug has harmed some patients. No one expects AZT to actually cure AIDS or to rid victims of the AIDS virus.

Almost every drug or antiviral treatment that has ever shown any prospect of combating any virus infection is being tested. The Federal drug agency has granted permission for early tests in patients of about 30 different substances that have demonstrated potential against the AIDS virus in test-tube experiments.

## The Search for New Drugs

Thousands of chemicals, synthetic and natural, are being screened for activity against the AIDS virus in the laboratory. But the drug search goes far beyond screening. Working on the frontiers of biology, chemists, virologists, immunologists and molecular biologists are trying to engineer new substances to attack the virus at every specific point in its life cycle.

The new collaboration among Government scientists, universities and drug companies is being sponsored by the National Institute of Allergy and Infectious Diseases, a unit of the National Institutes of Health in Bethesda, Md.

Dr. Anthony Fauci, director of the allergy and infectious disease institute, says there are five such consortiums now. He hopes to get 20 more started by Sept. 30, the end of this fiscal year, and 20 more next year, if Congress will provide the money. A separate effort is being developed to work out the complete three-dimensional structure of all the proteins the AIDS virus makes.

These studies should reveal more "little nooks and crannies of the virus" that may be good targets for drug designers, Dr. Fauci said. "Those are the kinds of approach that are going to yield results two or three years from now."

Viruses are organisms that exist on the very border between the living and the inanimate. A virus particle is a protein-coated package of genes wandering through the world of life, looking for living cells to infect. Its genes subvert the normal genetic apparatus of the infected cell and cause it to make a new crop of viruses, often killing the cell to do so.

In a recent article, Dr. Hiroaki Mitsuya and Dr. Samuel Broder of the National Cancer Institute listed eight points in its reproductive cycle at which the AIDS virus might be attacked.

The first is the actual contact between invader and victim—the binding of the virus to its target cell. From then on there are several opportunities to counterattack as the virus gets inside, sheds its coat and goes to work. The last stages are the assembly of virus particles within the infected cell and the budding of new viruses from the cell surface. Drugs are also being sought to hamper the action of key genes of the virus.

In addition, many studies are planned to test the effectiveness of combinations of antiviral drugs and substances known to strengthen the immune defense system. Many scientists believe that, in the end, such combinations will provide the best treatment for AIDS victims.

Dr. Lionel Resnick of Mount Sinai Medical Center in Miami Beach has noted that most of the drugs now used against the AIDS virus have some effects against a key viral enzyme, the reverse transcriptase, which acts inside an invaded cell to direct formation of DNA that encodes the virus's genetic message. Toxicity is a major problem with these drugs, he said, suggesting that they are not selective enough and therefore may interfere with normal cellular enzymes that assemble strands of DNA that the cell needs.

AZT and dideoxycytidine attack at the point at which the reverse transcriptase acts. They halt the production of the DNA strands that are normally manufactured from virus RNA with the enzyme's help. DNA and RNA are the principal genetic chemicals for all living things.

Suramin and HPA-23, drugs whose early promise has now faded, were designed to inhibit the action of the reverse transcriptase.

Ribavirin throws a chemical monkey wrench into the genetic machinery at a later stage, when the nucleus of the infected cell is sending out blueprints that the cell's production sites would use to begin assembly of new virus particles. Interferon alpha is believed to attack at the final stage of virus production, the point at which a new virus particle begins to bud from the surface of the infected cell.

Many other experimental drugs are being considered, including AL-721, thought to hamper the virus's ability to attach itself to cells; peptide T, which interferes with virus attachment in a different way; and Foscarnet, which attacks the action of a key viral enzyme. Other potential drugs are artificially produced pieces of DNA that glue themselves to key segments of the virus's genetic blueprints and take them out of action.

Doctors at several research centers are planning to try AZT in combination with other drugs, in AIDS patients and in people infected with the AIDS virus who have not yet developed AIDS. One new study will also test the drug in patients who have developed dementia or other symptoms of brain and central nervous system infection.

The question of possible drug benefit to patients who are infected by the virus but have no symptoms of AIDS is considered particularly important. Scientists see this strategy of early counterattack as probably the main hope for drugs against AIDS, whether the drug is AZT or something equally effective but less potentially toxic.

Few, if any, experts seem to expect to find a drug that will eliminate the virus from the patient's body altogether and cure the disease. Dr. William S. Robinson, a virologist and professor of medicine at Stanford University, for example, thinks a cure is "a slim hope."

For the present, at least, the hope is for a drug or combination of drugs that will keep the virus in check so that it neither kills the patient nor cripples the immune system. But the virus is known to be capable of lingering in the human body relatively inactive for years. In addition, some seemingly logical combinations of drugs may turn out to be deadly, or counterproductive. A recent study of ribavirin and AZT together, for example, found that in test-tube experiments the two drugs seem to cancel out each other's effectiveness against the virus.

Drugs to keep the AIDS virus under control would probably have to be taken for years, perhaps decades, and that goal implies the use of something harmless enough to the patient to be tolerated over long periods.

## Prospects for Treatment

In the immediate future, AZT will remain the best hope of many AIDS patients, experts say. By the end of the year, enough is expected to be available to treat at least 30,000 patients, although the drug is expected to be in short supply at the outset. And the manufacturer, the Burroughs Wellcome Company, has said that even after the drug, to be marketed under the name Retrovir, has been approved for prescription sale, its distribution will be restricted to patients in whom prior evidence indicates the drug is more likely to help than harm.

Two other drugs, dideoxycytidine and ribavirin, also show promise although they are in less advanced stages of clinical research than AZT.

In a clinical trial, ribavirin apparently helped prevent some patients with early signs of AIDS virus infection from progressing on to AIDS, according to the manufacturer, ICN Pharmaceuticals. But few data have been released and many experts have reservations about the drug.

The near-term prospect is that the lives of many patients afflicted with AIDS will be prolonged. But that is about as far as experts will go in predicting what lies ahead, even though the number of drugs that look promising in laboratory experiments is expected to increase substantially.

In laboratory experiments, dideoxycytidine, which is chemically related to AZT, has shown promise of being at least as effective as AZT but less toxic. The drug is now in early safety testing in patients and its therapeutic promise awaits confirmation.

As to AZT, scientists stress the potential dangers as well as the benefits. The chemical has a destructive effect on the bone marrow, the ultimate source of the blood and cells of the immune defense system. But the reaction to AZT seems to vary greatly from person to person. Some people with AIDS have tolerated the drug for many months. Others have been forced to stop using it.

The F.D.A., while considering the application for licensing of AZT, has permitted a special distribution to patients who fit the profile of those in whom benefits have been established—essentially, AIDS patients who have suffered pneumocystic carinii pneumonia, an indication of severe damage to the immune system. Since the beginning of October, the number of patients receiving the drug has grown by 30 to 50 a day.

The results have been encouraging. "We've had a handful of patients who have gone a year and a half," Dr. David W. Barry, research vice president of Burroughs Wellcome, said. "Several dozen over a year and several hundred over nine months."

But some patients have died despite the drug treatment and, in others, the inexorable course of the disease has begun again despite their treatment.

The original clinical trial of AZT began in the spring of 1986 with a division of patients into groups who received the drug and others who received a placebo, a harmless, ineffective substance. The use of the placebos was cut short last fall, however, and all patients were given the drug when scientists discovered that there had been only one death among 145 patients receiving the drug and 19 among an almost equal number who received the placebo.

As of last Jan. 12, the most recent date for which figures are available, there had been only eight deaths among the original 145 who took the drug from the start, and 32 deaths among the others. Among 3,247 patients involved in a subsequent, widespread research trial, there were 97 deaths through Jan. 12, but only 21 deaths among those who had used the drug for three weeks or more.

"I think there are a lot of things we don't know about AZT yet," said Dr. Martin

Hirsch of Harvard and Massachusetts General Hospital in Boston. "We know the short-term toxicities. We know the short-term ability to prolong life." But he added that there had not been enough time to analyze the long-term effects.

Cost is another problem; patients will presumably keep taking the drug for as long as they live, and the retail price is expected to be $8,000 to $10,000 a year for the needed doses.

Burroughs Wellcome, in justifying the price, says that production of AZT is complicated and expensive and that it has already borne enormous development costs. In January a company official said the company had spent more than $80 million developing the drug, with no assurance that it would ever reach the market.

Meanwhile, the spread of AIDS is increasing. Thirty-two thousand cases have been reported in the United States so far. The Federal Centers for Disease Control in Atlanta has estimated that there will be at least 21,000 new cases and 13,000 to 15,000 deaths during 1987. That averages out to three deaths every two hours.

As they search for drugs that attack the AIDS virus infection, doctors are also working feverishly to find better treatments for the related diseases that strike AIDS victims. These include a rare form of cancer, Kaposi's Sarcoma, and many infections that would not bother normal people but that attack patients whose immune defenses are ruined.

There has been progress against many of these diseases, but it is still unclear how much, if at all, the life expectancy of AIDS patients has been increased.

A common problem and one of the most fateful stages in the progression of any AIDS case is the first episode of one particular infection, pneumocystis pneumonia.

A few years ago, patients often died from the first attack of this infection. Today 70 percent to 75 percent survive, according to one expert, but it is crucial that further attacks be prevented. Studies have shown that only one patient in 20 lives 18 months after that first episode occurs. Sometimes the patient dies during another attack, sometimes from other complications of AIDS.

The treatment that seems to be best against the pneumonia, specialists say, is not a new frontier anti-infection drug, but dapsone, an old and respected substance that has been known since the 1940s as a treatment for leprosy.

A study is needed to determine whether dapsone actually increases the survival of patients, said Dr. Michael Grieco, head of immunology and infectious diseases at St. Luke's–Roosevelt. It appears to do so, but the data are not sufficient to be statistically significant.

## Conflict Over Access

Today the knowledge that there is no cure, that no patient has ever been known to survive AIDS and that there is a temporary shortage of many experimental drugs against the disease, has apparently generated a black market as well as amateur attempts at treatment. Some much-publicized patients, such as Rock Hudson, the film star, have made a futile journey to France for treatment with an unproved drug. More frequently, patients have gone to Mexico for ribavirin. Doctors in New York say there appears to a black market for both ribavirin and AZT in this country.

Some patients seeking AL-721 have evidently taken the matter into their own hands, making a crude version at home.

Some doctors, familiar with this self-treatment, say they do not really object to it. Others worry over any use of a "homemade" drug because the patient has no way of knowing just what it really is and whether it is safe to take.

The F.D.A. has established special procedures for evaluating and approving potential AIDS drugs much faster than usual. The process has led to wide, though controlled, distribution of AZT years earlier than normal procedures would have dictated. Federal officials have also established a network of 19 leading medical research centers around the country to coordinate clinical trials of promising drugs—controlled scientific experiments that offer the only way of determining whether a drug helps, scientists assert.

For many dying patients and their supporters, that has not been good enough. Health officials have faced constant, anguished pleas to let patients have access to drugs before their worth is proved.

Some officials admit to having suffered sleepless nights over the matter. But most scientists have concluded that controlled trials offer the only means of establishing the merits of new drugs. They also warn that potential AIDS drugs tend to be extremely toxic, akin to cancer drugs, and could rob victims of months of life as they offer a cruel false hope.

Without proper studies, Dr. Broder of the Cancer Institute said, "a good drug could be lost or a bad drug could be accepted as effective," causing immeasurable and perhaps irreparable harm.

## The Outlook

Many experts regard AIDS as the final stage of a long virus infection that advances at a different pace in different patients. If that is true, the damage may be close to irreparable by the time the full-scale disease appears.

Doctors who take this view tend to be much less pessimistic about the chances of learning how to cope with the early virus infection, perhaps keeping it at bay for years or even permanently if the right combination of drugs can be found. That is why there is much current emphasis on trying the new drugs in people who are infected with the AIDS virus but have not yet developed symptoms of serious illness.

In the search for drugs of this kind, it may be a source of hope as well as challenge that the AIDS virus is the most complex example known of the class known as retroviruses. The complexity offers many different points of attack because the virus life cycle involves so many different interrelated steps.

"Although the precise mechanisms are matters of future study," Dr. Mitsuya and Dr. Broder wrote in their review, "it is clear that this retrovirus has evolved an astonishingly complex system of genetic regulation."

"With luck," the two scientists said, "the very complexity of the virus could contribute to its defeat."

*March 17, 1987*

# New Picture of Who Will Get AIDS Is Dominated by Addicts

By GINA KOLATA

The AIDS epidemic, continuing its demographic evolution, is becoming ever more closely tied to the drug epidemic, a new study shows. Not only are intravenous drug users becoming infected, but so are crack addicts and other drug abusers, many of whom are women.

An extensive, unpublished analysis by researchers at the Federal Centers for Disease Control and Prevention in Atlanta has found that nearly three-quarters of the 40,000 new infections with H.I.V., the virus that causes AIDS, last year were among addicts.

Many of the addicts are IV drug users who share infected needles, but an increasing number are crack addicts who are contracting the AIDS virus through unprotected sex, often with multiple partners. Men and women alike often go on binges, having sex with many partners in exchange for crack or the money to buy it. "Maybe as much as half of the new infections among heterosexuals are occurring in relation to crack cocaine," said Dr. Scott Holmberg, a C.D.C. epidemiologist who conducted the study.

Data and analyses from the C.D.C. show that the people diagnosed with AIDS in 1993, the most recent year for which statistics on the disease are available, are a very different group from those the 1994 statistics show are now being infected with the virus. Development of AIDS generally occurs about a decade after infection.

Of those newly diagnosed with AIDS in 1993, who were probably mostly infected in the early to mid-1980s, about half were gay men and a little more than a quarter were intravenous drug users. Fewer than 10 percent were heterosexuals. The remaining cases were hemophiliacs and gay men who injected drugs.

Now, in his analysis of national data for new H.I.V. infections in 1994, Dr. Holmberg finds a very different pattern, which is continuing this year. Only a quarter of the most recent infections are in gay men. About half of the new infections are among drug users who shared needles. And about a quarter are heterosexually transmitted. Dr. Holmberg said that 70 to 80 percent of people who are getting H.I.V. infections through heterosexual transmission are women and the majority of those are women who had sex with men who got infected when they injected drugs. Many had sex with these men during crack binges, or while they were abusing other drugs or alcohol, when they were not inclined to think about safe sex, Dr. Holmberg said.

The crack addicts who are becoming infected, Dr. Holmberg said, are mostly young men and women who live in inner cities and are members of minority groups. They often have other sexually transmitted diseases, which is thought to make it easier for the AIDS virus to infect them.

Recently published statistics—that AIDS is now the leading killer of young adults and that the largest-percentage increases in new infections are among women—take on a different tone when read in the context of Dr. Holmberg's study. There are not many competing causes of death among those under 45. And although new infections are spreading fastest among women who acquire the infection through heterosexual intercourse, as many as half of these women are crack addicts.

Experts caution that the data do not mean that the virus is no longer a threat to Americans who do not use illicit drugs, and say that men and women should practice safe sex. Some researchers and advocates for people with AIDS are also concerned that the information carries another risk: that the nation will turn its back on these infected groups.

"That's a real worry," said Dr. Don C. Des Jarlais, an AIDS expert who directs the chemical dependency unit at Beth Israel Medical Center in New York. But, he said, fear of telling the truth about the epidemic is "one reason we have our priorities so out of order."

He added: "You're never going to have good public policy and stop an epidemic if you base your policy on misinformation or wrong information. You have to know where the disease is occurring and how to go after it."

Two years ago, Dr. Des Jarlais, a member of a committee of the National Research Council, argued that efforts to stamp out the epidemic should have a tighter focus. A report by the committee said that the epidemic was "settling into spatially and socially isolated groups and possibly becoming epidemic in them." The latest data provide a clearer picture of the characteristics of these isolated groups.

"It's a real dilemma," said Stephen Soba, communications director for the Gay Men's Health Crisis, an advocacy group for people with AIDS. "But we have to acknowledge that the face of the epidemic has changed and continues to be changing."

Mark Barnes, executive director of the AIDS Action Council, said: "These are tough issues. What this has meant for AIDS advocacy is that we have to not simply advocate around safer sex but for substance abuse treatment and for substance abuse treatment research, particularly for crack cocaine."

Others, however, fear that if the AIDS prevention message becomes a drug abuse prevention message, people outside the inner cities will falsely feel that they are not at risk.

"There is no magic ring around the inner city," said Dr. Mindy Fullilove, an associate professor of clinical psychiatry and public health at Columbia University in New York. "I think you can do targeting that makes people in the suburbs feel safe, and I don't agree with that."

But Dr. Des Jarlais said he feared more for the addicts, adding that the problem of redirecting AIDS prevention efforts hinges to a greater extent on the tendency of society to turn its back on addicts than on the dollars involved. He points out that it costs $3,000 to $4,000 a year to treat a heroin addict with methadone and that it costs $6,000 to $20,000 for residential treatment for a cocaine addict. But, he said, "The cost of just medical care for an H.I.V. infection is $120,000."

Perhaps the biggest surprise in the new image of H.I.V. infections is the rapid spread of the virus among crack users. Yet it makes sense, said Dr. James Yorke, a mathematician who has modeled the spread of AIDS and other diseases and who is director of the Institute for Physical Sciences and Technology at the University of Maryland. Dr. Yorke noted that transmission of H.I.V. differs from that of other sexually transmitted diseases in that it is riskier to have sex with many partners, only some of whom are infected, than to have sex the same number of times with one infected person.

The reason, Dr. Des Jarlais said, is that H.I.V. is transmitted more easily during two periods of the infection: when a person first contracts the virus and a decade or so later when the immune system is collapsing. If a woman, for example, has sex 100 times with a man who is infected with H.I.V. but is in the long latent stage when the virus is more difficult to transmit, she is much less likely to get infected than if she has sex just once with one man who may be in the infectious stage. So a woman is at much greater risk having sex once with 100 partners, most of whom are infected, than having sex 100 times with a man who is infected but in the latent stage.

Knowing who is becoming infected, and how, investigators say that they can envision strategies that could push down the rate of new infections. But, they say, it will take a shift of emphasis and resources. It means aggressively offering drug treatment and social programs, including jobs and support for addicts who often are homeless and have lost hope of being part of society. It means finding much better treatments for crack addiction. It means stopping transmission from infected heroin addicts, by supplying them with clean needles and by providing them with methadone. It means viewing AIDS as a consequence of the drug epidemic, and not as a separate entity.

The problem, said Dr. Sten Vermund, chairman of the department of epidemiology at the University of Alabama in Birmingham, is that to fight AIDS, "we have to have the political will to make investments in drug treatment and drug control." And to do that means giving inner city residents resources. "If we are hostile to drug treatment and job creation, then the epidemic will rage," he added.

Dr. Vermund said that he would like to see some money and effort diverted from the search for treatments and vaccines and put into prevention. "I, for one, think that the balance is distorted," he said. But, he said, at the very least, the way money is spent on AIDS prevention should be reconsidered.

AIDS prevention funds, "which are miserably inadequate to begin with, are largely spent on counseling and testing centers and in somewhat ineffectual mass media approaches," he said. To have an impact the money should be redirected to provide drug treatment. "I'm talking about removing the waiting lists for drug treatment," Dr. Vermund said. "Now a motivated addict who wants treatment in a city like New York is put on a waiting list for six months. That is a national disgrace."

Dr. Des Jarlais said that it is also crucial that "legal access to sterile needles should be implemented on a nationwide basis."

Mr. Barnes of the AIDS Action Council said that not only must advocates for people with AIDS start demanding research on substance abuse and substance abuse treatment, but they must also start insisting that education about AIDS prevention be incorporated into existing substance abuse treatment programs.

And those efforts, Mr. Barnes said, should include "everything from talking about issues of responsibility toward others and responsibility toward yourself to offering, even aggressively offering, partner notification strategies." Such efforts, he added, "are not something we have traditionally done as a nation," but that is in part because "we have separated prevention from treatment" of AIDS.

Dr. Vermund said, "It's a tough nut to crack." But he added: "We pay the price, and not merely in diseases like H.I.V. and sexually transmitted diseases and hepatitis, but also in our crime losses and correctional institutions."

As a society, he said, "we reap what we sow."

*February 28, 1995*

# New Studies Offer Powerful and Puzzling Evidence on Immunity to AIDS

By GINA KOLATA

Scientists have long suspected that some people might be immune to the AIDS virus. But now they are accumulating powerful, direct evidence of the extent and strength of such immunity. And many researchers are stunned.

The most recent study, published today in the journal *Science*, provides the most detailed and convincing evidence yet that 1 in 100 whites have complete immunity to infection by the AIDS virus and 1 in 5 whites have inherited a resistance to the progress of AIDS once infected with the virus.

Almost no blacks have the particular protective mutation investigated in this study, but scientists say that other forms of genetic immunity almost certainly exist in both blacks and whites.

The findings raise numerous questions and offer remarkable opportunities for research, scientists say. Among the puzzles are why some ethnic groups have such a mutation and others do not, how and when this mutation arose and what other genetic variants exist that protect against AIDS.

One of the study's surprises was that of 1,850 people, all of whom were at risk for infection, about 600 never became infected with H.I.V., the virus that causes AIDS. Since only 17 of them had the mutation identified as prevalent in whites, presumably the other people had some other form of genetic protection.

"The number that's impressive is the 1 in 5" who are resistant to the AIDS virus, said Dr. Michael Kaback, a geneticist at the University of California at San Diego. "Now you're getting up into the frequencies of blood group types or genes for eye colors," Dr. Kaback said.

A double dose of the mutated gene CKR5 confers complete immunity to AIDS, the researchers said. People who have inherited a single dose of the mutated gene can become infected with H.I.V., but AIDS progresses more slowly and they live on average three years longer than people who do not have the mutated gene.

In addition, the researchers who published in *Science*, directed by Dr. Stephen J. O'Brien of the National Cancer Institute's research center in Frederick, Md., found that much more genetic resistance was still to be understood. Although blacks, for example, virtually never have the mutated gene, they may have other genes that confer resistance to AIDS.

The 1,850 people in the study had been repeatedly exposed to H.I.V. because they were gay men who had sex without condoms, intravenous drug users who shared needles or hemophiliacs who injected themselves repeatedly with tainted blood products at the beginning of the AIDS epidemic. Since about 600 people in the study never became infected with H.I.V., the researchers report, the CKR5 mutation, as prevalent as it is, accounted for only 3 percent of the resistance.

The discoveries are making researchers ask why genes that confer resistance to AIDS are so common. Usually a mutation that knocks out a gene, as the CKR5 mutation does, would disappear from a population. It would only become common if it conferred a survival advantage.

Could it be, asked Dr. David Baltimore, a Nobel laureate molecular biologist at the Massachusetts Institute of Technology, that AIDS ravaged Europe centuries ago and that people with immunity today are the descendants of survivors? Or did the AIDS resistance genes also confer resistance to a different plague, like the Black Death?

Others researchers are asking how they can take advantage of the discoveries to develop new vaccines or drugs for AIDS and whether testing people to see if they are immune to AIDS is ethical.

It is, AIDS scientists say, an extraordinary time in the history of the AIDS epidemic, with new discoveries about AIDS coming so quickly that researchers' heads are spinning.

"In a way, this whole set of discoveries is really like an epiphany in AIDS research," said Dr. Jerome Groopman, an AIDS researcher at Harvard Medical School.

Last December, Dr. Robert Gallo, of the University of Maryland Medical School in Baltimore, a discoverer of the AIDS virus, identified mysterious substances in serum that could protect cells from infection with H.I.V. The substances were chemokines, chemicals used by the immune system to guide white blood cells to the sites of infection.

Researchers then asked why chemokines protected cells from H.I.V. Five groups simultaneously discovered last spring that H.I.V. uses a protein on the cell surface to slip into cells. That protein, CKR5, just happens to be the same protein that chemokines use to signal cells. Chemokines apparently protected cells from H.I.V. infection by tying up the CKR5 proteins on their surfaces, blocking H.I.V. from entering.

Finally, investigators asked whether there were people with mutations in their CKR5 genes that destroyed their cells' ability to make CKR5 proteins. If so, those mutations could prevent H.I.V. from entering cells and so provide immunity to AIDS. That led to papers published in August by Dr. Nathaniel Landau and his colleagues at the Aaron Diamond AIDS Research Center in New York, that identified two gay Manhattan men who had the CKR5 mutation and had never been infected with H.I.V.

In fact the two men had pushed researchers to explain their apparent immunity. The report published today extended those findings because researchers scrutinized the genetics of a large number of people clearly at risk for infection with H.I.V. The research on which today's paper was based was already in progress when the earlier papers were published.

The *Science* paper on genetic resistance to AIDS, whose principal authors were Dr. Michael Dean and Dr. Mary Carrington of the cancer institute in Frederick, involved analyses of stored blood from people who had been repeatedly exposed to the AIDS virus, including hemophiliacs, intravenous drug users, and gay men.

Many developed H.I.V. infections and so the researchers could ask if there were genetic differences between those who became infected and those who did not. They also could ask if there were genes that affected the course of the disease. Out of 200 genes they examined, only CKR5 mutations conferred resistance, Dr. O'Brien said.

As Dr. O'Brien and his colleagues were conducting their study, other groups pursued the CKR5 lead. Dr. Marc Parmentier of the University of Brussels studied a population of more than 700 Caucasians who were not at high risk for AIDS and found that 1 percent had two copies of mutated CKR5 genes. The group could not find the mutations in 124 Africans or in 248 Japanese.

The discovery of the CKR5 mutation, researchers say, opens doors to understanding AIDS and how to treat it. For example, Dr. Baltimore said, "it means that the receptor that has been identified is in fact the key receptor through which people get infected."

Secondly, he said, "people can live perfectly well without CKR5." And that means, he said, that "if you can develop a drug that blocks CKR5, it could block H.I.V. without serious side effects."

Stephen Soba, a spokesman for the Gay Men's Health Crisis, an advocacy group in New York, said there was something chilling, horrifying even, in the idea of testing for such a gene. Nonetheless, Mr. Soba said, a CKR5 test "would be an irresistible temptation."

Larry Kramer, the playwright and advocate of a gay rights, said gay men would want a CKR5 test.

"My lover and I each have buried a previous lover," Mr. Kramer said. "I'm H.I.V. positive and he's not." If a test disclosed that his lover was immune to AIDS, he said, it "would remove the sword of Damocles that's hanging over our heads."

But Dr. Norman Fost, an ethicist at the University of Wisconsin who is a visiting professor this year at Princeton University, urged caution.

"It's all very exciting and very promising," Dr. Fost said, but adding that with an AIDS immunity gene, the consequences of being wrong could be deadly. "You don't want someone to say, 'You have the gene so you don't have to practice safe sex anymore.'"

*September 27, 1996*

# The Genesis of an Epidemic: Humans, Chimps and a Virus

## By GINA KOLATA

Three years ago, Dr. Beatrice Hahn got a call from a colleague asking if she wanted some body parts from a chimpanzee that had died a decade ago.

The colleague said, "I have the spleen, the brain and the lymph nodes in my freezer. I need to clean my freezer, so before I throw it out, do you want to look at it?"

Then the scientist said the animal had antibodies in its blood very much like ones that people develop when they are infected with the AIDS virus.

Dr. Hahn leapt at the chance. It was a long shot, but it was possible that the long-dead chimpanzee could be a missing link in the search for the origins of AIDS. A few days later, Federal Express delivered a huge box of frozen chimpanzee parts, packed in dry ice, to Dr. Hahn's laboratory at the University of Alabama at Birmingham, where she is a professor of medicine.

Three days later, she had her answer. That chimpanzee, which had been healthy until she died in childbirth at age 26, held clues that eventually enabled Dr. Hahn and an international group of 11 others to unravel the mystery of the origin of the epidemic. It was a mystery that took years to solve and that had frustrated researchers and the public, stunned by the sudden emergence of such a terrible new disease.

Some said AIDS was caused by a mutant virus, a sort of Andromeda strain. Others favored conspiracy theories suggesting that H.I.V. had been created by scientists and escaped from germ warfare labs. There was a Western medicine disaster theory, which held that the virus was injected into Africans in bad batches of polio vaccine.

Then there was a more pedestrian idea—that people got H.I.V. from primates in Africa.

Scientists tended to favor the primate hypothesis because they knew that diseases can jump from animals to people. Dengue fever, Hantavirus, influenza and hepatitis B all originated in other species. But, researchers learned, it was not easy to trace the virus causing the human AIDS epidemic, H.I.V.-1, to an animal. And even when they started seeing provocative hints about the origins of AIDS, those hints soon turned contradictory.

The first evidence that H.I.V.-1 jumped to humans from primates came about a decade ago, when scientists isolated a virus from an African chimpanzee that

26

very closely resembled the AIDS virus now infecting tens of millions of people. The chimpanzee virus looked so much like H.I.V.-1 that it was almost irresistible to think that the animals had somehow given the virus to people. Its genes were arranged the same way, and it even had a distinctive gene, called vpu, that had never been seen in any other virus.

While AIDS-like viruses were starting to emerge in other primates and in other animals, none looked so much like H.I.V.-1 as this chimpanzee one did.

Adding to the evidence was a tantalizing snippet of another AIDS-like virus found in a tube of blood from a baby chimpanzee that had died. While the fragment was too small for anyone to be certain that it closely resembled H.I.V.-1, the genetic sequence from this second chimp lined up exactly with a piece of the first chimpanzee's virus.

But soon the picture became clouded. A few years ago, scientists found a third chimpanzee with an AIDS-like virus, but when they analyzed that virus, they discovered that it was only distantly related to H.I.V.-1. So, some asked, were chimpanzees really the source of the human AIDS epidemic? Or were chimpanzees, and humans, becoming infected by some other animals?

One way to find out would be to study wild chimpanzees and see whether they had a virus like the human form, H.I.V.-1, whether they had a different virus like the third chimpanzee's virus or whether they were infected with a variety of AIDS-like viruses. But the only way to find viruses was to look for them in blood. And researchers could not draw blood from the elusive animals without stunning them first with a tranquilizer gun, and the stunning effort was impractical.

To make matters worse, no one could show that the animal with a virus like H.I.V.-1 came from the region where the human epidemic first exploded.

That was when Dr. Hahn examined the frozen chimpanzee organs, and the mystery began to crack. That animal, she discovered, also had a virus in its tissues that looked like H.I.V.-1.

Suddenly, said Dr. Edward Holmes, an evolutionary biologist at Oxford University, he and others who had questioned whether chimpanzees really were the source of H.I.V.-1 in humans became convinced. While scientists had found only two, or possibly three chimpanzees that had the virus, Dr. Hahn's information, added to three other lines of evidence, was enough.

One line of evidence pointed to west-central Africa—a region where chimpanzees live—as the place where the human AIDS epidemic began.

Scientists, analyzing the genetic sequences of AIDS viruses found in patients from around the world, were discovering that the viruses in west-central Africa were the most diverse. And it is a general rule that the more diverse an organism's genes are, the longer it has been around. That is because as the years go by more and more variations accumulate in an organism's genes.

For example, Dr. Holmes said, human DNA is most diverse in Africa, supporting the idea that the human species originated on that continent.

The second line of evidence was a plausible way for the virus to get from chimpanzees to humans. People in west-central Africa eat chimpanzees. It was entirely reasonable to think that an infected animal's blood gave the virus to a person who was handling the chimpanzee meat, infecting the person and setting the stage for an AIDS epidemic.

"People eat chimpanzees," Dr. Hahn said. "We expect that transmissions occurred through the exposure to blood through hunting or preparation of meat."

Finally, researchers were discovering AIDS-like viruses in other animals and other primates in Africa, but none were as closely related to H.I.V.-1 as the viruses in the three chimpanzees.

The only species that fit all the evidence as the source of H.I.V.-1 was the chimpanzee, Dr. Holmes said.

A scientific paper that Dr. Hahn had published about the frozen chimpanzee "was extraordinarily important," Dr. Holmes said. "It really made people believe that chimps were the ancestral species."

Dr. Paul M. Sharp, a professor of genetics at the University of Nottingham who worked on the analyses of the viruses, said: "It had been a gradual shift in our perceptions. At first we had been saying that either chimps are the source or they are recipients, like humans." Dr. Hahn's chimp made all the difference, Dr. Sharp said.

Now, researchers say, they have found two more chimpanzees that were infected in the wild with a virus like H.I.V.-1. The animals were among a group of 29 captured in Cameroon, in the west-central region of Africa.

It would be ideal, of course, to find stored blood from the original people who contracted H.I.V.-1 and stored tissue from chimpanzees in the same area, and then show they had exactly the same virus, Dr. Holmes said. But, he added, that is not going to happen.

"You haven't got a smoking gun, but you're never going to have one," Dr. Holmes said. "The gun's long gone. You're never going to find it."

Yet, he said, there is the virus in chimpanzees, there is the geographical overlap between where chimpanzees live and where H.I.V. started, and there is a mechanism.

"That was it for us," Dr. Holmes said.

But knowing the virus came from chimpanzees left two pressing questions. When did the virus take hold in the human population? And how?

Dr. Bette T. Korber, a molecular geneticist at Los Alamos National Laboratory, and her colleagues had a way to get an answer to the question of when. They had the genetic sequences of viruses isolated from people and knew when those viruses were found, starting with the oldest human H.I.V. sample available. It was from a man in what is now Kinshasa, Congo, in west-central Africa, in 1959.

Since the viruses mutate at a roughly constant rate, the researchers could construct a path of how the virus had mutated and determine how long it would take to move from one virus to another one with the amount of genetic diversity found today. From those calculations, they found a date when the spark of the epidemic was lit: 1931, plus or minus 15 years.

"You might think, if the virus was present in 1930, how on earth did we not see it?" Dr. Korber asked. "But if it is only present in a few thousand individuals and it takes a decade to get sick, it could easily have been missed."

Researchers say the virus almost certainly infected humans repeatedly as they killed and ate chimpanzees over the years, but that it is hard to start an AIDS epidemic. For it to develop, the virus must be prevented from dying with its victims and a steady chain of transmissions must occur.

"We think that these transmissions have gone on forever and a day, for all the centuries that people hunted chimpanzees," Dr. Hahn said. "The rule is that these transmissions go nowhere. They just peter out, unless you have additional factors that promote subsequent spread in the new human host."

One possible explanation for the extensive spread of H.I.V.-1, several scientists said, was that people began congregating in cities in Africa. There, the conditions were ripe for an AIDS epidemic.

"If you look at the population of Kinshasa, it's an exponential curve going up," Dr. Sharp said. "During the 20th century, you have far more movement of people into urban areas and perhaps changes in behavior." In addition, doctors in clinics in Africa commonly reused needles without sterilizing them between patients, a practice that, he said, "would have played a role in getting the virus kick-started."

Another possible explanation is less comforting.

Dr. Korber asked if it was possible that nothing really special made the epidemic grow, other than an initial transmission that, by chance, did not die out. Could a very slow curve of exponential growth, starting around 1930, end up in an epidemic that finally caught the world's attention around 20 years ago?

Her mathematical models showed that it made sense. For the first 30 years, the number of cases would have climbed into the hundreds. As the web of infections grew, the numbers would jump, reaching large numbers in Africa by 1980. At that point, enough people would be infected that the epidemic would be noticed. That model is particularly troubling, Dr. Hahn said.

"If you say, 'I don't know how it got started; it could have been this, it could have been that,' and if all you need are a certain set of circumstances in the beginning so that it doesn't die out, then it could happen again," she said.

"People don't want to hear that."

*September 4, 2001*

CHAPTER 2

# Alzheimer's Disease

# Gene Mutation That Causes Alzheimer's Is Found

By GINA KOLATA

In a leap forward in the search for a cause of Alzheimer's disease, researchers have discovered that a pinpoint mutation in a single gene can cause this progressive neurological illness.

The discovery, by Dr. John Hardy of St. Mary's Hospital in London and his colleagues, is the first genetic cause for Alzheimer's disease that has been found. Although there are likely to be others that can cause the disease, the discovery of this gene will allow investigators to narrow their search for causes and treatments for the disease.

Alzheimer's, which afflicts an estimated two million Americans and is the nation's fourth-leading cause of death, is characterized by a gradual loss of memory and reasoning and eventually by severe disorientation. There is no treatment for it.

The finding is important for two reasons. It advances understanding of Alzheimer's disease by resolving a longstanding debate about whether a substance that accumulates in the brains of Alzheimer's patients is a cause of the disease or merely a byproduct. The defect discovered is in the gene that directs cells to produce this substance, a component of nerve cells called amyloid protein. And the finding of the defect in Alzheimer's patients but not in healthy individuals indicates that amyloid protein is indeed a cause of the disease.

Second, the search for treatments can now be focused on methods for removing the buildup of amyloid protein. Though such methods may lie far off, at least researchers will now have a strategy to guide them.

Dr. Hardy and his colleagues have found a distinctive mutation in the gene that directs cells to produce the amyloid protein, a crucial component of nerve cells. They found the mutation in members of two unrelated families who have Alzheimer's disease.

As further evidence that the mutation in the amyloid gene can cause Alzheimer's disease, the scientists reported they did not find the mutation in people who did not have Alzheimer's disease. Their paper will be published in Thursday's issue of the British journal *Nature*.

## Other Likely Causes

There are likely to be other genes that cause Alzheimer's disease because it is known that genes for the disease can lie on at least two different chromosomes. But it is also possible, researchers said, that these different genes bring on the disease in the same way, by causing the accumulation of amyloid fragments in the brain.

Researchers are also uncertain whether all Alzheimer's disease is inherited. If some cases occur by chance, there may be an infection or environmental cause that could possibly be traced back to accumulations of the same protein fragments.

For weeks, news of Dr. Hardy's discovery has been whispered among researchers, who are astonished that a possible gene for Alzheimer's could have been found so quickly—within a few years of the time that a search began in earnest—and that the discovery fits so well into a leading hypothesis of how and why the disease occurs.

"It really is important," said Dr. Dennis Selkoe, a researcher at Brigham and Women's Hospital in Boston. "I'm quite excited about it and a lot of other people are, too."

Dr. Rudy Tanzi, a researcher at the Massachusetts General Hospital, agreed, calling the finding a "breakthrough."

Alzheimer's disease, which afflicts at least one in five Americans by the age of 85, has baffled generations of investigators since it was described in 1901. It is characterized by a progressive and unrelenting death of neurons in areas of the brain that are used for memory and reasoning and, eventually, areas that control the personality.

In studying the disease, many investigators have focused on amyloid, a protein found in every nerve cell but whose synthesis seems to go awry in Alzheimer's disease. But researchers have not known which was the cause and which was effect. Did the nerve cells, in dying, spit out pieces of amyloid or did pieces of amyloid pile up and kill the nerve cells?

Some, like Dr. Tanzi, put their money on amyloid. "I would bet you a great deal of money that if you could prevent the accumulation of amyloid, you could stop dementia," he said.

Others were not so sure.

At the same time, a search for an Alzheimer's gene was going on in earnest as researchers looked for families in which there were clear patterns of inherited disease. Such families can help narrow the search for a defective gene among the 23 pairs of chromosomes that carry the genetic information that directs all activities of human cells.

The Alzheimer's mutation, a change in a single chemical, was found on chromosome 21. Many researchers had suspected that a gene might lie on that chromosome because people with Down syndrome, who have an extra copy of chromosome 21, almost always develop Alzheimer's disease. So it looked like an extra dose of some gene or genes on chromosome 21 could cause the disease. In addition, the gene for amyloid was on chromosome 21.

Two years ago, Dr. James Gusella and his colleagues at Massachusetts General Hospital found that some families who develop Alzheimer's disease in their 40s and 50s, a very young age for the disease, have an aberrant gene on chromosome 21. Other families, they found, did not have such a gene there.

Recently, Dr. Allen Roses of the Duke University School of Medicine reported that another Alzheimer's disease gene was on chromosome 19, and investigators suspect there may be still other genes. Dr. Timothy Bird of the University of Seattle, for example, has found families in which Alzheimer's disease is inherited but who do not have Alzheimer's disease genes on chromosome 21 or chromosome 19, indicating there is yet another location.

But, Dr. Selkoe said, the finding by Dr. Hardy indicates that amyloid must play a fundamental role in causing the disease.

*February 16, 1991*

# Landmark in Alzheimer Research: Breeding Mice With the Disease

### By GINA KOLATA

After years of false starts, false claims and false hopes, researchers say they have finally produced the hallmarks of Alzheimer's disease in laboratory animals.

Researchers at Athena Neurosciences Inc. of South San Francisco, in collaboration with Eli Lilly & Company of Indianapolis, report that they have inserted a human Alzheimer's disease gene in mice. The mice seem fine when they are young but, starting in middle age, the areas of the animals' brains involved in learning and memory became riddled with plaque, the characteristic Brillo-like balls of protein that are found in the brains of patients with Alzheimer's disease. Nerve cells in the mice degenerated in these areas of the brain just as they do in Alzheimer's patients.

The researchers' report, being published today in the journal *Nature*, is being hailed by scientists as a landmark achievement. Although the disease in the mice is not a perfect reflection of human Alzheimer's disease, the animals provide a way to screen and test drugs that might prevent plaque formation and that could enable crucial hypotheses to be tested.

Scientists can use the mice to study how and why the plaques develop and how other risk factors for Alzheimer's disease might exacerbate the brain deterioration.

Alzheimer's disease is the fourth-leading cause of death in the United States. It affects four million Americans and costs the nation $100 billion a year, said Dr. Leonard Berg, chairman of the medical and scientific advisory board of the Alzheimer's Association. He also directs Alzheimer's research at Washington University in St. Louis.

A person afflicted with Alzheimer's disease gradually loses his memory and ability to think and reason, eventually becoming completely incapacitated. There is one drug on the market for Alzheimer's, Cognex, made by the Warner-Lambert Company, but it does not stop the disease. Dr. Berg called it "mildly helpful for a minority of people who try it."

For years, scientists have tried to find laboratory animals with Alzheimer's symptoms, an important tool to speed research. "There have been many attempts, partial successes, intrigue and detours," said Dr. Zaven Khachaturian, who directs Alzheimer's disease research at the National Institute on Aging in Bethesda, Md. But until now, the efforts have failed.

Dr. Khachaturian acknowledged that experts might be leery of claims of yet another Alzheimer's mouse. In fact, some said, and Dr. Khachaturian agreed, the failures have made it essentially impossible to get Federal money to finance such risky research. But he added that the newly reported finding "looks like the real thing."

Dr. John Hardy, who directs research on Alzheimer's disease at the University of South Florida in Tampa, said he was "very, very excited about it."

And Dr. Steven Younkin, a professor of pathology at Case Western Reserve University in Cleveland, said the discovery "will obviously galvanize the whole field."

Dr. Ivan Lieberburg, vice president for research at Athena Neurosciences, said the company had not yet begun the complex tests required to see whether the mice had impaired memories. But he added that because the mice had lost brain cells and connections between neurons, he would be surprised if their memories were intact.

The mice are not exactly like humans with Alzheimer's disease, however, because they do not have tangles, twisted proteins inside the brain cells of Alzheimer's patients that look like tangled wire. But some researchers say that it is plaques, not tangles, that are the crucial features of Alzheimer's disease.

Dr. Lieberburg said that fully 20 percent of people with Alzheimer's disease did not have tangles. Dr. Hardy said that because the mice had plaques and lost brain cells, the work shows that "tangles aren't particularly important."

The mice reported by Athena today were actually created by another company, the Exemplar Corporation of Waltham, Mass., which has gone bankrupt. Athena bought the company last December for $100,000 and 420 shares of Athena stock, which was then trading at about $6 a share, Dr. Lieberburg said. Exemplar's main asset was its mice.

Dr. Lieberburg said the mice have a mutated gene, found by Dr. Hardy in 1991, that causes Alzheimer's disease in some families. The mutation alters beta amyloid, a fragment of a normal protein that is the major constituent of plaque. Researchers have focused on beta amyloid ever since Dr. Bruce Yankner of Harvard Medical School found in 1990 that shards of beta amyloid alone can kill brain cells in the laboratory.

The researchers linked the mutated gene to a piece of DNA that forces cells in the brain to make large quantities of it. In particular, this DNA segment turns on the added gene in the hippocampus and cerebral cortex, areas of the brain used for learning and memory.

Because of the troubled history of research on Alzheimer's mice, Athena scientists showed their data and slides to leading pathologists to prove they had what they said they had.

One who examined the data was Dr. Donald Price, a professor of pathology and neurology at Johns Hopkins University School of Medicine in Baltimore. He said he saw "bona fide amyloid deposits in the brain in regions that are also vulnerable to Alzheimer's disease."

Dr. Price applauded the decision to allow experts to see the slides. "In contrast to other companies and some other investigators who refused to let anyone see their slides, Athena has been very forthcoming," he said.

But many investigators are concerned that Athena has not yet shared its mice. Dr. Lieberburg said the company was breeding hundreds of animals a month for its own research. He said he hoped to make the mice available to scientists at academic centers, but also said that would "require Athena and Lilly to come to an agreement, and we have only begun our discussions."

Meanwhile, some researchers say they will definitely try to make their own mice, repeating the methods Athena uses. But Dr. Yankner said it will probably take as long as two years to make such mice, and "there are no guarantees."

*February 9, 1995*

# Promise Seen for Detection of Alzheimer's

By GINA KOLATA

D r. Daniel Skovronsky sat at a small round table in his corner office, laptop open, waiting for an e-mail message. His right leg jiggled nervously.

A few minutes later, the message arrived—results that showed his tiny start-up company might have overcome one of the biggest obstacles in diagnosing Alzheimer's disease. It had found a dye and a brain scan that, he said, can show the hallmark plaque building up in the brains of people with the disease.

The findings, which will be presented at an international meeting of the Alzheimer's Association in Honolulu on July 11, must still be confirmed and approved by the Food and Drug Administration. But if they hold up, it will mean that for the first time doctors would have a reliable way to diagnose the presence of Alzheimer's in patients with memory problems.

And researchers would have a way to figure out whether drugs are slowing or halting the disease, a step that "will change everyone's thinking about Alzheimer's in a dramatic way," said Dr. Michael Weiner of the University of California, San Francisco, who is not part of the company's study and directs a federal project to study ways of diagnosing Alzheimer's.

Still, the long tale behind this finding shows just how difficult this disease is and why progress toward preventing or curing it has been so slow.

Ever since Alzheimer's disease was described by a German doctor, Alois Alzheimer, in 1906, there was only one way to know for sure that a person had it. A pathologist, examining the brain after death, would see microscopic black freckles, plaque, sticking to brain slices like barnacles. Without plaque, a person with memory loss did not have the disease.

There is no treatment yet to stop or slow the progress of Alzheimer's. But every major drug company has new experimental drugs it hopes will work, particularly if they are started early. The questions, though, are, who should be getting the drugs and who really has Alzheimer's or is developing it?

Even at the best medical centers, doctors often are wrong. Twenty percent of people with dementia—a loss of memory and intellectual functions—who received a diagnosis of Alzheimer's did not have it. There was no plaque when their brains were biopsied. Half with milder memory loss, thought to be on their way to Alzheimer's, do not get the disease. And with such a high rate of misdiagnosis, some who are mistakenly told that they have Alzheimer's are not treated for conditions, like depression or low levels of thyroid hormone or drug side effects and interactions, that are causing their memory problems.

Brain scans that showed plaque could help with some fundamental questions—who has or is getting Alzheimer's, whether the disease ever stops or slows down on its own and even whether plaque is the main culprit causing brain cell death.

Dr. Skovronsky thought he had a way to make scans work. He and his team had developed a dye that could get into the brain and stick to plaque. They labeled the dye with a commonly used radioactive tracer and used a PET scanner to directly see plaque in a living person's brain. But the technology and the dye itself were so new they had to be rigorously tested.

And that is what brought Dr. Skovronsky, a thin and eager-looking 37-year-old, to his e-mail that recent day.

Five years ago, Dr. Skovronsky, who named his company Avid in part because that is what he is, had taken a big personal and professional gamble. He left academia and formed Avid Radiopharmaceuticals, based in Philadelphia, to develop his radioactive dye and designed a study with hospice patients to prove it worked.

Hospice patients were going to die soon and so, he reasoned, why not ask them to have scans and then brain autopsies afterward to see if the scans showed just what a pathologist would see. Some patients would be demented, others not.

Some predicted his study would be impossible, if not unethical. But the F.D.A. said it wanted proof that the plaque on PET scans was the same as plaque in a brain autopsy.

The Avid study was designed to provide that proof. And the full results, contained in the e-mail message sent that day, May 14, were the moment of truth. When he saw them, Dr. Skovronsky said they were everything he had hoped for.

"This is about as good as it gets," he said that day.

He went into a rotunda that serves as Avid's lunchroom to tell the company's 50 employees. "This is a big day for us," he continued. "I thought about what I would say, but I have totally forgotten it."

His employees applauded. Then they had champagne in blue plastic cups.

## A First Dye

The type of scans used in this study, PET scans, are expensive and patients have to go to a scanning center, get injected with a radioactive dye, wait for the dye to reach their brain and then have a scan.

Other tests are being studied—ones that look for amyloid in cerebrospinal fluid that bathes the brain; MRI scans that look for shrinkage of the brain in areas needed for memory and reasoning; PET scans that look for uptake of glucose, a cellular fuel, to show areas where the brain was active and where it was not. The tests, though, were not necessarily specific for Alzheimer's and none had been studied to see if they accurately predicted plaque on autopsy.

Earlier this decade, two scientists at the University of Pittsburgh developed an amyloid dye that, while not practical for widespread use, stunned scientists by showing it seemed possible to see amyloid in a living brain.

The researchers, Chester Mathis and William Klunk, began their work two decades ago, persevering even though they had no research money. In the first 10 years, they tested more than 400 compounds. When they finally found one that seemed promising, they tested more than 300 variations.

"On and on it went," Dr. Mathis said.

Finally, in late 2001, they began working with collaborators in Sweden to test their dye in humans.

On Valentine's Day 2002, the Swedish researchers injected the first Alzheimer's patient with the dye, known as Pittsburgh Compound B, and scanned the patient's brain.

It worked, the Swedish doctors told Dr. Mathis in an excited phone call.

A PET scan showed amyloid exactly where it would be expected. The Swedish doctors were convinced they were seeing actual plaque. They told Dr. Mathis it was time to celebrate.

But Dr. Mathis worried. What if the same pattern occurred in people without Alzheimer's?

Two weeks later, he got another call from Sweden. His colleagues had scanned a person without Alzheimer's. There was no sign of telltale plaques.

His sweet reward came in July 2002, when the scans were shown to an audience of 5,000 scientists at an international conference on Alzheimer's.

"There was an audible gasp," Dr. Mathis said. "The field was taken aback."

"The rest is history," he added.

Yet there was a problem. Pittsburgh Compound B used carbon 11 as its radioactive tracer. And its half-life is 20 minutes. Researchers have to make it in a cyclotron in the basement of a medical center, quickly attach it to the dye, dash over to a patient lying in a scanner, and inject it.

And a critical question remained: Was a PET scan with the Pittsburgh dye really equivalent to a brain autopsy?

Meanwhile, others, including Dr. Skovronsky, had another idea—use fluorine 18, with a half-life of about two hours. It could be made in the morning, and used that afternoon. And fluorine 18 is made routinely for two million cancer PET scans each year.

Dr. Skovronsky, starting at the University of Pennsylvania and then at Avid, worked with a University of Pennsylvania chemist, Hank Kung, for nine years to find and develop the radioactive dye. The university had the patent; Avid licensed it. Finally, on June 8, 2007, a patient at Johns Hopkins had a scan with their compound. Plaque lit up.

Most of the time, the scans were as expected—those with Alzheimer's had lots of plaque, those with normal memories had little if any and those with mild memory impairment were in between.

But about 20 percent of people over 60 with normal memories had plaque.

"Then we looked more carefully," Dr. Skovronsky said. "The 20 percent who had amyloid, though they were still statistically in the normal range, did worse on every memory test than the control group."

What, Dr. Skovronsky asked, did that mean? Were they starting to develop Alzheimer's? If so, could dementia be stalled if there were drugs to stop amyloid from accumulating?

The definition of Alzheimer's is plaque plus memory loss and other symptoms of mental decline. But what is not known because no one could follow the development of plaque before a person died, was whether people with plaque and normal memories were developing Alzheimer's.

"We've always assumed the pathology has been there, that the plaque has been there years before symptoms," said Dr. Steven T. DeKosky, an Alzheimer's researcher who is vice president and dean at the University of Virginia School of Medicine. "But we never had a way to detect plaque in living persons," he said. And so plaque in the brains of people with normal memories has been a puzzle.

"Over the next couple of years, we will find out what it means."

## A Request of the Dying

On Oct. 23, 2008, Avid and two other companies, Bayer and General Electric, that are developing fluorine 18–based dyes for amyloid scans, got a pointed question from an advisory committee to the F.D.A.: How do you know that what you are seeing on scans is the same as the amyloid you see on autopsy?

It seemed impossible to answer. If researchers wait for their subjects to die before comparing scans with autopsies they can be waiting a long time.

But Avid had a plan, and the committee agreed in principle that it would work. Hospice patients would be study subjects, some with dementia, some without. All would have memory tests and brain scans. After death, their brains would be autopsied. Avid suggested that after the first 35 died, there should be enough data to know if the scans gave a true picture of the pathology. Then the F.D.A. could decide if the results were convincing enough to approve the dye for marketing.

Some doctors had misgivings, wondering how they could ask people who were sick and dying to be scanned just to help Alzheimer's research. But, they found, most patients and their families agreed and said they were grateful to have been asked.

That was evident on May 19, when Dr. Skovronsky gave a lunch for patients' families in Sun City, Ariz., to thank them for participating.

They thanked him.

"It really touched my heart to be in this," said Dorothy Wall, whose husband, Claude E. Wall, died of liver cancer in Sun City on March 3.

"Something bad happens, and now something good happens."

## Answers

Late last year, Avid saw the initial results of its hospice study—data from the first six patients. Then, as more patients were studied, the data from them were held by a company that would analyze it. Avid did not see the results until the study was completed. But those first six were encouraging.

A man diagnosed with Alzheimer's and cancer had a scan showing no plaque. His autopsy did not show it, either. The diagnosis was wrong. Another man with Parkinson's disease and dementia had been diagnosed as having dementia solely due to Parkinson's. His scan showed amyloid. So did the autopsy. He had Alzheimer's. A woman with mild memory loss had a scan showing no amyloid.

Her autopsy also found none. Three others had clinical diagnoses of Alzheimer's, confirmed by scans and autopsies.

Finally, on May 14, 35 patients had been scanned and autopsied. The Avid study was complete, and the full data will be presented at the meeting next month. Other companies, still doing their studies, did not yet have data to examine.

And Dr. Skovronsky got that e-mail message.

"This is going to have a big impact on Alzheimer's disease, guys," he told his staff that day.

*June 23, 2010*

# Rules Seek to Expand Diagnosis of Alzheimer's

By GINA KOLATA

For the first time in 25 years, medical experts are proposing a major change in the criteria for Alzheimer's disease, part of a new movement to diagnose and, eventually, treat the disease earlier.

The new diagnostic guidelines, presented Tuesday at an international Alzheimer's meeting in Hawaii, would mean that new technology like brain scans would be used to detect the disease even before there are evident memory problems or other symptoms.

If the guidelines are adopted in the fall, as expected, some experts predict a two- to threefold increase in the number of people with Alzheimer's disease. Many more people would be told they probably are on their way to getting it. The Alzheimer's Association says 5.3 million Americans now have the disease.

The changes could also help drug companies that are, for the first time, developing new drugs to try to attack the disease earlier. So far, there are no drugs that alter the course of the disease.

Development of the guidelines, by panels of experts convened by the National Institute on Aging and the Alzheimer's Association, began a year ago because, with a new understanding of the disease and new ways of detection, it was becoming clear that the old method of diagnosing Alzheimer's was sorely outdated.

The current formal criteria for diagnosing Alzheimer's require steadily progressing dementia—memory loss and an inability to carry out day-to-day activities, like dressing or bathing—along with a pathologist's report of plaque and another abnormality, known as tangles, in the brain after death.

But researchers are now convinced that the disease is present a decade or more before dementia.

"Our thinking has changed dramatically," said Dr. Paul Aisen, an Alzheimer's researcher at the University of California, San Diego, and a member of one of the groups formulating the new guidelines. "We now view dementia as a late stage in the process."

The new guidelines include criteria for three stages of the disease: preclinical disease, mild cognitive impairment due to Alzheimer's disease and, lastly, Alzheimer's dementia. The guidelines should make diagnosing the final stage of the disease in people who have dementia more definitive. But, the guidelines also say that the earlier a diagnosis is made the less certain it is. And so the new effort to diagnose the disease earlier could, at least initially, lead to more mistaken diagnoses.

Under the new guidelines, for the first time, diagnoses will aim to identify the disease as it is developing by using results from so-called biomarkers—tests like brain scans, M.R.I. scans and spinal taps that reveal telltale brain changes.

The biomarkers were developed and tested only recently and none have been formally approved for Alzheimer's diagnosis. One of the newest, a PET scan, shows plaque in the brain—a unique sign of Alzheimer's brain pathology. The others provide strong indications that Alzheimer's is present, even when patients do not yet have dementia or even much memory loss.

Dr. Aisen says he foresees a day when people in their 50s routinely have biomarker tests for Alzheimer's and, if the tests indicate the disease is brewing, take drugs to halt it. That is a ways off but, he said, but "it's where we are heading."

"This is a major advance," said Dr. John Morris, an Alzheimer's researcher at Washington University in St. Louis who helped formulate the guidelines. "We used to say we did not know for certain it was Alzheimer's until the brain is examined on autopsy."

Dr. Ronald Petersen, an Alzheimer's researcher at the Mayo Clinic in Minnesota and chairman of the Alzheimer's Association's medical and scientific advisory council, said adding biomarkers to a diagnosis would be a big improvement.

Today, he says, when a patient comes with memory problems, doctors might say that the person has a chance of developing Alzheimer's in the next decade, a chance of not getting much worse for several years, and a chance of actually getting better.

Tests like brain scans, Dr. Petersen said, "will allow us to be much more definitive." If the tests show changes characteristic of Alzheimer's disease, a doctor can say, "I think you are on the Alzheimer's road."

That can be a difficult conversation, but it can allow patients and their families to plan. "At least it's a conversation the physician can have with the patient," Dr. Petersen said.

Alzheimer's experts welcomed the new criteria.

"Overall, I think this is a giant step in the right direction," said Dr. P. Murali Doraiswamy, a psychiatry professor and Alzheimer's disease researcher at Duke University who was not involved with making the guidelines. "It moves us closer to the cause of the disease rather than just looking at symptoms."

But, he added, it also is a huge change.

"This has implications for everybody alive, anybody who is getting older,"

Dr. Doraiswamy said. Among other things, he said, it will encourage a lot more testing. And, Dr. Doraiswamy said, "diagnosis rates, like testing rates, only go in one direction—up."

Doctors will have to learn new terms—preclinical Alzheimer's; prodromal, or early stage, Alzheimer's. Patients going to see a doctor with memory problems might be offered biomarker tests, which can be expensive.

The ripple extends beyond doctors and patients, Dr. Doraiswamy said. The new diagnostic criteria also have consequences for lawyers, insurance companies and workers' compensation programs.

And, he said, people have to be prepared for unintended consequences, which always occur when the diagnosis of a disease is changed. For now, he said: "We ought to be cautious that we don't stimulate all this testing before we can give people something to manage their disease. There is no point in giving them just a label."

*July 13, 2010*

# Three Drugs to Be Tested to Stave Off Alzheimer's

By GINA KOLATA

Scientists have selected three different types of Alzheimer's drugs to be tested in the first large-scale international attempt to prevent the disease in people who are otherwise doomed to get it.

It is one of three studies with the same goal that will start early next year. This one involves 160 people from the United States, Britain and Australia with a variety of gene mutations that cause Alzheimer's with absolute certainty. Most of the test subjects will have no symptoms yet of the degenerative disease that ravages the brain, destroying memory and thought. But they would be expected to start showing signs of problems with memory and thinking within five years unless the drugs work. The hope is that by intervening early, the disease might be headed off.

Another study starting next year involves an extended family in Colombia that shares the same mutation. Anyone who inherits that mutated gene gets Alzheimer's disease. A third study will involve people in the United States age 70 and older who seem perfectly healthy and who do not have any known Alzheimer's mutations but in whom, brain scans show, the disease is starting to manifest itself.

In recent years, as studies involving people who already have Alzheimer's have failed, researchers increasingly have called for studies in those who do not yet have the disease, arguing that the time to intervene is before the brain is irreversibly damaged. So the new study with people who are destined to get Alzheimer's unless a drug can stop it is a way to test that idea.

"It's an exciting opportunity," said Dr. Ronald Petersen, director of the Alzheimer's Disease Research Center at the Mayo Clinic, who is not involved with the study.

Maria C. Carrillo, vice president of medical and scientific relations at the Alzheimer's Association, said the results would come quickly. Within a few years, as researchers simultaneously compare the three approaches to stopping the disease, they should know which drug, if any, is going to work. The association contributed $4.2 million to the study, more than twice as much as it has ever spent on a grant, Dr. Carrillo said.

The announcement comes at a time of transition for Alzheimer's research. In recent years, investigators have discovered methods of spotting and tracking the progression of the disease before any clinical symptoms appear, using brain scans and spinal taps and sensitive tests of memory. They have led to what many think is the start of a new era in which drugs can be assessed without waiting for effects on profound symptoms.

That is a goal of the study whose drugs were announced on Wednesday. Known as DIAN TU, for Dominantly Inherited Alzheimer's Network Trials Unit, it was designed to get the most information possible in as short a time as possible. Three-quarters of the subjects will get one of three drugs aimed at beta amyloid, a protein that forms the hard, barnaclelike plaques on the brain that are the hallmark of Alzheimer's.

The drugs were chosen from among 15 that drug companies offered, said the study's principal investigator, Dr. Randall Bateman of the Washington University School of Medicine in St. Louis. A committee assessed them, looking for drugs with the best evidence of effectiveness and the least likelihood of dangerous side effects. One concern is something called ARIA, for amyloid-related imaging abnormality. People with the abnormality may have no signs that anything is wrong, but brain scans show what looks like a change in neural connections. ARIA is a rare side effect of some experimental Alzheimer's drugs, and it is not clear what it means, but it is a concern and will be monitored closely, Dr. Bateman said.

For the first two years of the study, researchers will follow the subjects with scans and memory tests, looking for signs that the drugs are working. If one or more seems clearly effective, they will switch all the subjects to it and continue the study, looking for clinical benefits.

The drugs to be tested are gantenerumab, made by Roche, which binds to clumps of amyloid and allows it to be removed from the brain, and two drugs by Lilly. One, known as LY2886721, blocks an enzyme, beta-secretase, used to make amyloid. The other, solanezumab, attaches itself to amyloid that is floating free in the brain before it clumps into plaques, facilitating its removal.

Solanezumab was recently tested in people with mild to moderate Alzheimer's and appeared to have no effect on the disease. But Lilly also handed over all of its data to a group of academic researchers, giving them complete control of the presentation of their analysis and publication, and the group noticed something interesting. The investigators pooled data from the company's two large clinical trials of the drugs. In their extensive analysis, presented Monday at the American Neurological Association meeting in Boston, they reported that it improved Alzheimer's dementia, particularly in mild cases.

"This is the best news we've had in a decade," said Dr. Paul Aisen, an Alzheimer's researcher at the University of California, San Diego. Dr. Aisen helped analyze the Lilly data and is also a member of the DIAN TU committee that helped select the drugs for the clinical trial.

DIAN is hoping that the same sort of exquisitely sensitive cognitive tests will provide the first sign that one of the drugs is working.

If any of the drugs come to market, they will be expensive, which raises issues of how patients will ever be able to pay for them.

Researchers said they would face that issue when they come to it.

"Right now we have to get treatments that work," said Dr. Rachelle S. Doody, director of the Alzheimer's Disease and Memory Disorders Center at the Baylor College of Medicine. "Then we can put pressure on to bring down the cost."

*October 10, 2012*

CHAPTER 3

# Antibiotics

# "Giant" Germicide Yielded by Mold

## By WILLIAM L. LAURENCE

A new chemical substance elaborated by a special strain of mold in bread and Roquefort cheese that has proved itself in tests on animals and in preliminary clinical trials on human beings as the most powerful non-toxic germ-killer so far discovered, thousands of times more potent than any of the drugs of the sulfanilamide family, was described here today.

Hundreds of leading physicians from the United States and Canada, attending the annual meeting of the American Society for Clinical Investigation, heard Dr. Martin H. Dawson, Associate Professor of Medicine at the College of Physicians and Surgeons, Columbia University, New York City, report on the new germ-killer.

Associated with Professor Dawson in this work, which physicians here hailed as opening a new chapter in the fight of medical science against bacterial infections caused by the vast host of deadly microorganisms known as gram-positive bacteria, were Drs. Gladys L. Hobby, Karl Meyer and Eleanor Chaffee.

## Not Available in Pure Form

The new substance, not yet available in pure form, is known as penicillin, after the family of molds known as penicillium. Only one specific strain of it can elaborate the new giant among germ-destroyers, and its final isolation, Professor Dawson said, would depend on a larger supply of the starting material than is now available. However, even in its present crude form, Dr. Dawson reported, minute doses have proved remarkably effective in protecting animals against enormous doses of deadly bacteria of various types.

Recent experiments have shown, Professor Dawson reported, that penicillin is "extremely active" in a dilution of one to 500,000. Mice infected intraperitoneally (through injection of bacteria directly into the peritoneum) with a highly virulent strain of hemolytic (blood destroying) streptococci in amounts up to two cubic centimeters of whole culture, containing from 50,000,000 to 100,000,000 organisms, were protected with a dose of about seven milligrams of a "soluble, impure preparation," given subcutaneously. Control animals receiving the same bacteria in dilutions of one part in 10,000,000, Dr. Dawson reported, died within forty-eight hours.

"In further experiments," Dr. Dawson reported, "it has been shown that penicillin is effective intravenously and intraperitoneally as well as subcutaneously. Animals have also been treated successfully as long as eight hours after infection. Experiments on oral administration are as yet incomplete."

Penicillin, Professor Dawson reported, has been administered to four patients suffering from that deadly form of bacterial heart disease known as sub-acute bacterial endocarditis. "Sufficient material was not available for adequate therapy in these cases," he said. "However," he added, "no serious toxic effects were observed."

"It would appear," Professor Dawson concluded, "that penicillin is a chemotherapeutic agent of great potential significance. Penicillin probably represents a new class of chemotherapeutic agents which may prove as useful, or even more useful, than the sulfonamides."

It was originally observed by [Alexander] Fleming in 1929, Dr. Dawson told the physicians, that staphylococci failed to grow on plates in the neighborhood of a colony of penicillium mold.

## New Light on Gramicidin

Last year Dr. René J. Dubos startled the scientific world with the announcement that he had extracted from a special strain of soil bacteria a chemical substance he named gramicidin that had proved the most powerful microbe-killer until then known to man. Unfortunately, gramicidin was found to be highly toxic to animals as well as to bacteria.

At the meeting today there were presented two reports, from the Mayo Clinic, Rochester, Minn., and from the Massachusetts Memorial Hospital, Boston, respectively, announcing studies on the gramicidin that have made it possible to apply it successfully in a number of human infections that had not responded to any other treatment.

Dr. Wallace E. Herrell and Dr. Dorothy Heilman of the Mayo Clinic, set out to determine, by methods of tissue culture, the manner in which gramicidin produced its toxic effects on animals. They found that along with its powerful bactericidal action it also possessed the power to break down red blood cells by the process called hemolysis. This at once indicated that the chemical might be used safely in local infections where it was not necessary to introduce it into the blood stream.

Tests on animals proved that this was the case, and that the gramicidin could be used safely in local applications, as it did no harm at all to tissues. It has been used effectively, the Mayo and Boston physicians reported, in the treatment of sinus infections, infections of the bladder, infected but not bleeding wounds, ulcers and empyema from pneumonia.

The Boston report was presented by Drs. Charles H. Rammelkamp and Chester S. Keefer.

Sinus infections were cleared up within forty-eight hours, Drs. Herrell and Heilman reported. Severe bladder infections that the sulfa drugs did not affect were cured within one week.

Infected wounds were freed of all bacteria within twenty-four hours after gramicidin treatment, following which the wounds rapidly healed, Drs. Rammelkamp and Keefer reported.

*May 6, 1941*

# Discoverer Stresses Penicillin War Boon

The prospect that if sufficient penicillin becomes available battle wounds might be prevented from becoming infected or, if infected, they might generally be cured in a month was held out today by Sir Alexander Fleming, discoverer of the wonder drug.

Preaching a hospital Sunday sermon at the Savoy Chapel Royal, he recalled that in the last war there were many soldiers whose wounds remained open six months. Sir Alexander said that penicillin now "has already done a great deal to help wounded soldiers and is going to do far more as the supply increases."

Although the United States has already far outstripped Britain in the production of penicillin, and Canada, Australia and Russia have entered the field, "civilians must wait just a little longer," he said, before supplies became sufficient for them.

Penicillin was first used in the treatment of war wounds in Tunisia.

*June 12, 1944*

# New Drug Is Used to Treat Typhoid

Streptomycin, the germ-killing qualities of which were revealed only a year ago, has been used successfully in the treatment of typhoid fever, a disease for which to date there has been no known positive cure, it is disclosed in the current issue of the *Journal of the American Medical Association*.

Of five persons treated who had been infected with typhoid through a germ carrier reportedly stemming from a bakery, three were completely cured, and in the two other cases the authors suggested that certain human body substances were present that inhibited the influence of the streptomycin.

These new experiments with streptomycin, which indicate its effectiveness in combating Gram-negative bacteria, against which penicillin has been used without success, were conducted last December by three Philadelphians. Their studies are the first publicly reported successful experiments in treating typhoid with streptomycin.

The scientists are Dr. Hobart A. Reimann of the Jefferson Medical College and Hospital, who directed the clinical studies, assisted by Dr. Alison H. Price of the same institution and Dr. William P. Elias of the Wyeth Institute of Applied Biochemistry, who handled the laboratory tests.

While purely in the experimental stage, streptomycin was nevertheless said to present the first good approach to a cure for typhoid, which scientists have sought for ages, but thus far they have developed only a conservative fever treatment.

The experiments also indicated a probable superiority of streptomycin, originally discovered by Dr. Selman A. Waksman of Rutgers University, over penicillin in the long-range treatment of such diseases as tuberculosis. With few exceptions, penicillin has proved of little value in the treatment of these diseases.

In the Philadelphia experiments, the five individuals were treated over a period of one to two weeks each and received daily dosages of streptomycin.

The patients were treated with streptomycin orally as well as intravenously and intramuscularly with success, although the oral treatment alone was ineffective. The report suggested, however, that oral treatment with streptomycin in typhoid areas might prove useful in preventing the disease in the same manner that atabrine is successful in preventing malaria.

Streptomycin is available in limited quantities and is provided for experimental uses only. It was described by one scientist not connected with the Philadelphia experiments as in approximately the same stage of development for general public use as penicillin was two years ago.

Streptomycin has been used successfully in the treatment of tuberculosis in guinea pigs in experiments at the Mayo Clinic by Drs. W. H. Feldman and H. C. Hinshaw, but results of the treatment of tuberculous patients with streptomycin have not yet been reported publicly.

*May 24, 1945*

# Drug Is Effective for Tuberculosis

"Definitely and consistently encouraging results" have been obtained with streptomycin treatment of tuberculosis in 100 patients during the past two years.

This is reported by a group of scientists who pioneered in the treatment of tuberculosis with the chemical from bacilli found in soil. They are Drs. H. Corwin Hinshaw and William H. Feldman of the Mayo Clinic and Foundation and Dr. Karl H. Pfuetze of Cannon Falls, Minn.

Streptomycin should have more extensive trials in treatment of many forms of tuberculosis, they recommend in the forthcoming issue of the *Journal of the American Medical Association.*

Large doses must be given for prolonged periods; they caution against starting streptomycin treatment unless enough of the antibiotic drug is likely to be available for two to four months. This would be close to one pound of the drug.

Most of the patients who get this prolonged treatment will develop toxic symptoms. Their sense of equilibrium is likely to be disturbed, and this will continue for several weeks after the drug has been stopped.

Streptomycin is not a substitute for other and proved effective forms of treatment of tuberculosis, the scientists state. It should not be given to patients who are getting better with other treatment or who are likely to recover under usual treatment.

Actual healing in tuberculosis, they point out, must be accompanied by the slow processes of resorption, fibrosis and calcification, during which the germs are walled off in a calcified area of tissue. The role of streptomycin is to block paths for extension of the disease while the healing forces are operating.

*December 1, 1946*

**CHAPTER 4**

# Blood Pressure

# To Retard Old Age With Electricity

In the current issue of *The Medical Times* Dr. Samuel G. Tracy of this city describes a method by which, he says, old age can be retarded. He uses electric currents to lessen blood pressure, thus modifying the results of arterio-sclerosis, or hardening of the arteries which is characteristic of advancing age.

Dr. Tracy says in part:

"A celebrated French clinician claims that a man is as old as his arteries. In other words, beginning arterio-sclerosis is the starting point of senescence irrespective of the number of years the patient may have lived. A man or a woman may be young in years but old in his or her arteries, hence the importance of avoiding conditions and habits of life which are likely to produce a high blood pressure with hardening of the arteries.

"Senility is a natural process, and it should come on gradually and painlessly; however, owing to inheritance or predisposition, as well as the strenuous life we live in our struggle for existence, senescence creeps on us before we are aware of it. This is the time for the physician to exercise his functions and protect his patient before he is actually senile.

"When a man begins to get old much can be accomplished by proper medical advice and treatment to retard the symptoms which are an accompaniment of the inevitable decline in years.

"It is admitted by many of our profession that arterio-sclerosis (with loss of elasticity in the walls of the arteries) is really the beginning of old age. The changes in the wall of the blood vessel are said to be due to hypertension and to vitiated blood. The condition of the blood is due to auto-infection, and the floating in the blood stream of waste materials."

## Danger in Over-Eating

"The waste material found in the blood is due to over-eating, excessive drinking of alcohol, and auto-intoxication. In the latter case the chemistry of the system is unbalanced, there is faulty metabolism, and waste and repair do not take place equally. There is more waste than repair, and the organs which preside over elimination of waste material being overtaxed, are unable to efficiently take care of the excess, and consequently some waste material floats in the blood stream, acting as a poisonous substance, vitiating the 'rivers of life,' and degenerating the 'river beds.'

"Degeneration in old age takes place by two methods, fatty degeneration and calcareous degeneration. Fatty degeneration is the increased production of unhealthy fat, due to defective nutrition, and when the fatty degeneration affects the liver, kidneys or heart we have serious pathological conditions.

"Calcareous degeneration is an unnatural increase of lime deposit in the tissues. These products are often found as true incrustations. When calcareous degeneration takes place in the walls of an artery the vessel becomes hardened, loses its elasticity, and its calibre becomes smaller. At this time the resisting powers of the system are lessened and a long train of symptoms, particularly those pertaining to the circulatory system, are in evidence, and fatal results from apoplexy, heart or kidney disease are likely to follow.

"When arterio-sclerosis has manifested itself by hypertension in the blood vessels, strong emotions, excessive mental excitement or physical strain is likely to endanger life by a sudden rupture of a small vessel in the brain.

"An artery of the body can be compared with a flexible rubber tube used for a drop light and filled with illuminating gas. Continual overpressure of gas within the tube will affect the walls of the tube and diminish its elasticity. If the tube is slightly damaged or obstructed, increased pressure of gas may cause a fissure in the inner wall of the tube. To make the tube to do good practical work it is absolutely necessary to moderate the pressure of the gas. So it is with our arteries. When arterio-sclerosis first makes its appearance we must reduce the pressure in the blood vessel.

"While old age cannot be prevented, we have agencies at our disposal which will materially assist in retarding it, and in making its symptoms more comfortable. These agencies are high frequency electric currents, diet and hygiene. The physiological effects of a high frequency current are due to the spark or condenser effect which produces mechanical effect on the tissue, an increased heat in the body, and the formation of ozone and ultra violet light. The local action is accomplished by a general reaction, the blood pressure is lowered, and combustion through the lungs is increased. The eliminative processes are generally stimulated."

## Treatment by Electricity

"Formerly I obtained high frequency currents by the use of a transformer attached to a static machine, but recently I have been using the Hyfrex coil.

"Treatment by the Hyfrex coil: A senescent patient with arterio-sclerosis may be placed in a solenoid and connected with the high frequency apparatus, or he may be placed on a condenser couch or chair. In the latter case he may lie or sit without removing his clothing, and be subjected to a bombardment of millions of oscillations per second. In from twenty to thirty minutes his blood pressure will be reduced from ten to fifteen millimeters, and his temperature raised one to one and one-half degrees. This séance may be repeated three or four times a week. While subjected to the electric action, the system is energized, the circulation of the blood equalized, the blood pressure is reduced, the general nutrition is improved, functional activity stimulated, the proper relationship between waste and repair is better sustained, and at the same time the elimination of poisonous products takes place more rapidly. After repeated applications nature assumes her normal functions, or as near normal as the case will permit, and performs her own work without the electrical stimulus.

"At this point I wish to say that I do not depend entirely upon high frequency currents in the treatment of arterio-sclerosis or senility, for diet and hygiene play an important part. As one grows older he requires less food. An old man requires one-fifth less than an adult. In a general way most people eat too much, especially in our large cities, and they take too little exercise.

"As one writer on this subject has well said, there are few of us who are muscularly and cerebrally well balanced. We live too much in the brain and too little in the body.

"The old man or woman should eat little at a time, often as necessary, and chew much. A large rich meal should never be taken, particularly in the evening, because under the influence of the digestion the circulation of the blood becomes more active and the blood pressure increases. Tea, coffee and alcoholic beverages should not as a rule be taken; however, habit has much to do with this. My advice on the subject, generally speaking where arterio-sclerosis exists in the aged with the accompanying full pulse, distilled and fermented drinks should be given up entirely. However, in the old man of the opposite type, who has a weak pulse and is easily exhausted, wine and even whisky or brandy may be taken in small doses, preferably at mealtime. I have no doubt in many cases of the aged with hardened arteries, that alcoholic beverages are responsible for attacks of apoplexy, angina pectoris and acute bladder and kidney diseases.

"The old man with cold skin should have plenty of fresh air, but the surface of his body should be well protected with suitable clothing. He should wear light but warm clothing, with frequent massage of the body. For those who are approaching old age, or are actually senile, moderate but not violent exercise is very important."

*February 2, 1908*

# Blood Pressure Lowered in Tests

By WILLIAM L. LAURENCE

A derivative of adrenalin, which can be prepared synthetically in the laboratory in unlimited amounts, has been discovered to be highly effective in reducing high blood pressure in animals, it was reported today before the semi-annual meeting of the American Chemical Society.

The report of a new advance in the quest for means to combat man's greatest natural enemy, responsible for more than 375,000 deaths annually in the United States, and striking largely among the most useful members of the community, was presented by Dr. K. A. Oster, physician, and Dr. Harry Sobotka, chemist, of the Mount Sinai Hospital in New York City.

This marks the first discovery of an artificially prepared substance effective in reducing high blood pressure. Previously, extracts from kidneys and a natural substance, known as tyrosinase, extracted from mushrooms, had been reported as capable of producing similar effects. However, the kidney extract and the mushroom tyrosinase can be obtained only in very small amounts, and both are impure in form and likely to produce toxic effects.

## Tested on Rats and Dogs

The synthetic substance, known as adrenochrome, it was reported, has been found to be non-toxic when given to animals. It was given to rats in doses as high as 100 milligrams and to dogs in doses twice as high. In all cases the high blood pressure in these animals was reduced to normal in a few hours, and remained normal as long as the chemical was provided at the proper intervals, the Mount Sinai scientists reported.

It was emphasized, however, that no trials on human beings with high blood pressure had been made and, furthermore, that no conclusions as to the possible applicability of the chemical to human cases would be justified at present. But the fact that the chemical has produced the same results in two different species of animals, rats and dogs, is regarded by the scientists as a hopeful indication that it may also act in a similar manner in human applications.

The chemical in its present form, it was found, is rather unstable, losing its activity as an anti-pressor substance within a week. Efforts are now being made to produce it in a form which would be more stable, Drs. Oster and Sobotka stated.

Adrenalin, secreted by the medulla (inner part) of the adrenal gland, is by itself a blood-pressure-raising substance. It is converted into adrenochrome, the blood-pressure-lowering substance, by oxidation, in the course of which four hydrogen atoms are removed from its molecules. The new substance belongs to a large chemical family known as ortho-quinones.

## Derivative of Recent Origin

Adrenochrome was first prepared in England about five years ago. Not until the Mount Sinai Hospital investigators began their tests, however, did its properties as a reducer of high blood pressure become known. Oddly enough, the substance will not reduce the blood pressure in normal animals.

There are two types of chemicals, Drs. Oster and Sobotka explained, exerting an effect on blood pressure. One type they described as anti-pressor substances. These lower pressure only where it is high but do not affect the pressure in normal animals. Adrenochrome belongs to this group. There is another group named depressor substances, which lower the blood pressure even when it is normal.

High blood pressure, it is believed, is produced when substances known as "pressor amines" are present in the blood stream as the result of an insufficient blood supply to the kidney, or other causes as yet unknown. The adrenochrome, it is likewise believed, produces its effect by oxidizing, or burning up, these pressor amines.

Substances which raise blood pressure, Drs. Oster and Sobotka stated, can be converted within the body into closely related compounds which have the opposite effect. This was demonstrated by them, they reported, by means of "a most delicate method" which they devised and in which the transition of a noxious substance to a protective one in individual cells of the kidneys of healthy animals was observed by a color reaction under the microscope.

The adrenochrome is a dark brown powder insoluble in water, and must be kept in the absence of air. It is injected intramuscularly in rats and intravenously in dogs in a suspension of olive oil or propylene glycol.

## Tests with Adenine Reported

Adenine, a compound found in yeast, liver and other natural foods, and para-amino-benzoic acid, an anti–gray hair vitamin, may, if taken in excess, be detrimental to the body's ability to protect itself against bacterial infections, it was reported at the meeting by Dr. Gustav J. Martin and C. Virginia Fisher of the Warner Institute for Therapeutic Research.

"These compounds increase the growth potential of bacteria in the body," Dr. Martin declared. "These are indications that they also render useless sulfonamides which are commonly used in the treatment of many bacterial diseases.

"Adenine, present in yeast and in liver and playing a role in human nutrition, as demonstrated by Dr. Tom Spies of the University of Cincinnati, has been demonstrated by use to be detrimental in three ways in any instance in which sulfonamides are used. It greatly increases the toxicity of the sulfonamides while diminishing their therapeutic action, and it increases the growth rate of bacteria in the body. Thus adenine has a profound effect on the course of bacterial infections.

"Compounds like para-amino-benzoic acid and adenine, both of which occur in yeast, should not be taken during the course of any bacterial disease; if they are, the patient's chances will be materially diminished. This danger cannot be overemphasized, particularly as para-amino-benzoic acid is now being marketed as a cure for gray hair. Great caution and good judgment should be used before proceeding with any type of vitamin therapy containing compounds such as adenine and para-amino-benzoic acid in significant amounts.

"Adenine, closely related to uric acid, is a purine base found in the nucleic acids of plant and animal origin, and is therefore present in products such as yeast and liver. It can be extracted from many glandular organs and from tea. It is known to have a diuretic action, to influence muscle action, and to affect the nervous system."

## "Differential Diet" Involved

The dietetic aspects of therapeutics are now being approached from an entirely new angle, which might be labeled "the differential diet in disease," Dr. Martin said.

"The problem is simply one of supplying the body with its vitamin requirements, and yet keeping the bacteria from getting adequate amounts of their vital food factors," he explained. "This assumes differences in nutrient requirements, which have been demonstrated to exist. Feed the body and starve the bacteria. The best diet for a normal animal with no disease is not necessarily the best diet for an animal with an infection, even assuming equal intake."

The general problem of sulfonamide therapy has recently undergone a radical change, due to the appearance of many strains of bacteria not susceptible to sulfonamides, Dr. Martin continued.

"Specifically, some pneumococci, the organism causing pneumonia, were isolated which could not be inhibited in their growth by sulfonamides," he explained. "It was a phenomenon occurring with other organisms, such as gonococci, streptococci, etc. This seemed to indicate that a time would come when the sulfonamides would be useless as modes of therapy against bacterial diseases.

"It became necessary to explain how bacteria developed a resistance to the sulfonamides. A theory was advanced which suggested that the sulfonamides acted by starving the bacteria, preventing certain food substances necessary for their growth, from getting to the organisms. One of these food substances was para-amino-benzoic acid, another was methionine, an amino acid.

"It is necessary to know all of the substances which counteract the known sulfonamides in order to find a sulfonamide which would be resistant to these anti-sulfonamides. It was also apparent that an oversupply in the diet of the patient of any of these compounds would not only counteract the sulfonamide but would stimulate the growth of the bacteria in the body, thus being detrimental for two reasons."

*September 11, 1942*

# New Drug Hailed at Heart Meeting

### By ROBERT K. PLUMB

The American Heart Association heard praise today of the new drug chlorothiazide as potent and apparently safe. It is used against high blood pressure, so-called "dropsy" of waterlogged tissues and allied conditions.

A third group of investigators gave that report at the final session of the association's thirtieth scientific meeting. They termed chlorothiazide potent in enhancing the power of other drugs to lower blood pressure as well as a powerful agent itself.

The finding came from Dr. Edward D. Freis, Dr. Ilse M. Wilson and Dr. Alvin R. Parrish of the Veterans Administration Hospital in Washington.

Previously the heart men heard from Dr. Robert W. Wilkins, the president of the association, and his associate, Dr. William Hollander, both of the Massachusetts Memorial Hospitals in Boston, that chlorothiazide worked against high blood pressure.

Dr. John H. Laragh and Dr. Felix E. Demartini of Presbyterian Hospital and the Columbia University College of Physicians and Surgeons reported Saturday that chlorothiazide was effective in eliminating water and salt from the tissues of victims of congestive heart failure and those suffering from allied kidney and liver disorders.

## A Problem for Physicians

Chlorothiazide is the chemical name for a compound of a substituted benzothiadiazine and a free sulfonamide group. It has been known as a diuretic, or agent to stimulate the elimination of fluids. It is not yet on the market. It will be sold as diuril, a product of Merck & Co.

Diuretic agents, now in use, apparently lose their potency after they have been injected over a period of time. Chlorothiazide can be given orally, in contrast to injections by physicians or nurses that are necessary with other diuretics.

When tried against both high blood pressure and congestive heart failure, Dr. Freis reported, the compound appears to be free of disagreeable side effects.

*October 29, 1957*

## CHAPTER 5

# Cancer

# "Cundurango"

The victims of cancer who have been anxiously looking forward to a time not far distant when they would be able to procure a supply of the South American specific "cundurango," will be pleased to learn that Dr. D. M. Bliss, of Washington, expects very soon to obtain a sufficient quantity to furnish all who may be in need of it. Hon. A. H. Laflin, Naval Officer at this port, made application a few days ago, in behalf of a friend, for some of the specific, and in reply Dr. Bliss wrote, on the 15th inst., that he had none to spare. He says, "I receive but a small quantity at a time, and it being my purpose to treat a few cases here, where they can be under my own observation, it will be impossible for me to send any of it away. The remedy, as well as myself, having been attacked. I desire to demonstrate to the public what it will do, which necessitates the above course." In a circular note, however, the doctor says he expects to receive a sufficient quantity by the 1st, or the 15th of August at the furthest, to supply the profession or the public as they may desire. He says that enough has been developed by its use to assure him that it is the most powerful alterative ever in the hands of the profession, and that it possesses a specific influence over the poison of cancer. "From the statements of the physicians of Quito, and my own experience in its use, I am convinced that the 'cundurango' is quite as reliable as a specific in cancer, scrofula and other blood diseases as cinchona and its alkaloid have proved to be in zymotic diseases."

*July 18, 1871*

# The Cause of Cancer Probably Discovered;
## Its Cure Possible

Malaria, diphtheria, smallpox, yellow fever—these are diseases known to be caused by microbes preying upon the human system. But cancer, whose victims are counted by the tens of thousands every year, has been a complete mystery to the scientist. Now, however, a discovery has been made which promises to trace to its source this deadly scourge of the human race and to find a cure for it. This discovery is the result of seven years of the most careful investigation by the State Cancer Laboratory at Buffalo, of which Prof. Gary N. Calkins of Columbia University is the biologist. If it is borne out to its logical conclusion by future investigations, it means that cancer is to be classed with such diseases as malaria and diphtheria in having a living microbe, or germ, for its cause; if further investigations confirm the results obtained thus far, not only is it proved that cancer is a germ disease, but the germ, the bacillus itself, has been actually found, seen and identified. Furthermore, with the cause of cancer thus known, it is a reasonable hope that its cure will soon be found. Indeed, a serum of apparently specific remedial action has already been found.

The popular theory of cancer today is a modification of the one which was first given by the famous German pathologist Cohnheim, who died in 1884, and whose conclusions on the subject have recently been elaborated by Prof. Beard of the University of Edinburgh. This theory accounts for cancer as a sort of unused tissue remaining undeveloped in the human embryo, and subsequently appearing as disease tissue in the adult organism. It is upon this theory that Prof. Beard has founded his system of treatment by trypsin and amylopsin, the apparent success of which has recently been attracting the attention of the medical profession.

The work of the State Laboratory at Buffalo, however, has not concerned itself, as yet, with any system of medical treatment, although it has incidentally found a serum which, in the tests made with inoculated mice, showed a specific curative action. The microbe, or parasite, revealed by the experiments in the laboratory has been found to be invariably present in all the cancerous growths shown by the animals under observation. Under microscopic analysis this parasite proves to be one of the spirochaetes, of the same genus, although not the same species, as the germ which is now recognized as the cause of lues, relapsing fever, and other diseases in man and the lower animals. This parasite, which is only the five-thousandth part of an inch in length, or a spirochaete very similar to it, was observed last year by Loewenthal of Berlin in human cancer, but neither do the experts of the State Laboratory nor does Loewenthal claim, as yet, that it is the cause of cancer. More experiments along the same line will have to be made before that can be definitely announced, the inference in the meantime being that cancer is a disease whose germ has been discovered, a disease that is perhaps infectious, possibly yielding to serum treatment, and not due in any way to the embryological cause given by Prof. Cohnheim and later by Prof. Beard.

In reviewing the work which has been done in the study of cancer in the Buffalo Laboratory Prof. Calkins said to a *Times* reporter:

"Throughout the world there are hundreds of scientifically trained investigators who, with proper equipment and carefully educated assistants, are striving to get some light, some positive knowledge, regarding cancer, perhaps the subtlest of human diseases. From such men the public hears little or nothing, for familiarity with the subject breeds with them only the deeper sense of its subtlety, and with it a keen appreciation of the false hopes aroused and the disappointments that will surely follow the premature publication of hasty and unproved conclusions. Fed only on the popularized conceptions which science exploiters furnish, it is small wonder that the general reader grows to accept ill-timed and unbalanced theories of cause or cure, which, being afterward refuted, awakens in him a distrust of any theory whatsoever. But the methods of science, if rigorously followed, are bound to produce accurate and reliable results which are sure of an ultimate acceptance that will displace the crude theories by which the popular mind has been more or less misled.

"The scientific investigations now carried on in many different parts of the world in connection with the search for the cause and cure of cancer are based upon experiments with the lower animals. Ever since carcinoma was found to be transplantable from mouse to mouse, laboratories devoted exclusively to the study of this disease have sprung up in Frankfort, in Heidelberg, and in London, while numerous commissions, under public or private endowment, have been established in many cities, both in this country and abroad, all of them using thousands of mice annually in the prosecution of cancer study.

"Although the majority of cancer laboratories have sprung up since the development of the experimental method, one at least, the State Cancer Laboratory at Buffalo, was conceived and established long before the transplantation of mouse tumors was recognized as an adequate, although indirect, means of studying human carcinoma. It is gratifying that the Legislature of New York should have been the first official body to recognize the importance of a special laboratory for cancer research, and that it should have had sufficient faith in the undertaking to support the institution for seven years, in spite of the few visible, practical results that have been obtained.

"This laboratory was founded largely through the efforts of Dr. Roswell Park of Buffalo, and has ever had his hearty interest and support. The work is done in a well-equipped building, given for the purpose by Mrs. Gratwick, also of Buffalo. Dr. Gaylord, as pathologist, and Dr. Clowes, as chemist, have devised the experiments and have followed them out to some brilliant conclusions. From the outset the staff has been in perfect agreement with Dr. Park in the idea that a parasite lies at the bottom of the cancer process. Pursuing the line of inquiry indicated by this theory and going over the field in various directions, it was found necessary to run down many false leads. Cell inclusions of various kinds were discovered, regarded for a time as a possible cause of cancer, and as many times abandoned. Discouragement and hope alternated with persistent regularity, as is usually the case in the minute and laborious course inevitable in all strictly scientific research."

*

"A great step forward was made in our work in the Spring of 1904, when Dr. Gaylord returned from Europe bringing two mice which had been inoculated with carcinoma in Jensen's laboratory in Copenhagen. These mice remained alive until Dr. Gaylord reached New York; but they died from exposure during the trip from the latter city to Buffalo. Inoculations were made from the dead mice, however, and one set proved successful. The strain of cancers thus started, known as the Jensen tumor, is still carried on in the Buffalo Laboratory, and many important conclusions in connection with spontaneous recovery, with natural and acquired immunity, with cage infection, and with the possible cause of the disease have followed.

"Statistics of mouse tumors in the Buffalo Laboratory show that about 22 per cent of the mice in which transplanted tumors develop recover from the disease. Using the blood from such spontaneously recovered mice Dr. Clowes found, by injecting it into mice with new, developing cancers, that small tumors can be made to disappear and that larger ones can be retarded in growth—in other words, that mice with cancer, if taken in time, can be cured by serum treatment.

"Another important and significant discovery made in the Buffalo Laboratory throws a new light on the subject of cancer infection. The case to which I allude had to do with an interesting tumor development in certain rats with which we were experimenting. The original rats had a peculiar fibro-sarcoma, and were brought by Dr. Loeb to the laboratory in 1900, where they were kept for some months, after which they were removed. The smaller cages in which they had been confined were sterilized, but the larger ones were put aside and not used for a period of two and a half to three years. A number of healthy rats were finally put into one of these larger and unsterilized cages, and three of them developed sarcoma of the same type as that which had been confined in the same cage three years before. The rarity of fibro-sarcoma in rats, and the large percentage of primary tumors which developed in the infected cage is regarded by the experts connected with the laboratory as strong evidence of the parasitic theory of cancer.

"All of our attempts, however, to demonstrate the existence of a parasite in either mouse carcinoma, or this rat sarcoma which is still successfully transplanted in the Buffalo Laboratory, had been futile, until June of last year, when a most important discovery in this direction was made. As a result of this discovery, and as Dr. Gaylord reported before the State Medical Association at its one hundred and first meeting at Albany last week, it now seems probable that a specific parasite accompanies carcinoma in mice. Using a method of demonstration which Dr. Levaditi of the Pasteur Institute devised for demonstrating the characteristic organism, or germ, of lues, Dr. Gaylord found last summer that peculiar spirally wound organisms, belonging to the genus *Spirochaeta*, are present within and around every mouse tumor that has been examined. These spirochaetes are present in a young, rapidly growing, non-ulcerated primary tumor in a mouse obtained from Massachusetts, and in every strain of transplantable tumors now in the Buffalo Laboratory. This discovery would appear to be of the utmost importance in the future study of the cause, development and possible cure of cancer. It is premature to say, however, that these organisms are the cause of mice carcinoma; but their presence in and around the cancer cells, and their absence elsewhere, is a sufficient justification for continuing research and experimentation along the lines of the parasite hypothesis of human cancer.

"To the lay reader it may seem singular that in all the microscopical examinations which have been made of cancerous tissue heretofore the presence of the spirochaeta has eluded expert analysis until now. It must be remembered, however, that these infinitesimal organisms are extremely difficult to see even under the most powerful of microscopes except with the use of certain stains and acids in the preparation of the tissues containing them. Thus, in demonstrating the existence of the spirochaetes in the cancerous tissue of mice, the impregnation was made with silver nitrate and the reduction with pyrogallic acid. This leaves the organism black, while the cells and surrounding tissue are unstained. Ordinarily, mounted for observation on the slide of a microscope, the spirochaetes are, of course, without life or movement. Dr. Gaylord, however, has seen and studied these organisms alive."

\*

"There are altogether about twenty known species of *Spirochaeta*, the majority of which are not supposed to be disease producing. Five of them, however, are admittedly pathogenic. These are *Spirochaeta pallida*, the cause of lues; *Spirochaeta obermeieri*, the cause of relapsing fever; *Spirochaeta duttoni*, the cause of tick fever in Africa; *Spirochaeta gallinarum*, the cause of disease in chickens; *Spirochaeta anatifera*, the cause of a disease in ducks. It is somewhat difficult to classify these organisms with absolute exactness. The spirochaetes found in the diseased tissue of mice at the Buffalo Laboratory are about five microns in length—something like the five-thousandth part of an inch—and are undoubtedly independent organisms. But these organisms are on the very border line between animals and plants. Their animal relatives are protozoa, such as *Trypanosoma*, one species of which is known to be the cause of sleeping sickness, and another causes a disease in horses. Their plant relatives are the spiral bacteria. The evidence, however, so far as we have been able to collect it, is mainly in favor of the animal nature of the spirochaetes.

"Of course, during the past ten years many supposed cancer germs have been discovered and described. All of these, however, have turned out to be false leads—that is, in every case it has been demonstrated that the so-called germ is not a true organism. But there is no question as to the organic nature of the spirochaetes found in the Buffalo Laboratory. All who have seen it agree that it is a true organism. If it is ultimately found in all cancers, the only conclusion will be that this organism is the cause of the disease."

*February 3, 1907*

# Erysipelas Germs as Cure for Cancer

Following news from St. Louis that two men have been cured of cancer in the City Hospital there by the use of a fluid discovered by Dr. William B. Coley of New York, it came out yesterday that nearly 100 cases of that supposedly incurable disease have been cured in this city during the last few years, all through the use of the fluid discovered by Dr. Coley.

This fluid, which is known to medical men as "mixed toxins of erysipelas and bacillus prodigiosus," has saved many lives all over the world, medical men say. It has in recent years come to be used in almost every country where the medical profession is in an advanced state of progress. A peculiarity of its effect is that it gives the patient a mild form of erysipelas, and the system in struggling against the new disease, throws off the other and more serious disease. There is no secret about the remedy, for, following his discovery, Dr. Coley gave its benefit to the medical world at large. That was about fifteen years ago. Since then the fluid has been improved upon and its effect is now more sure and safe than in its earlier use.

The fluid is now made at the Collis P. Huntington Research Laboratories in Germantown, Penn., of which Dr. Martha Tracey, a woman physician, is the head. The Collis P. Huntington Fund for Cancer Research in this city also handles the fluid and distributes it. The formula used at the laboratories in Germantown was discovered by Dr. Coley, and the latter has more cancer cures to his credit than any other surgeon in the world. Dozens of cases have been treated and cured free of charge by Dr. Coley in the General Memorial Hospital at 106th Street and Eighth Avenue. Many other sufferers from cancer have been cured at his private sanitarium.

Dr. Coley is the attending surgeon at the General Memorial Hospital, and associate surgeon at the Hospital for the Ruptured and Crippled. He is also a clinical lecturer at Columbia, and has written a number of works on surgery and the cure of cancer.

## Probably 150 Cases Cured

In speaking recently of the work accomplished here through the use of the mixed toxins, Dr. Coley said:

"The use of the toxins has been followed by complete disappearance in 47 personal cases and nearly 100 cases reported by other surgeons and physicians. If, however, we count as cures only those cases in which there is known to have been no recurrence for at least three years, there have been 28 cures in cases under my own treatment, and upward of 80 cures in cases treated by other medical men.

"Although sufficient time has not yet passed to justify us in counting the total figure of about 150 successful cases as cures, the effect of the toxins in destroying the disease and in preventing metastases warrants the conclusion that in the great majority of those cases the disappearance of the tumor will prove to have been final and the cases will eventually have to be classified as cures.

"My 28 cases of cures, already of over three years' standing, include sarcomas of every kind, except melanotic, and in all parts of the body ordinarily subject to the disease. They include cases primary in the skin, muscle and fascia; cases originating in the bone, periosteal and myeloid; cases primary in the neck, tonsil, pelvis, long bones (femur and tibia), spine and breast, and they include small round-celled, large round-celled, giant-celled and mixed-celled sarcoma."

## Unknown to Many Physicians

In the great majority of the cases the diagnosis of sarcoma was confirmed by microscopical examinations made by the leading pathologists of the United States, and in the few remaining cases the concurrent opinions of independent surgeons left no reasonable doubt as to the correctness of the diagnosis. In several cases there was also a history of recurrence after primary operation.

"Although the cases show that the mixed toxins have already been used with success by a very large number of surgeons and physicians besides myself, it is constantly being brought to my notice that the possible benefit to be gained by the use of the toxins, in inoperable and apparently hopeless cases and as a prophylactic against recurrence after primary operation, is still unknown to the majority of medical men. I also frequently receive letters from surgeons and physicians in this country, as well as in other parts of the world, who are aware of the use of the toxins, but are unacquainted with the recent developments in their preparation and application, or are in doubt as to the method of treatment in particular cases."

Dr. Coley says that he has personally treated about 430 cases of sarcoma, which is the medical term for cancer, with mixed toxins. In 47 of these cases, he says the tumor completely disappeared.

"And in 28 cases a period of from three to fifteen years has passed since the disappearance," says Dr. Coley. "Twenty-six patients have remained well from five to fifteen years. Moreover, these figures cover a period of fifteen years, and during this period important improvements have been made, from experience, in both the preparation of the toxins and the method of administration. The proportion of successes is therefore higher now than in the whole past period.

"Furthermore, the cases treated include cases brought to me in the last stages of the disease, cases of melanotic sarcoma in which I have had no successes, and many desperate cases which had become inoperable after one or more extensive operations. In these desperate cases the percentage of successes from the use of the toxins is necessarily extremely low, while in other cases, not involving the long bones, the percentage of successes is considerably higher than is indicated by the figures given above.

## Chance of Permanent Cure Good

"When the growth is slow, the patient is in good general health, and the case is treated at a comparatively early stage of the disease, before the involvement of any important organs or the development of metastases, the chances of success are certainly much higher than the general percentage of 11 per cent, derived from the total figures of my own cases. The cases, however, vary so much and in so many features that no pretense can be made to accuracy in estimating the chance of success in any particular case, or even in any particular class of cases.

"It can, however, be safely said that in a very large number of cases there is a very fair prospect of permanent cure, while no case is so desperate that the possible benefit from the use of the toxins should be withheld."

Dr. Coley says there is no risk from the treatment of sarcoma by the mixed toxins. He says that out of the 430 cases treated by him only in three instances could death possibly be attributed to the toxins. And these three cases were in the last stages of the disease.

*July 29, 1908*

# Starving Cancer, a New Treatment

D r. William S. Bainbridge of the New York Skin and Cancer Hospital delivered the annual clinical lecture in the assembly room of the hospital yesterday afternoon. In the course of the clinic, the subject of which was "Ligation," the process of cutting off the blood supply upon which cancerous affections feed, he exhibited several apparent cures which aroused the keenest interest. For instance, Dr. Bainbridge introduced first a man and then a woman, both of whom had suffered from serious cancers of the face. In each case nearly the whole side of the face had been removed and a new cheek created by grafting skin, taken from the patients' legs and arms, on the side of the head where the cancer had been.

The clinic drew an attendance of physicians and others which taxed the capacity of the hall. These, many of them women, rose and cheered several times following the introduction of some man or woman who had been benefited by the surgery of Dr. Bainbridge and his corps of assistants, who, Dr. Bainbridge said, must share with him the credit of any work that had been done in the war on cancer which the hospital is making.

Dr. L. Duncan Bulkley, who as the representative of the hospital Trustees introduced Dr. Bainbridge, said, incidentally, that the hospital now has plans ready for the construction of a twelve-story building on the site of the present small structure, and that as soon as the necessary $1,000,000 is forthcoming work on this much-needed building will begin. He asked everybody present to aid in the work of making possible the proposed new hospital, and said that there were wealthy men in New York who, he thought, could well give the hospital consideration in the distribution of their wealth.

Dr. Bainbridge, who was then introduced, enjoys the reputation of being the youngest-looking medical man in New York for his age. He is over 40, yet he looks not a day over 30. Several who had never seen him before were not certain that it was "Bainbridge, the cancer specialist," when he got up to talk, and asked their nearest neighbor if this really was the man whose prominence in investigations of the disease is recognized throughout the world.

Dr. Bainbridge began by referring to the clinic as one of the happiest days in his struggle against one of the most horrible of diseases, since it enabled him to show some results. He went on to state the subject of the clinic, ligation, which he defined as the starving out of the death-eating growth. Near Dr. Bainbridge at this time was an elderly man, over the left side of whose face was spread a piece of antiseptic cloth. The man looked happy. Presently Dr. Bainbridge turned to him, and calling him by name asked him to come forward.

The man walked briskly up to the side of Dr. Bainbridge, and the latter put his arm around him and removed the cloth which obscured his face. Even some of the doctors present shuddered at what they saw. Nearly half of the man's face was gone, but the hole was healing, as everybody could see.

The man came to Dr. Bainbridge several weeks ago, he said, apparently in a dying condition. An operation was performed, the blood vessels leading to the cancer being closed so that it had nothing to feed upon.

"This man," said Dr. Bainbridge, "was operated on five weeks ago. He tells me now he has no pains, that he has gained eight pounds in weight, and he is feeling fine."

The next man who came forward was a middle-aged citizen of Westchester County. He wore glasses, the left lens of which was made of darkened glass such as blind men wear. Dr. Bainbridge told him to remove the glasses. Those present looked at a man who had once been in exactly the same condition as he who had just appeared before them. But there was no gap in his face. The skin was clear and healthy in appearance, only the cicatrix and the depression in the cheek showing that he had once undergone a serious operation.

"This man," said Dr. Bainbridge, "two years ago was in just as bad a fix as the one you have just seen. Then he came to us. An operation was successfully performed and skin taken from his leg and grafted on the cheek. Now he looks all right, doesn't he? My friend came to New York this morning to tell his only daughter—"

"Excuse me, it was my oldest, Doctor," the man from Westchester laughingly interrupted.

"All right, old fellow, your eldest daughter then. She sailed for Bermuda this morning, and he just stopped in to show you what can sometimes be accomplished."

Seated in the rear of the room while Dr. Bainbridge was talking was a little German woman, only 23 years old. She came to the hospital only last month. The doctors found that she had long been suffering from cancer in its most malignant form. Ligation was performed and the growth isolated. Yesterday, just thirty-eight days after she left the operating table, she was in the room. No one there would ever have thought she had been a victim of the disease.

Since she was operated upon the color has come back to her cheeks, she has gained 10 pounds in weight, and is able to attend to most of her household duties.

When the woman had gone, Dr. Bainbridge turned around and asked Sergeant Shea of the New York police force to come up.

"A year ago last Christmas." said Dr. Bainbridge, "Sergeant Shea was eating his dinner when he felt a severe pain in his stomach. He did not know what it was, but when we examined him we found that he was suffering from a terrible cancer. It was one of the worst cases, but we operated and the diseased parts were removed. That was a year ago last January. Today Sergeant Shea is feeling fine and he is still one of the good men who are guarding your persons and your property in this city."

Next was a middle-aged woman, a happy-faced little creature, who looked at Dr. Bainbridge with an expression that showed more plainly than words that the youthful-looking surgeon was not less than a saint, in her opinion. She had undergone the same operation that the Westchester man had, and she, too, had a new left cheek. Dr. Bainbridge put his arm around her and asked her how she felt.

"Fine, doctor," she said.

"And you are glad to be alive, aren't you?" the doctor asked.

"Indeed I am," she answered smilingly.

Then Dr. Bainbridge, his arm still around her, told how near death she was when she went to the hospital many months ago.

"I don't know whether I have a brain or not, Mrs. _____." Dr. Bainbridge said gently, "but I know that you have, for I have seen it."

The skin for the new cheek that this woman has was grafted from her arm. Like the Westchester man, she is happy, and apparently completely cured.

"This dear little lady," said Dr. Bainbridge, "was in just as bad a fix as was the man you have seen. Now she does her work, can go wherever she wants to, takes care of her home and is happy and contented."

A dapper-looking young man, stylishly dressed and looking as if he never had a care in the world, came forward next.

"What hospital is this?" Dr. Bainbridge asked him.

"The New York Skin and Cancer Hospital," the man answered in a clear voice, enunciating the words perfectly.

"Let's hear you say 'Dr. Bulkley,'" said Dr. Bainbridge.

The reply was clear and distinct. Then Dr. Bainbridge told the man to show his tongue. There was but a little of it left. Today, to all appearance, he is cured.

The man himself says he never felt better in his life.

These were only a few of the remarkable cases that Dr. Bainbridge showed yesterday. All of them owe their present improved condition to the system of surgery known as ligation. Dr. Bainbridge does not pretend that all are cured. He does say, however, that all have been greatly benefited and that in many cases they are apparently cured.

After the lecture Dr. Bainbridge was overwhelmed with congratulations, many of the physicians present declaring that what they had seen could be described by one word, and that word was "wonderful."

*April 21, 1910*

# Says He Has Found Cancer Microbe

PARIS—Dr. Gaston Odin of this city makes the announcement that he has discovered the microbe of cancer and has succeeded in isolating and cultivating it. He hopes before long to supply tubes containing a vaccine which will cure cancer or act as a preventive.

In an interview with *The New York Times* correspondent today, Dr. Odin said his researches dated back ten years. Only six months ago were they crowned with success. He added that Prof. Matruchot, who occupies the Chair of Botany at the Sorbonne, had verified his discovery and asserted its genuineness, and that Prof. Lannois of the School of Medicine had pronounced it important.

"I succeeded," said Dr. Odin, "in cultivating the microbe in conformity with the most rigorous Pasteur methods, and I have in my tubes of cultures formal proof of my claim. The cancer microbe is a parasite blood amoeba, that is to say, a protoplasmic mass, an inferior living organism, which transforms, develops, and reproduces itself. The variety of its forms surpasses imagination. The cancer amoeba is flat and gelatinous in composition, with irregular torn edges surrounding a central kernel—that is, when it is in a static or primitive form. When, in consequence of the modification of its environment, the amoeba is able to develop, it spreads and shoots forth in all directions."

Questioned as to the consequences of his discovery, Dr. Odin said he hoped that his vaccine would enable him to do for cancer what Dr. Roux did for diphtheria and Jenner for smallpox. "Whether or not I have discovered a means to prevent or cure cancer," he remarked, "it is already established that by the aid of my discovery we can tell with certainty whether an individual is cancerous or not. An examination of his blood will reveal the fact. The active element already at my disposal enables me to kill the cancer microbes when the disease is not too far advanced, and a culture of cancer microbes which I obtained a few days ago results in the attenuation of cancerous lesions."

Dr. Odin closed his statement with the assertion that his vaccine might be applied with beneficial results in cases of smoker's cancer.

*

A physician of the New York Skin and Cancer Hospital, to whom the foregoing dispatch was shown last night, said:

"The importance of this announcement for physicians in the United States will depend on the medium through which it was made. If it was made to a reputable medical society, and properly authenticated, it is in a position to be investigated by the medical fraternity. Its merits may then be determined by investigation and debate. But if it was made simply through a newspaper in Paris, its value is problematical.

"Announcements of cancer cures, cancer vaccines and cultures, and the isolation of the cancer microbe have been very frequent recently. Any number of physicians in Europe have made assertions that they have isolated the cancer microbe and made cultures of it. One of the points of uniformity among these various announcements is that the cancer microbe is a low form, a protoplasmic degenerate, or an undeveloped form of cell life, and that it may exist harmlessly, in a static state, or in an active and reproductive and expanding state, creating pathological conditions in the body where it lives.

"That cultures of the germ may be used for diagnosis is interesting if true, and has an analogy in a similar form of diagnosis now generally in use for another group of maladies."

The names of the French physicians mentioned in the dispatch, he added, were not known to him.

*August 14, 1912*

# Cause of Cancer Found at Last by Boston Scientist

By VAN BUREN THORNE, M.D.

Dr. Howard W. Nowell, instructor in pathology in the Boston University School of Medicine, has achieved a notable triumph in the domain of medicine by discovering a cause of cancer. The active agent which he has succeeded in isolating, after years of patient laboratory work, is an inorganic poison and is derived from human carcinoma, the latter being the name by which true cancer is designated in scientific nomenclature.

The reason Dr. Nowell is sure he has really found a cause of cancer is that a solution of this inorganic chemical substance produces carcinoma, or true cancer, when injected into the bodies of healthy animals.

The writer of this article visited the Robert Dawson Evans Department of Clinical Research and Preventive Medicine in Boston, where the experiments destined to attract world-wide attention by their brilliant results have been conducted, on Monday last, and, through the courtesy of Dr. Nowell, was permitted to examine animals which were the subjects of experimentation. They presented the clinical evidences of cancer. Tumors which had been removed in autopsy from rabbits presented the usual macroscopic appearance of malignant growths taken from human beings. Sections of these tumors, stained and mounted on glass slides, were revealed under the microscope as true carcinomatous growths, differing in no respect from similar sections of cancerous tumor as found in the human subject.

Dr. Nowell has done a good deal more, however, than isolate an inorganic trade agent from human carcinoma as the result of his long series of bio-chemical studies, although he wishes it to be distinctly understood that he does not assert that he has found a cure for cancer. By the repeated injection of small quantities of a solution of the toxic agent into the bodies of healthy rabbits, antibodies or immunizing agents have been developed in the blood of these animals and subsequently, when other animals have received injections of a mixture of the toxic agent and the blood serum containing the antibodies in properly graduated proportions, cancer has not developed.

The only inference that scientists are likely to draw from this fact is that the serum from immunized animals may prove of value in preventing cancer in human beings, and that it may be efficient in the treatment of persons afflicted with cancer. These possibilities are still the subject of speculative inquiry, but are already engaging the attention of research workers in this country and in Europe.

In any event, Dr. Nowell is sufficiently sure of the logical basis of his deductions (and his work has been checked up at each stage of the experiments by every means known to science) to proceed with the treatment of human patients. He began the treatment of a proposed series of 600 men and women last week. As a matter of fact, he has classified the 600 selected typical cases into three subdivisions of 200 each.

Realizing the tragedy that might result if time should show that he had been in error, he announces that he will refuse to receive a patient at this time who can be benefited by operation. He holds with the belief of surgeons throughout the world that the knife is still the only known and tried remedial agent for cancer in the early stages. Consequently he will inject the serum into 200 patients immediately after operation in the attempt to immunize them against a secondary development of malignant disease; the second 200 will be patients in whom malignant growths have developed following operations, while the third series will consist of 200 patients who cannot be operated upon because of the advanced state of the disease, the location of the tumor, or for other reasons. The selection of the cases is in the hands of a committee of physicians. Reports of all these cases will be issued from time to time through the medium of the medical press. It will take at least two years to determine the value of the treatment.

It may be stated here that Dr. Nowell will announce, in the course of a few weeks, the results obtained in animals in which cancer had been induced by the injection of the toxic agent he has isolated by treatment with the immunizing serum he subsequently prepared.

Dr. Nowell's announcement, which, whether or not it results in the discovery of a cure for cancer, cannot be regarded as other than a milestone in bio-chemical experimentation, was made in Boston on Tuesday evening, April 8, at the seventy-third annual meeting of the Massachusetts Homoeopathic Society. It was stated there that Dr. Nowell's results represented three years of work, but they really represent much more than that, as Dr. Nowell explained to the writer in his splendidly equipped laboratory in the Evans Memorial Building, the gift of the widow of Robert Dawson Evans to the Boston University School of Medicine. It may be mentioned that there is a motto, in raised letters, over the entrance to the Evans Memorial. It reads, "Truth Above Everything."

"As a boy," said Dr. Nowell, "that is, as a student in the School of Medicine, it was a part of my duty in the routine of laboratory work to analyze the contents of stomachs of persons afflicted with cancer. The quantities of lactic acid in these contents led me to speculate as to whether or not the acid was evolved as a protective agent, or whether it was simply thrown off as a product of the malignant growths. This speculation was really the incentive to acquire further knowledge regarding malignant neoplasms, and such has been my aim ever since."

The experiments described by Dr. Nowell to the Massachusetts physicians constitute a practical achievement. They constitute as well the ideal consummation of scientific research. Nearly every one will concede the romantic element in the study of astronomy. This element is perhaps as obvious a factor in the pursuit of chemical and bio-chemical research. Can this be the reason that so many women nowadays are fascinated by the lure of laboratory work? Whatever the answer may be, it is a fact that a very large number of women in the United States are devoting their energies to scientific research. In addition to their scientific knowledge, they bring to the laboratory a precision, a deftness, a natural manipulative skill, which the man scientist can only acquire by long and patient practice. In any event. Dr. Nowell is greatly indebted to his assistant, Dr. Gladys Howard Brownell, who was graduated from the Boston University School of Medicine last year. She carried on a great many of the experiments under his direction, and prepared the beautifully stained and mounted specimens for microscopic examination.

Before proceeding with the elaboration of the experiments as described by Dr. Nowell to the gathering of physicians, this summary of his conclusions is given:

"1. A procedure has been developed whereby a substance or mixture of substances may be isolated from carcinomata (cancer), the method precluding the presence of organic life in the end product.

"2. This end product has been shown to be of a highly toxic character.

"3. The intoxication with the tumor substance probably stimulates an intense and pernicious cell activity since the peritoneal exudate of a guinea pig thus poisoned is far more toxic than is the original tumor substance, the course of the symptoms in both instances differing only in degree and not in kind.

"4. The tumor substance produces well-defined, well-characterized carcinomata, the site of the primary lesion being different from and independent of that of the injection.

"5. The appearance of the first tumor is followed by the appearance of numerous growths in neighboring glands in different parts of the body, and the characteristic loss of weight, loss of appetite, &c. manifests itself.

"6. The poisonous tumor preparation is characteristic of carcinomata, since similar preparations from benign tumors and other preparations, including the introduced metallic base, have been shown to be wholly incapable of reproducing any of the observed phenomena.

"7. By the repeated injection of very small doses a large number of rabbits have been immunized.

"8. The serum from the animals thus immunized contains a substance or mixture of substances which possesses the power of antagonizing the toxic action of the tumor substance. This has been demonstrated by injections of the serum, either previous to or simultaneous with that of the tumor poison. In both events no effects are observed from quantities of the poison which if injected alone would produce a rapidly fatal intoxication.

"9. With the simultaneous injection of the poison and antibody it has been shown that one part of the latter will effectually antagonize ninety-nine parts of the former.

"10. Many of the developments suggested by this preliminary work are already in process of investigation in the laboratory of the Dawson Evans Memorial, connected with the Boston University School of Medicine."

After a few preliminary remarks relating to the metabolic changes in the body and the decrease in functional activity in advancing years, Dr. Nowell proceeded to the discussion of the etiology of cancer. He stated that only three factors were known which had to do with the origin of carcinoma. These are heredity, advanced age, and irritation of some sort. As in some other diseases, the part that heredity plays is probably only an inherited tendency or inherited weakness of the tissues which alone is insufficient for the development of the malady. From the age of forty years on there is a retrogression of many tissues in the body, and hence it is likely that advancing age favors the development of cancer in persons who have an inherited disposition to vulnerability of tissue. These two factors enter into the problem of the development of carcinoma in a most important manner when the third factor—namely, irritation—appears. That irritation, which comes under the surgical classification of trauma or injury, is a factor in the production of cancer has been proved many times by clinical experience and microscopic examination.

Every physician is familiar with the so-called smoker's cancer of the lip, cancer of the stomach resulting from gastric ulcer, and the cancer that develops in scar tissue that has been subjected to mechanical irritation.

Dr. Nowell then entered upon a discussion of the location of the first changes in the tissues at the beginning of carcinomatous growths, and of the efforts that had been made to produce cancer of the skin artificially by long-continued irritation. The details of this discussion will be omitted here. The speaker then proceeded to outline his chemical theory, and then described the procedure to demonstrate the presence of toxic compounds in carcinomatous growths. This is the experiment which resulted in the isolation of the inorganic poison.

"From cases of operable tumor where a diagnosis of carcinoma had been positively established, both by clinical and microscopical findings, the freshly extirpated growth was carefully freed from fat and extraneous tissue adhering to it, the material itself was cut into very small pieces and the mass digested with water at 100 degrees for many hours. When the digestion was complete, the mass was filtered to remove the exhausted residues, the clear filtrate containing those portions of the tumor which were soluble in water.

"By acidifying this filtrate and again boiling, the soluble proteins were coagulated and the precipitate thus formed removed by a second filtration. The protein-free filtrate was exactly neutralized, and the solution evaporated on the water bath to a syrupy consistency. This syrup was carefully extracted with pure alcohol, and the extract, after the removal of the alcohol by distillation, repeatedly treated with ether.

"This time the ethereal extracts were collected, the solvent removed by distillation and the final residues again dissolved in water. The aqueous solution was rendered alkaline, boiled for half an hour and again filtered.

"On the spontaneous evaporation of the filtrate, long, white, needle-shaped crystals separated, and these were purified by repeated recrystallization from water. These crystals in their purified form are the basis of the subsequent investigations.

"Up to the present, their exact chemical nature is not known, and extensive and exhaustive investigation will probably be required to determine their exact chemical constitution. The author is pleased to be able to announce that this part of the work has been undertaken by an expert organic chemist and that the investigation is already well under way.

"Whatever the exact chemical constitution of this compound may be, this much is evident, that the substance or substances secured by this method of procedure have been freed from all organic life, and any results obtained by its use must be referable to its own inherent chemical nature and not to the presence of organized life in any of its manifold forms.

"The crystals show a sparing solubility in water—about 4 parts in 100; and for convenience sake, carefully sterilized aqueous solutions were used in all the subsequent investigations."

As soon as Dr. Nowell had succeeded in isolating this chemical product, he proceeded to determine its physiological effect. For this purpose be selected rabbits, chiefly for the reason that they are not, as he explained, "normally subject to tumor growths." As far as he knows they have never given positive results in the experimental production of tumors. On the contrary, he asserted, rabbits show a very high degree of resistance to pathogenic influences along this line.

Eight rabbits were used in the first series of experiments. Ten milligrams of the poisonous substances were injected into each of four of the animals under strictly aseptic conditions. The other four were used as controls, and each of them received an injection of a sterile saline solution under exactly the same conditions. Each rabbit which received an injection of a solution of the toxic agent developed a local disturbance at the point of inoculation, and there was also a rise in temperature accompanying general constitutional symptoms. There was a period of restlessness, followed by a quieter period and a dulling of the senses.

These general symptoms lasted for a day, when three of the rabbits resumed their normal activity and for several days thereafter appeared to be in good health. The fourth rabbit died in three days, apparently as the result of the development of a septic condition which Dr. Nowell ascribed to a possible fault in the technique of administration of the toxic agent.

Following the period of apparent health, the three remaining rabbits gradually lost weight, became anemic, and finally developed a condition which presented the usual clinical manifestations of malignant disease. The three animals died in less than three months.

Dr. Nowell explained to the writer that he counted one month of a rabbit's life as corresponding to a year of human life. It is customary for physicians to speak of the probable duration of human life after carcinoma has developed as two years. It will be noted, therefore, that the duration of the lives of rabbits subjected to the influence of the toxic products of human malignant disease corresponds quite exactly to the ratio established.

The investigator gave the case histories of each of the four rabbits in detail. They will not be repeated here, but these comments by Dr. Nowell regarding the initial experiments are interesting:

"The results obtained from this preliminary experiment indicated that the tumor extract possessed, first, a marked toxicity, and, second, the power to reproduce in healthy tissue growths similar to, that from which it was itself derived. In the course of the subsequent experiments the latter point was still more strikingly illustrated and these observations may well be described at this point."

The fifth animal subjected to experimentation was a Belgian hare that weighed 2,800 grams. A solution of the toxic agent containing four milligrams of the active substance was injected under the skin of the abdominal wall. At the end of ten days a second injection of ten milligrams was made. Ten days later twenty milligrams more were administered in the same manner. By the time this last injection had been made a hard swelling had appeared on the under surface of the neck. This increased in size gradually. Another interval of ten days passed, when a fourth injection, of ten milligrams, was made. In one month the animal had received forty-four milligrams of the toxic agent.

The tumor which had been observed under the neck of the hare kept on growing until at the time of the animal's death it was as large as a hen's egg. It died on the fortieth day after the first injection. In the meantime, the clinical picture of carcinoma had been manifested in the general constitutional symptoms.

The post-mortem examination revealed beyond doubt that the animal had developed carcinoma of the thyroid gland. This was shown by microscopic examination. There were also malignant foci in the liver and in various glands throughout the body.

Four other rabbits in this second series showed similar results.

"These experiments," Dr. Nowell remarked, "in connection with the histological findings leave no question that the substance prepared by chemical means and in a manner which wholly excludes organic life is capable of producing a general carcinomatosis when injected under sterile conditions into healthy adult rabbits.

"Experiments will be shortly undertaken to ascertain if the same or a similar substance can be prepared from the rabbit tumors. That this investigation should give positive results seems highly probable."

While the experiments described were in progress others were being carried on to find out just the degree and character of toxicity of the substance derived from the human carcinoma. Twenty milligrams of the poison injected into a guinea pig killed it in two hours, and the symptoms resembled those of tetanus. Autopsy showed a venous engorgement of the body and an increase in fluid in all the cavities. A brownish exudate was found in the peritoneal cavity. Ten cubic centimeters of this fluid was removed, under strictly aseptic conditions, and put in a sterile tube. As small a quantity as 0.2 cubic centimeter of this substance produced an intoxication in a healthy guinea pig, and this indicated that the toxic property of this substance was much greater than that of the original chemical agent. Dr. Nowell discussed this feature of his discovery later.

A similar series of experiments to determine the toxicity of the agent was conducted with rabbits. An injection of 0.5 cubic centimeter of the solution was sufficient to kill a rabbit in twelve hours. The symptoms preceding death were similar to those observed in the guinea pigs.

The increase in toxicity in the exudate obtained from the guinea pigs prompted the investigator to inoculate rabbits with it. An injection of 0.5 cubic centimeter of the exudate resulted in the death of a healthy adult rabbit in one hour. This was sufficient to demonstrate to the investigator that the tumor extract is responsible for a cell activity which results in the formation of more toxic material. Inasmuch as "one-twentieth of the peritoneal exudate from the guinea pig causes death in the rabbit in one-twelfth of the time which the same volume of the pure extract requires," it is obvious that the production of fresh poisonous material must progress at an extremely rapid rate.

The next question that presented itself to the mind of Dr. Nowell was whether or not the poison contained in the peritoneal exudate of the guinea pig was the same as that contained in the toxic agent isolated from human carcinoma. He asserted that the same clinical picture resulted from the injection of the two substances, but it was evident from the increased virulence of the guinea pig exudate that the original toxin was either powerfully concentrated by its temporary sojourn in the body of the guinea pig, or that the result of the inoculation of the guinea pig with the original toxic agent had resulted in the production of a new and more powerful substance, similar to that derived from human cancer.

Another series of experiments is in progress to determine, if possible, which of these hypotheses is the correct one.

It was obvious to Dr. Nowell, his assistants, and the physicians connected with the School of Medicine who were keeping in close touch with the experiments that further investigations must be made to determine the specific action of the toxic agent isolated. Doubt might arise as to whether the poison could result from chemical action involving the bases used in the experiments; or, on the other hand, the toxic agent might result from similar chemical treatment of non-malignant tissue. A new series of experiments was undertaken to determine the truth of these possibilities.

A salt was prepared from the base used and lactic acid. Injections of large quantities of this material produced only temporary irritation. In brief, the results were negative. Next, non-malignant tumors were subjected to the same treatment as the original carcinomatous tissue. A crystalline material was obtained which differed from that isolated from cancer. The injection of a solution of this material (in quantities ten times as large as those of the carcinomatous product used) into rabbits and guinea pigs failed to produce any more serious reaction than was obtained by the injection of normal salt solution. These results also must be classed as negative. Hence, Dr. Nowell reaches this conclusion:

"Carcinomata contain some substance or substances which are susceptible of isolation and which when injected into healthy tissue produce results which are dependent upon the inherent chemical nature of the material itself."

Dr. Nowell's conclusion warranted the assumption that it might be possible to produce a so-called antibody, that is, a substance whose effect would be to antagonize the poison exactly. In other words, the next step was to attempt the production of an immunizing serum.

The theory of the production of such a serum is well understood at present, and is illustrated in the familiar diphtheria antitoxin which is everywhere in practical use today. The theory, briefly, is this: If small doses of the toxic products of bacteria are injected into healthy animals, other chemical compounds antagonistic to the first are produced, forming in the blood and capable of isolation from the coagulated serum. These substances are the antibodies. A serum prepared from the antibodies when mixed with the original poison in certain chemical preparations nullifies the action of the poisonous agent. This mixture can be injected into animals without producing disease. In fact, in the case of several diseases a serum prepared in this manner is used either as an immunizing or curative agent, or both, in the treatment of the ailment from which the toxic product was originally obtained.

"In the case of poisons of relatively simple structure," Dr. Nowell remarked to his colleagues, "up to the present time, at least, the usual procedure for the production of antagonistic antibodies has been unattended by success."

Complex toxins, the investigator observed, produced from bacteria as well as from complex vegetable poisons, are capable of stimulating the organisms that receive them to produce specific antibodies. Although the chemical nature of the cancer extract has not been learned, Dr. Nowell proceeded along the lines of the theory outlined above and began a series of immunization experiments.

A large number of rabbits were used in these experiments. A small quantity of the toxic agent in solution was injected into the abdominal walls of the animals. Ten days later a larger dose was given, and at the end of a second ten-day period a dose large enough to kill a rabbit in twelve hours, if it were the initial administration of the poison, was given. Symptoms of general intoxication followed, but the animals were able to tolerate the poison. The symptoms were of a severity, however, to indicate the necessity for the administration of smaller doses. Three other immunizing doses were given at intervals of ten days. In fifty days each of fifty-three rabbits received 64 milligrams of the toxic product. Five of the animals died, ten others became ill, while thirty-eight remained perfectly healthy.

These healthy animals were used for the purpose of obtaining the serum. Blood was removed under strictly aseptic conditions, the animals suffering no discomfort, and all of them recovered. The serum was obtained from the blood by the usual laboratory methods.

Guinea pigs were used as the subjects of the subsequent experiments in immunization. One cubic centimeter of the rabbit serum was injected into one guinea pig, and the same quantity of a sterile salt solution into another. Two days later one cubic centimeter of the original cancer poison was injected into each of the guinea pigs. The one which had received the salt solution died in 80 minutes; the one treated with the rabbit serum showed no effects whatever and is alive and well at the expiration of several weeks. The latter animal undoubtedly had been immunized by the serum against the attack of the toxic agent of a malignant growth.

The strength of the cancer antitoxin was determined later by another series of experiments.

In addition to his assistant, Dr. Brownell, Dr. Nowell accords a large share of credit for the success of his experiments to Dr. Allan Winter Rowe, Professor of Chemistry at the School of Medicine; Dr. William H. Waters, Professor of Pathology; Dr. William O. Mann and Dr. Frank C. Richardson, who are also connected with the school.

Dr. George R. Southwick, the retiring President of the Massachusetts Homeopathic Society, who is Professor of Clinical Gynecology in the School of Medicine and is interested in the raising of a $1,000,000 endowment fund for the benefit of the institution and the development of original research work, commenting on Dr. Nowell's experiments, said:

"Dr. Newell's bio-chemical product undoubtedly produces cancer. His experiments form the first reasonable basis for the hope that a cure for cancer may be found."

"Those interested in this work," said Dr. Richardson, who is the Medical Director of the laboratory in which the experiments were carried on, "wish to guard against an impression that a cancer cure has been found. But a most important step has been taken toward ascertaining the cause of cancer, a step which must necessarily precede the hope of cure."

Dr. John P. Sutherland, Dean of the Boston University School of Medicine, said: "Dr. Nowell has absolutely displaced the old parasitic theory of cancer. He has done his work faithfully and conscientiously. The applicability is yet to be determined. His material promises to be as effective as the diphtheria antitoxin."

In the last ten days Dr. Nowell has received telegrams and cable messages from all over America and Europe relative to the results of his experiments. He has placed himself in the hands of a committee of physicians, and none of the 600 patients selected for treatment will receive injections of the serum until five physicians have declared the patient to have suffered or to be suffering from malignant disease.

Dr. Nowell himself discusses his work with a quiet enthusiasm, employing the language of the laboratory with a facility indicative of patient study and intense application. He was born in Merrimacport, Mass., and has just turned 40 years. He is a graduate of Lyndon College and the Boston University School of Medicine, and is pathologist to the Massachusetts Homeopathic Hospital, a large, up-to-date institution adjoining the School of Medicine and the Evans Memorial Building in East Concord Street.

*April 20, 1913*

# Removal of Lung Applied in Cancer

By WILLIAM L. LAURENCE

PHILADELPHIA—The lives of many patients suffering from cancer of the lung, until recently impossible to cure, are now being saved by modern surgical technique that makes it possible to remove an entire lung.

This was reported here tonight before the annual clinical congress of the American College of Surgeons by Prof. Evarts A. Graham of the Washington University School of Medicine, St. Louis, who delivered the annual oration of surgery at the presidential meeting and convocation held at the American Academy of Music.

Nearly 5,000 leading surgeons and hospital executives from all parts of the United States, as well as delegates from Canada and other countries, are taking part in the congress, which also included the hospital standardization conference.

Professor Graham told the dramatic story of a fellow-physician whose ailment had been diagnosed as cancer of the lung, then the equivalent of a death sentence as the patient knew only too well. There being no hope, the surgical removal of the lung was decided upon. This was the first time that such an operation had been performed.

## Technique Spread Over World

The operation, the first of its extent, was a complete success, Dr. Graham reported, adding that recently, six years after the operation, this one-lunged physician was the only one who did not get winded after walking up several flights of stairs in the company of a group of two-lunged physicians.

The operation has now been performed over the world several hundred times and Dr. Graham said that he had performed it about forty times for lung cancer and in many other cases for non-cancerous conditions.

"In suitable cases, where the cancer is not too far advanced, the operation can be done with a mortality of only 10 per cent," Dr. Graham stated.

"When the cancer is advanced, however, the mortality jumps to 40 or 50 per cent. A very discouraging feature is that about 80 per cent of those patients who come for the operation are too far advanced to have a chance.

"The whole medical profession needs to be educated to the necessity of early diagnosis and early radical treatment of this condition."

## Advances in Diagnosis

Cancer of the lung, Dr. Graham stated, nearly always arises in the large bronchial tube. Accounting for about 8 to 10 per cent of all cancers of the body, it is most common in males at about or soon after middle age. Characteristic symptoms are a persistent cough, a feeling of tightness or pain in the chest and bloody sputum.

With modern methods, employing the X-ray and bronchoscope, Dr. Graham said, it was now possible to diagnose the condition, positively in 80 per cent of the cases.

Such technique, he added, also enabled diagnosis of both benign and malignant tumors of the mediastinal spaces between the lungs.

"Thoracic surgery has improved so greatly that it is now possible to remove the benign tumors with an operative mortality of only 10 per cent," he went on.

"But more striking than the low operative mortality is the fact that these operations can be performed without creating any deformity of the chest and without even removing a rib.

"To make a sufficient opening in the chest two or three ribs can be divided and then sewn together again. The scar gradually becomes invisible.

"Some of the tumors, especially those which arise in the lymphatic tissue, are better treated by X-ray than by operation.

"For the most part the malignant tumors of the mediastinal spaces cannot be removed by operation. Many of them, however, have a long period during which they are non-malignant, only to become malignant later. For that reason, in most cases they should be treated early before there is a chance of malignant degeneration."

## Record in Approved Hospitals

At the hospital standardization conference in the morning, Dr. Howard C. Naffziger of San Francisco, retiring president of the college, made public the list of approved hospitals in the United States and Canada for 1939.

A total of 2,720 hospitals, out of 3,564 registered with the college, are on the approved list this year, fifty-six more than last year, and the largest number ever to meet the college's rigid requirements.

Of those approved, 2,371 received a rating of fully approved, while 349 were rated as provisionally approved.

The navy had sixteen hospitals approved and the Veterans' Administration, eighty-two hospitals, out of an equal number surveyed. The United States

Public Health Service received full approval on twenty-five hospitals out of twenty-six surveyed.

The army, out of forty-one hospitals surveyed, received a rating of full approval on thirty-four, provisional approval on two, while five failed to receive approval.

The college also made public a plan for post-graduate training of 500 surgeons annually, the object being to provide skilled surgery for the patient of average means. For this purpose 381 hospitals throughout the country have been approved as training centers.

## Other Sciences Called Upon

Dr. Naffziger, in his retiring presidential address tonight, advocated encouraging men trained in other scientific disciplines, such as physics, biology, biochemistry, psychology and physiology, to study medicine.

Medical science, he said, needed men with such training, as they could bring their knowledge to bear upon the specialized advancement of medical art.

"The advance of medicine depends upon the contributions made by the application of fundamental knowledge coming from the basic sciences," he said.

"Many of us can recall occasional instances in which an engineer or chemist became interested in medicine and, with his eyes thus opened, his energies permitted vast dividends in accomplishment which are impossible to those not so prepared."

## Dietary Factor in Surgery

Professor Charles B. Puestow of the University of Illinois College of Medicine and Graduate School, who discussed the relations of dietary deficiencies to surgical convalescence, told the conference that a patient's state of nutrition "was a very important factor in surgical mortality and morbidity."

Patients, he stated, should be carefully prepared for a sufficient time before operation to correct dietary deficiencies and to establish adequate reserves of food, vitamins and fluids.

Except in emergency surgery, he added, hospital regulations "should require adequate pre-operative hospitalization to permit proper study and preparation; this will enable us to render better service to our patients and to improve surgical results."

*October 17, 1939*

# Science Winning Fight on Cancer

An increase of nearly 30 per cent in fifteen years in cures of breast cancer was reported last night by Dr. Frank E. Adair of Memorial Hospital, chairman of the executive committee of the American Society for the Control of Cancer.

The increase, according to Dr. Adair, is the result of the educational campaign by the society and its Women's Field Army on the importance of early diagnosis of cancer through periodic physical examinations and the avoidance if delay in reporting to a qualified physician any suspicious lump on the breast as soon as it is discovered.

The data cover cases of women who have had no recurrence of the disease in five years.

"Women have been told that cancer must be taken in its early stages to be cured, and they are taking advantage of this information," Dr. Adair said. "In 1920 the average delay in a breast case from the time a patient noticed a lump until she came to the hospital was eleven months and seven days. In 1940 this lapse of time had been cut more than in half, to four months and four days.

"In primary operable cancer of the breast in 1920 we secured 37.4 per cent five-year cures; in 1935, the latest year which we may use as a basis for calculating our five-year cure, we had raised the rate to 47.5 per cent, a gain of nearly 30 per cent in fifteen years."

## More Clinics Approved

Another important advance in the battle against cancer, the society announced, has been the growth in the number of cancer clinics approved by the American College of Surgeons. These increased from 272 in 1938 to 307 in 1939 and to 345 in 1940.

Physicians throughout the country, according to the society, also report wider use of the gastroscope (new apparatus for looking into the stomach) and esophagoscope (device for examining the gullet) for the detection of early cancer in these organs, improvement in X-ray diagnosis, and the reduction of the cost of X-ray film from 60 cents to 6 cents by a refinement in technique that makes it possible to use a much smaller film, only 4 by 5 inches.

The physicians questioned by the society, it was added, also reported improvement in the treatment of cancer. There is a better preparation of patients for surgery, while newer anesthetics and newer surgical techniques increase operability, thus decreasing the number of cases hitherto regarded as inoperable and therefore hopeless. More experienced surgeons, the report declared, are now doing surgery on cancer of the lung.

"In New York City," it went on, "there are excellent facilities available for men and women to get themselves examined for cancer and be treated at modest fees. Specifically, at the Strang Cancer Prevention Clinics at the New York Infirmary for Women and Children (321 East Fifteenth Street) and at the Memorial Hospital (444 East Sixty-eighth Street) any one may arrange for a periodic physical examination."

## Schedule of Fees

"Fees are arranged as follows: If the patient is a private one, with, for example, an income of $5,000 or more, the charge is $5. If the patient has an income of $1,500 to $2,500 and a small family, he would be regarded as semi-private and would be charged $3. For those of smaller income, clinic examination charges may be $2, $1, 75 cents, 50 cents, or nothing, depending on the clinic and the status of the patient. Examination and diagnosis are never refused. Free diagnosis is also available at the city hospitals and health centers in New York.

"These clinics only examine patients, they do not treat them. However, if cancer is found, and the experience of the last three years demonstrates that the disease is discovered in around 10 per cent of the cases, the patient is referred either to his or her personal physician or to an appropriate clinic, of which there are many."

Tomorrow will mark the beginning of a thirty-day intensified educational campaign throughout the country by the American Society for the Control of Cancer, in line with a proclamation by President Roosevelt designating April as Cancer Control Month.

*March 31, 1941*

# Cigarette Filter Held Ineffective

F ilter-tip cigarettes have not proved effective in materially reducing the hazard of lung cancer in smokers, Dr. Leroy E. Burney, Surgeon General of the Public Health Service, said today.

Writing in the *Journal of the American Medical Association* Dr. Burney emphasized that no method of treating tobacco had reduced the peril, either. Some cigarette brands have advertised a reduction in tars and nicotine.

In the article, Dr. Burney examined evidence of the relationship of smoking to lung cancer.

## Smoking "Principal" Cause

The Public Health Service, he concluded, "believes that the following statements are justified by studies to date:

"1. The weight of evidence at present implicates smoking as the principal etiological (causative) factor in the increased incidence of lung cancer.

"2. Cigarette smoking particularly is associated with an increased chance of developing lung cancer.

"3. Stopping cigarette smoking even after long exposure is beneficial.

"4. No method of treating tobacco or filtering the smoke has been demonstrated to be effective in materially reducing or eliminating the hazard of lung cancer.

"5. The nonsmoker has a lower incidence of lung cancer than the smoker in all controlled studies, whether analyzed in terms of rural areas, urban regions, industrial occupations or sex.

"6. Persons who have never smoked at all (cigarettes, cigars, or pipe) have the best chance of escaping lung cancer.

"7. Unless the use of tobacco can be made safe, the individual person's risk of lung cancer can best be reduced by the elimination of smoking."

## Death Rise Cited

Dr. Burney wrote that the Public Health Service was deeply concerned with the increasing death rate from lung cancer in the United States and in other parts of the world. Cancer of the lung is increasing more rapidly and causing more deaths than any other form of cancer in the adult male population, he said.

In little more than a quarter century the death rate from lung cancer among white men has risen from 3.8 to 31 for each 100,000 persons. This rise occurred between 1930 and 1956. In the latter year 29,000 persons died of lung cancer.

Dr. Burney pointed out that until 1926 lung cancer death rates among men and women in Massachusetts were about equal. As the disease increased the mortality distribution by sex changed until 1956, when the death rate in men was five times that in women.

Dr. Burney suggested that there might be a true sex difference in susceptibility between men and women, but said the data were not conclusive.

A number of investigators, the article pointed out, have suggested that "increased volumes of automobile exhaust fumes and industrial vapors polluting the air are to a great part responsible for the causation of lung cancer."

"The possibility that there are other factors yet unknown has also been suggested," it said. "Since carcinoma of the lung is also a disease of nonsmokers it is evident that factors other than tobacco contribute to its etiology."

Filter-tip cigarettes, which accounted for 1.4 per cent of the market in 1952, now constitute approximately 50 per cent.

"Present knowledge," Dr. Burney wrote, "indicates that it is not possible to filter, selectively, specific components such as carcinogens. Since the evidence from both human and animal studies shows that the risk of developing cancers is related to the amount of exposure to tar, the problem is to design a filter that will permit the minimum flow of whole tobacco smoke to pass, consistent with smoking satisfaction. "The filters presently in use do not eliminate, but merely reduce, the tar. It is questionable whether, from a health point of view, any so-called minimum exposure to such a hazard should be accepted."

## Conclusions "Unwarranted"

Two organizations supported by tobacco manufacturers took issue with Dr. Burney's statement yesterday.

James P. Richards, president of the Tobacco Institute, said it was difficult to understand how the Surgeon General could have come up with such "extreme and unwarranted conclusions."

Mr. Richards said:

"By largely ignoring the balanced evidence reviewed in his [Dr. Burney's] own scientific paper and summarizing his opinions with so little regard for that evidence, he has performed a real disservice, not just to the 65,000,000 smokers and the millions of Americans engaged in the tobacco business in one way or another, but to the public a whole."

"During the months we have been hearing about this new study of old findings by the Surgeon General's Office," Mr. Richards said, "we had hoped that repeated assurances of fair play would be borne out. It is obvious they have not."

Dr. C. C. Little, scientific director of the Tobacco Industry Research Committee, which makes grants for independent medical research, said:

"Today, more than ever before, scientific evidence is accumulating that conflicts with or fails to support the tobacco smoking theories of lung cancer. Many of these have been omitted from or glossed over in the Public Health Service article and press release."

Within recent months, Dr. Little said, new evidence has been presented that:

1. Finds that people described as the world's heaviest cigarette smokers have low lung cancer death rates compared with people who smoke less but have been long exposed to urban air pollution.

2. Shows that direct inhalation of tobacco smoke by laboratory animals over long periods of time has not resulted in causing lung cancer in these animals.

3. Reveals that human lung tissues undergo changes, considered suspicious by some, that are found among both young and old, in nonsmokers and smokers, while lung tissues "may be perfectly normal in heavy smokers."

4. Confirms that long established but little publicized fact that lung cancer occurs more frequently in people who have a medical history of previous serious lung ailments, such as tuberculosis, pneumonia and influenza, indicating a relationship of possible significance.

*November 27, 1959*

# New Cancer Treatment View Scored

By JANE E. BRODY

Los Angeles—Surgeons attending a meeting here on breast cancer took sharp issue today with the contention of some colleagues that the standard treatment for the disease is more drastic than necessary.

The standard treatment, called radical mastectomy, involves removal of the entire breast, the lymph nodes in the armpit, the muscles of the chest walls and the lymph nodes under them.

In recent months, several surgeons, writing in popular women's magazines, have contended that this extensive surgical procedure produces no better results than a simpler operation involving only removal of the breast (simple mastectomy) and sometimes only removal of the cancerous lump (lumpectomy).

The appearance of the articles in the lay press has led many women with suspicious breast lesions to "shop around" for a surgeon willing to perform the simpler type of operation.

"Many women are coming in waving the articles in their hands, demanding that we do that kind of operation," one breast surgeon remarked at the American Cancer Society's second national conference for breast cancer here. "Yet the claim that their chances of survival are as good with the simple operation as with the more radical one is based on very flimsy evidence."

One advocate of simple mastectomy, Dr. George Crile of the Cleveland Clinic, whose work has been widely quoted in the lay articles, has reported that he gets the same 70 per cent survival at five years after surgery with simple mastectomy as with the radical procedure. Among 56 patients who had only lumpectomies, 59 per cent were alive five years later, he told a recent surgical conference.

## Finds Sample Too Small

However, Dr. James A. Urban of Memorial Hospital in New York City said here that a bias was built into Dr. Crile's study. "The group he treated with radical mastectomy had larger tumors than the patients who underwent simple mastectomy," he said, adding that a breast cancer patient's chances of survival are known to be better if the tumor is smaller.

A similar bias appears in other studies claiming the same results with simple and radical mastectomy, Dr. Urban said. Still other reports are based on such small numbers of patients as to be totally meaningless, said Dr. Arthur Holleb, a former breast cancer surgeon who is now a vice president of the American Cancer Society.

Dr. Holleb agreed that in some cases, in which the cancer is confined to within the milk duct, simple mastectomy might be an adequate procedure.

"But, as presently detected, 90 per cent of breast cancers have already broken through the duct wall and are potentially invasive—capable of spreading," he pointed out. "For these, you need the more radical procedure to be sure you get out all the nodes to which the cancer might have already spread."

Dr. Holleb added that he hoped the debate would be at least partly resolved as more women underwent periodic screening for breast cancer. Screening, especially with special breast X-rays, can detect at an early, noninvasive stage when simple mastectomy may be all that is needed, he said.

Too often, however, women delay in seeking treatment even after they have noticed a lump in the breast. Part of the delay was attributed by Dr. Holleb to the "tremendous psychological impact of mastectomy to women living in this breast-oriented culture—it is a great trauma to the female psyche when a breast is removed."

Breast cancer is the most common cancer that can be fatal to women. Patients who die of breast cancer are those whose disease has spread beyond the local region of the breast.

## Second Operations

Dr. J. Englebert Dunphy, surgeon at the University of California Medical Center in San Francisco, said that, even in early cases of breast cancer, some 25 to 30 per cent of patients who underwent simple mastectomy would later show signs of cancer in the underarm lymph nodes and would require a second operation.

Dr. Dunphy said that in most cases he preferred a modified version of the radical mastectomy, one that leaves the major chest muscle intact but removes the lymph nodes likely to be diseased. This approach, he said, is easier on the patient and produces a better cosmetic result.

A major problem in deciding what kind of operation will produce the best survival results, Dr. Dunphy remarked, is that doctors cannot tell in advance which cancers are going to spread and which are not.

*May 20, 1971*

# The Doctor's World: Mastectomy: The Unanswered Questions

By LAWRENCE K. ALTMAN, M.D.

An operation first done by Dr. William S. Halsted in 1882 in New York and repeated millions of times since then has become one of the most debated procedures in the history of medicine. The operation—known as the Halsted radical mastectomy—was devised only 36 years after the introduction of anesthesia, when surgery was just beginning to become more science than magic.

For almost a century, the Halsted radical mastectomy reigned as the standard treatment of breast cancer. Rarely in surgical history has an operation lasted as long as Halsted's. Now its dominance has been challenged by the advances in cancer biology as well as by other forms of surgical, radiation and drug therapies. Its role in treating breast cancer has been highly controversial for some time.

A marked shift away from Halsted radical mastectomies to modified radical mastectomies has occurred recently, according to a study by Dr. Josef Vana and his team at Roswell Park Memorial Institute in Buffalo in the Aug. 15 issue of *Cancer*. The conclusion was based on a comparative study of almost 30,000 cases of breast cancer in 670 hospitals in the United States in 1972 and 1977. That shift raises several questions, among them:

- Why did the Halsted radical mastectomy survive for so long when almost all other operations devised at the same time have since been either refined several times or discarded entirely?

- Why did it take doctors so long to seek alternatives to the Halsted radical mastectomy operation in the face of advancing knowledge about tumor biology?

- Did the public play a greater role than the medical profession in bringing about the newer studies that suggest that other treatments can be as effective as Dr. Halsted's operation?

We must recognize that scientifically controlled trials are a relatively new form of human experimentation. Still, the specific answers to these questions are important because they affect the treatment of breast cancer as well as many other

104

common diseases. Yet the answers are not known with the exactitude that would persuade scientists and historians and would validate or refute the many theories that have been developed.

Among the alleged reasons: individual surgeons have chosen the technique more for emotional than scientific reasons; data that was obtained from poorly executed reviews of case records from multiple sources rather than from meticulous analyses of prospective studies that record a change in treatment and follow the patient for a long period of time to see if it changed the outcome.

*

Recently I looked up Dr. Halsted's papers again in an attempt to answer the questions that I first asked myself in medical school. There, we heard about a controversy set off in Edinburgh by Dr. Robert McWhirter, who suggested that simple mastectomy combined with postoperative radiation was equally effective as Dr. Halsted's radical mastectomy. During specialty training, we also heard the benefits of less radical breast operations argued by Dr. George Crile Jr. and Dr. Oliver Cope.

But most surgeons I knew persisted in a blind faith in the operation designed by Dr. Halsted, a Yale football captain who went on to become one of America's most illustrious surgeons.

Dr. Halsted was the first to put rubber gloves on members of the surgical team in the operating room. His superior results were attributed to his extraordinary antiseptic techniques as well as his meticulous handling of human tissues and control of bleeding during surgery. These were details to which few other surgeons paid attention and were crucial in improving surgical results.

Dr. Halsted also pioneered in developing regional anesthesia by injecting cocaine into his nerves. However, those self-experiments nearly ended his professional career. He became addicted to cocaine, and, in turn, the morphine he took to combat the cocaine dependence.

Yet Dr. Halsted became a founder of Johns Hopkins Medical School in Baltimore. There he developed new techniques for hernia, thyroid and other operations. He perfected his most famous operation—the radical mastectomy—by expanding on the work of German surgeons. In it, the surgeon removes the entire breast, the muscles in the chest wall beneath the breast and the axillary lymph nodes in the armpit. Of course, the tumor is removed, but this is one of the most mutilating operations because it often leaves a sunken chest wall and a weakened, swollen arm.

A re-reading of Dr. Halsted's unorthodox original papers is a striking reminder of how much medicine has changed in the last century. His first report of 13 cases was buried in a long paper on the treatment of wounds. His subsequent reports on breast surgery were anecdotal and lacked the statistical analyses and long-term follow-up that are considered standard today. Accordingly, there was no firm evidence that Dr. Halsted's operation enhanced patient survival.

Most important, the breast cancers that Dr. Halsted considered small measured about three inches by three inches and are huge by today's standards. As a result of mammography, patient education and self-examination—techniques developed in the last two decades—breast cancers now can be detected when they are only a few millimeters in size. The startling fact is that many of the first patients to undergo Halsted radical mastectomies would not be considered candidates for the operation today because the cancer was too advanced.

Dr. Halsted's radical mastectomy was in keeping with his understanding—contemporary but incomplete—of the nature of the spread of breast cancer. He believed it spread primarily through the lymph system, a theory that persisted until after World War II, and therefore the more radical surgery was the best defense. Doctors now believe that the spread of breast cancer through the blood stream is more important than its spread through the lymph system.

*

It was not until the late 1950s that doctors began the experimental studies to determine if other therapies were equally effective, or even better than Halsted's radical mastectomy. And there are few studies trying to provide the answers as to why they were so long in coming.

The answers are beginning to come from those continuing experiments. But because breast cancer is a complex disease—cases sometimes reappear after being dormant for 20 years—it will take several more years for final results.

Meanwhile, we can learn from our experience with the Halsted operation to be more critical about standard therapies. Otherwise, who knows what will be said a century from now about the therapies that we accept so dogmatically today?

*September 8, 1981*

# Scientists Pinpoint Genetic Changes
# That Predict Cancer

By GINA KOLATA

Researchers are well on their way to determining the precise genetic changes that must occur to make a normal cell cancerous, an achievement that could make it possible to identify people susceptible to particular kinds of tumors.

The latest findings, which have been reported or privately discussed in the last few months, could also lead to tests that would tell a cancer patient whether the disease is likely to spread or will remain confined to a specific site in the body.

Some experts say that within three to five years doctors will be able to test the genes in patients' cells and tell them, for example, whether they have already suffered one of the four to six genetic changes that lead to colon cancer, or two of the 10 to 15 genetic changes that lead to lung cancer. Such information could offer clues to early treatment and warn susceptible individuals to avoid increasing their risk. A smoker who realized he was already well on the way to lung cancer, for example, would have a powerful incentive to quit.

In patients who have already developed cancer, gene tests are expected to allow doctors to determine whether a tumor will remain confined to a local site, where it can be removed entirely by surgery and radiation, or whether genetic changes make it likely that the tumor has spread its seeds elsewhere in the body, making it necessary to administer highly toxic chemotherapy.

The new genetic research began with very rare tumors in children that are caused by fewer genetic alterations. It has now moved on to the common cancers, where the alterations are more difficult to decipher. Among the common cancers, the work has progressed fastest in studies of colon cancer, lung cancer and, to a lesser extent, breast cancer. Experts say similar approaches are expected to work against a wide variety of other cancers.

Excited about the new findings, Dr. Samuel Broder, director of the National Cancer Institute, has formed a committee to help bring the new gene research to clinical practice as quickly as possible.

"There is so much information and so much excitement in the field," Dr. Broder said. He added that the recent findings are "one of the real astonishing success stories of the national cancer program over the past 18 years." Dr. Broder said he formed the committee because "we want to eliminate any bureaucratic or organizational issues" that could impede the clinical applications.

The imminent clinical applications "are not a pipe dream," said Dr. John Minna, who heads the cancer institute committee. Dr. Minna is the chief of the National Cancer Institute–Navy Medical Oncology Branch and professor of medicine at the Uniformed Services University of the Health Sciences in Bethesda, Md.

But some researchers urged caution in predicting when the results will be put to clinical use. "I'm enthusiastic but my enthusiasm is tempered by many experiences where things don't turn out as rapidly as we might like," said Eric Stanbridge, a professor of microbiology and molecular genetics at the University of California at Irvine who studies cancer genes in human cancer cells.

Cancer experts say they also are very aware of the ethical issues in cancer risk assessments. "The obvious question is: should we really be genetically typing people?" Dr. Minna said. People who learn they are highly susceptible to a particular type of cancer might find it difficult to get health insurance, for example, or may not be hired or promoted. But Dr. Minna said he thinks the health implications are so overwhelming that society will have to use the new genetic information.

## Sporadic Damage to Genes

In recent months, Dr. Bert Vogelstein of Johns Hopkins University and researchers there and at the University of Utah Medical Center in Salt Lake City have found that colon cancer occurs only after four to six genes are altered. Dr. Minna and his colleagues have found that one type of lung cancer, called small cell lung cancer, appears to occur as the culmination of a sequence of about 10 to 15 genetic alterations in a cell. Small cell lung cancer now accounts for about 20 percent of all lung cancers, or 35,000 to 40,000 new cases a year, Dr. Broder said, and the percentage has inexplicably been growing in recent years.

Dr. Dennis Slamon of the University of California in Los Angeles said breast cancer is also likely to be caused by an accumulation of genetic alterations. He and his colleagues have found that the extent of genetic alterations in cells from breast cancers seems to predict whether the cancer will spread. Although breast cancer researchers have not found a specific sequence of genetic changes that occur as normal cells become malignant, "we are heading that way," Dr. Slamon said.

Among all the common cancers, research on colon cancer is the farthest along. Dr. Vogelstein and his colleagues have identified the genetic events that occur as colon cells go from being normal to forming a benign polyp to becoming cancerous.

The alterations probably occur as a result of sporadic damage to the genes in a single cell caused by carcinogens in food or water, for example. Each alteration of a single gene is harmless, but multiple genetic changes make a cell cancerous.

One of the first steps in the development of colon cancer is the loss of part of chromosome 5, one of the 46 chromosomes in human cells. That means that a gene is deleted, and Dr. Vogelstein and others suspect it must be a gene that normally keeps a cell from growing too rapidly. When it is gone, the cell loses one of its brakes on growth.

In the next steps, the cell suffers an alteration in a gene that turns on growth, making the cell grow more rapidly than ever, and it loses genes from chromosomes 17 and 18, which also have genes that are used to slow cell growth. By now, the cell has become cancerous. The exact sequence of the alterations that occur after the initial chromosome 5 deletion does not appear to be important, Dr. Vogelstein said, but if they all accumulate the result is cancer. He added that he cannot be sure that every colon cancer occurs in exactly this way, but that certainly "the great majority" do.

## Decisions on Treatment

If a cell accumulates even more genetic alterations, the cancer seems to be more likely to spread elsewhere in the body, Dr. Vogelstein and his colleagues, including Ray White of the University of Utah School of Medicine, have found. The two research groups collaborated in the studies.

Dr. Vogelstein said he and his colleagues have tested their ability to predict the spread of colon cancer in only about 60 cancer patients so far. "We need several hundred to gain confidence that we could use it in making clinical decisions," he said. He expects to have studied that many patients in 12 to 18 months.

If the results hold up, it should be possible to analyze a patient's tumor, see how many genes are altered, and then use that information in deciding whether the patient needs chemotherapy or radiation in addition to the surgery that removed his tumor, Dr. Vogelstein said. If only four genes are altered, the tumor is apt to remain localized. If more than six genes are altered, the tumor is likely to spread.

In order for a cancer to spread, or metastasize, it needs additional genetic alterations that enable it to break loose from the tumor and get into the blood stream.

These alterations also might help cancer cells set up their own blood supply when they take up residence elsewhere in the body.

Dr. White and his colleagues have also found that people with an inherited condition, called familial polyposis, which almost always leads to colon cancer, are born without the same part of chromosome 5 that is lost when healthy colon cells in other people start to turn cancerous. People with this condition can develop hundreds of thousands of colon polyps.

## Determining Inherited Risk

Dr. White recently reported at meetings that he had studied a family whose members have a strong predisposition to develop colon cancer but do not have familial polyposis. Yet they too lack a part of chromosome 5. This supports the hypothesis that people who inherit a predisposition to cancer are born with cells that have already taken the first cancer step.

Dr. Vogelstein said it may be possible to look at the genes in blood cells of a person with a strong family history of colon cancer and determine whether that person inherited the increased risk.

Eventually, Dr. Vogelstein said he hopes to develop a test for aberrant proteins that leak from colon cells that have cancer genes activated; the proteins appear in the blood or stool. But in the meantime, he expects that researchers will examine polyps, which can be precursors of cancers, and look for gene changes in those cells.

Dr. Minna and his colleagues, in their studies of small cell lung cancer, made gene findings similar to Dr. Vogelstein's. But this lung cancer, they found, only occurs after 10 to 15 genes have been altered. "That was the big surprise to us, the sheer number of genetic lesions," Dr. Minna said. He added that it may explain why lung cancer is so hard to get—a person almost always has to be a smoker or exposed to asbestos for years in order to get lung cancer—and why it is so hard to cure. The lung cells that finally make it along the path to cancer "are Olympic champions of a sort," Dr. Minna said. Stopping them is not easy.

"If you have all these lesions, do you get them all by smoking or do you inherit some, or do you get some during embryonic development?" Dr. Minna asked. He said he suspects that the people who get lung cancer are born with at least one of the necessary genes altered.

"We would not want these people to smoke," Dr. Minna said. "It may be that we can't cure lung cancer—only 10 percent of all patients with lung cancer can be cured even with the best possible diagnosis and treatment. But if we could tell people that they have a 100 percent chance of getting lung cancer if they smoke, we could focus our anti-smoking, anti-radon, and anti-asbestos efforts on them."

## Same Genes, Different Cancers

Another possibility, Dr. Minna said, would be to take lung cell samples from bronchial washings from smokers and look for cells that are starting to develop the sequence of alterations that lead to cancer. Those patients whose cells are already on their way to becoming cancerous may benefit from cancer therapy, Dr. Minna said.

As molecular biologists probe the genes of cancer cells, they are finding that the same genes show up in different cancers. This may explain why people at risk for one type of cancer also may be at risk for other types. These people may be born with one of the cancer genes already damaged.

"If you have lung cancer or someone in your family has lung cancer, you have a two- to threefold increased risk of getting other cancers, including cancer of the bladder and breast," Dr. Minna said.

The new cancer findings also suggest that it may eventually be possible to cure cancer by stopping just one of the errant genes. "If it took five hits to get a cancer, if we correct one of them, that might be sufficient," Dr. Stanbridge said. He showed last year that he can reverse at least one sort of cancer in laboratory experiments by correcting one missing gene. He took cancer cells from children with Wilms tumor, a rare kidney cancer, and added back a chromosome that was partly deleted in these cells. The cells reverted to normal. This is not a practical treatment, but it shows, Dr. Stanbridge said, that it may not be necessary to reverse all the cancerous genetic changes in a cell.

*May 16, 1989*

# How Demand Surged for Prostate Test

By GINA KOLATA

Dr. Joseph E. Oesterling, a urologist at the Mayo Clinic in Rochester, Minn., recently polled practicing doctors in his state to ask whether they were using a widely promoted screening test for prostate cancer. Ninety-two percent said they routinely used it on men over 50.

But the blood test, which costs $50 to $80 per patient, has not yet been approved by the Food and Drug Administration as a screening test and no data yet exist to show that it has an effect on long-term medical outcome.

The test, known as the P.S.A. test, for prostate-specific antigen, also has a high rate of false positive results, meaning that a positive result leads to other, more expensive follow-up tests and treatments to confirm it. Almost 1 in 5 people with high P.S.A. levels does not have cancer, and nearly 1 in 4 with prostate cancer has normal P.S.A. levels.

Some economists estimate it would cost the nation $28 billion a year if all men 50 and over have the test, along with subsequent tests and treatments for those with positive results.

## Effectiveness of Test

A study reported this summer in the *Journal of the American Medical Association* found the test to be twice as effective as a physical examination in finding early cancer, and many doctors and patients are convinced of its usefulness.

But the question remains, in this time of national agony over health care costs, how did an unapproved test with potentially astronomical costs become entrenched as part of the nation's medical system? Despite the lack of F.D.A. approval, the test is recommended for screening by the American Cancer Society and the American Urological Association. But it has not been endorsed for that purpose by the National Cancer Institute or the United States Preventive Services Task Force, a federally sponsored but independent group that draws up medical guidelines.

Doctors and health care analysts say the story of the P.S.A. test's rise to prominence and acceptance shows the power of the pharmaceutical and device industry to create and increase demand for a product. Even doctors who say they are convinced that the test is saving lives say it would never be so popular today were it not for aggressive promotions.

112

For example, proponents and opponents of the test agree that much of the public demand was elicited by the enthusiastic advertising of the annual Prostate Cancer Awareness Week, paid for by the makers of drugs to treat the cancer and by makers of the P.S.A. test. The ubiquitous public service advertisements featuring celebrities like the baseball star Stan Musial are paid for by TAP Pharmaceuticals of Deerfield, Ill., a maker of a prostate cancer treatment.

The companies also support a patient group, Us Too, which sent a representative to a recent meeting held by the National Cancer Institute to discuss the merits of the test and to an F.D.A. advisory committee meeting last spring to discuss an application by Hybritech of San Diego, a division of Eli Lilly & Company, to market the P.S.A. test as a screening test. The committee asked for more data than the company had supplied and said that if the test received approval, it should be used to screen only men at high risk.

## Drumming Up Demand

"To me, the whole issue of P.S.A. testing is, in a microcosm, what's wrong with our health care system," said Dr. Peter Albertson, a urologist at the University of Connecticut in Farmington. "Industry is pumping a lot of money into this and creating a demand for a product."

Urologists benefit because the test has made the prostate "the biggest money-maker for urologists, a large part of a urology business," he said. Hospitals benefit because prostate patients fill many beds. So, he said, even though the test has limitations, "sometimes people don't want to look too hard at a gift horse."

Dr. John Wasson, director of the Center for Aging at Dartmouth College, agreed. Now that the test is so widely accepted, he added, "the scary thing is, this will happen with other tests in the future."

Dr. Oesterling, a proponent of the test who is nevertheless critical of the marketing tactics, explained how the test's makers persuaded doctors to use it. "They marketed the heck out of it," he said. "They went around the country saying, 'Doctor, you need to get a P.S.A. on your patients. Start using it, start using it.' The next thing, patients started coming in and saying, 'Doctor, check my P.S.A.'"

The test detects a protein, P.S.A., that leaks into the blood from the prostate, a walnut-size gland that produces fluid that nourishes sperm. Prostate cancers can lead to high levels of the protein, but so can innocuous enlargements of the gland. Sometimes men have high P.S.A. levels with no apparent cause. The F.D.A. approved the test in 1986 as a way of following the progress of cancer in men in whom the cancer had already been diagnosed. But once a test is on the market, doctors can use it for other purposes, at their own discretion.

Prostate cancer is the leading cancer among men and the second leading cause of cancer deaths among men. After the cancer spreads outside the prostate there is little that doctors can do to treat it. Proponents of the test say that it can find prostate cancers while they are still small and potentially curable.

Opponents say that it has never been shown that P.S.A. screening has an effect on the ultimate outcome of the disease for most men. As many as 70 percent of all men in their 80s have early prostate cancer, but in a vast majority these cancers remain undetected and unthreatening. No one knows which cancers will turn out to be deadly and no one can say whether early treatment with surgery or radiation cures them. And the treatment has its own risks, often resulting in impotence and incontinence.

The P.S.A. test, as Dr. Albertson recalls it, came to prominence in the late 1980s, spurred by several developments. Reports in medical journals about the success of the P.S.A. in detecting tumors brought it to the attention of urologists and other doctors. Then the follow-up test, which had required a hospital visit, suddenly became a quick and easy office procedure when makers of transrectal ultrasound machines began selling them to urologists, complete with a spring-loaded biopsy gun, to obtain tissue samples.

## "A No-Brainer"

"Overnight, a procedure that required booking in the hospital became basically a no-brainer," Dr. Albertson said. "It became a test that takes 15 minutes, with no pain, and is relatively risk-free."

At the same time, the marketing of prostate cancer screening began. In 1989, the first Prostate Cancer Awareness Week was held, with a campaign engineered by the New York public relations firm of Burson-Marsteller, and paid for by the Schering-Plough Corporation.

Last year, said Dr. Stephen Rubino, senior product manager at Schering Laboratories in Kenilworth, N.J., the pharmaceutic company paid $1.2 million for this campaign. For this year's campaign, which began on Sept. 20, other companies and the American Cancer Society have joined to share the burden with Schering-Plough, whose share of this year's $240,000 campaign is $100,000. The campaign is under the auspices of the Prostate Cancer Education Council, a group of doctors, health educators and patient support groups.

The campaign has been "extremely successful," said Dr. E. David Crawford, a urologist at the University of Colorado Health Sciences Center in Denver who is head of the education council. Dr. Crawford said that when it began in 1989, the group hoped to draw a few thousand men for screening. Instead, he said: "We had an overwhelming response. Fifteen thousand men came to 91 sites for screening. The next year we had 150,000. The years after that, we had over half a million."

Dr. Stephen Brenner, an internist who has a private practice in New Haven, said that he got many requests for the test, and that he felt he could not refuse to do it, even though he had reservations about its usefulness as a screening tool.

## "An Avalanche" of Requests

"It's an avalanche," he said. "It's really snowballed. The overwhelming majority of my male patients are aware of the test. They'll either ask about it or request it." He also worries about malpractice suits. And, he added: "I feel it can be helpful, but I don't know when."

Dr. Brenner said he felt the Prostate Cancer Awareness Weeks were "pretty transparent." He added: "I'm opposed to industry promoting products to patients. I am opposed to demand coming from industry. We ought to have firm scientific evidence that a test is useful before we start using it."

Last year, the American Cancer Society recommended that all men over 50 have an annual P.S.A. test and digital rectal examination. It recommended that men with a family history of the disease or who are black, placing them at higher risk, have the tests every year starting at 40.

JoAnn Schellenbach, a spokeswoman for the cancer society, said the reason for the screening recommendation was that "men were having the test anyway."

"Doctors were doing it," she said. "We needed to spell out some very distinct practice guidelines. That is more useful than debating and riding the fence."

Now, some researchers question whether it will ever be possible to learn if the test saves lives. The only definitive way to do that would be to enroll men in a study, randomly assigning some to have it and others not to and then see which group benefited most. This is a study that the National Cancer Institute hopes to do.

But, Dr. Oesterling said: "That study will never get done. You are never going to find in the United States any more a control group of people who will not get a P.S.A."

*September 29, 1993*

# Stand on Mammograms Greeted by Outrage

By GINA KOLATA

Dr. Leon Gordis, the chairman of the expert panel that advised the National Institutes of Health on mammograms last week, is a veteran of controversy.

He was a member of a panel that examined medical complaints by veterans of the Persian Gulf war, another that looked into allegations that food additives make children hyperactive and one that evaluated the safety of the nation's blood supply in the early days of the AIDS epidemic.

But Dr. Gordis, an epidemiologist at the Johns Hopkins University School of Medicine, said nothing had prepared him for the venomous reaction his panel got when it said in a report that it had no reason to recommend routine mammograms for women under 50. The reaction, he and others said, says more about the politics and psychology of breast cancer than it does about the science behind the committee's decision.

The panel was asked whether routine mammograms could prolong the lives of women in their 40s. There is abundant evidence that when women who are 50 or older have mammograms every one to two years, they reduce their chances of dying from breast cancer by about 30 percent. But whether women under 50 would benefit from similar screening has been uncertain.

After spending six weeks reading more than 100 scientific reports and then hearing 32 presentations in a two-day meeting, the group decided that there was not enough evidence that women in their 40s would benefit to advise them to have the X-ray test as part of routine health screening. The panel said women should weigh the risks and benefits of the test and decide for themselves if they want it.

Barely had the words come out of Dr. Gordis's mouth on Thursday morning when the audience began muttering and people began rushing to the microphones to rebuke the group, whose members sat looking stricken under the barrage. Prominent radiologists castigated the committee, with some accusing it of bias and others saying the panel was condemning American women to death. One of the radiologists, Dr. Daniel B. Kopans of Harvard Medical School, said the committee's report was "fraudulent" and should not be released to the public until it was "corrected."

Dr. Richard D. Klausner, who, as director of the National Cancer Institute, had asked that the panel be convened, rushed to the hallway to use a public telephone after Dr. Gordis read the statement. In an interview there, he said he was "shocked" by the conclusions, adding that he disliked their negative tone. He said an advisory board to the cancer institute would review the decision next month.

Some breast cancer patients who are convinced that their lives were saved by mammograms said they felt betrayed by a report that questions the usefulness of these X-rays of the breast in younger women.

People who were not at the meeting have also chimed in. Dr. Bernadine Healy, dean of the College of Medicine at Ohio State University and a former director of the National Institutes of Health, said that although she had not read the report, she was shocked by the panel's conclusion. "I am very disturbed that a group of so-called experts challenged the notion of early detection," she declared. "What they are saying is that ignorance is bliss."

Before the week was over, Dr. Gordis said, he had been summoned by Senator Arlen Specter of Pennsylvania to testify before Congress on the panel's report.

Panel members and some who attended the conference were stunned by the reaction. "I didn't have a clue" that people would respond so angrily, said Dr. Leslie R. Laufman, a cancer specialist at Hematology Oncology Consultants in Columbus, Ohio. The arguments, Dr. Gordis said, "have gotten so one-sided that people are unwilling to listen." Dr. Suzanne W. Fletcher, a professor of ambulatory care and prevention at Harvard Medical School and an invited speaker at the two-day meeting who commended the panel on its report, said the reaction was "very scary, frankly."

Constance A. Rufenbarger, a breast cancer survivor and consumer advocate who was on the panel, said that its members would have been eager to endorse the use of screening mammograms for women in their 40s but that the studies simply did not support such a recommendation.

The studies show that somewhere between zero and 10 women out of 10,000 in their 40s who were screened by mammograms would have their lives prolonged—but not necessarily saved. Some studies found no effect of regular mammography for women in their 40s, while a few found a small beneficial effect a decade after the women had first started having mammograms. None found anything like the 30 percent drop in the death rate from breast cancer that occurs in a few years in women over 50 who have regular mammograms.

Dr. Donald A. Berry, a panel member who is a statistician at Duke University, said that another way to look at those data was to say that, at best, 98.5 percent of the women who have annual mammograms throughout their 40s got no benefit.

"The other 1½ percent have their lives extended by 200 days," he said. It is not clear "how we parcel out those 200 days," he said—one woman might get 199 extra days of life while another might get one day, for example.

At the same time, the panel noted, mammography carries risks of its own.

Overall, women who have mammograms every year from age 40 to 49 run a 30 percent chance of being told that the test has found an abnormality even though their breasts are normal. Such women then need additional tests—including, in some cases, surgery—to be sure that no tumor is present. The mammography also tends to find tiny indeterminate lumps. To play it safe, doctors treat such tumors as if they were cancers. Forty percent of the tumors detected in younger women are of this type, called intraductal carcinoma in situ. And 40 percent of the women in their 40s who have these tumors have mastectomies. The rest have lumpectomies, with or without radiation.

Moreover, the panel said, mammography cannot even give women peace of mind. Mammograms miss one-fourth of the invasive breast cancers in women in their 40s, compared with 10 percent in older women, perhaps because of the density of the younger women's breasts.

"We're dealing with healthy young women," Dr. Berry said, "and we're doing things that have a potential for harm." He added that the "data suggest that the benefits are not sufficiently great" to make up for the harm caused.

Dr. John H. Wasson, a panel member who is a professor of geriatrics at Dartmouth Medical School, said it was "unfair" to ask the committee to work without pay to analyze these data and stay up all night writing its report only "to face a pack of hungry wolves."

But some women's health advocates and panel members said that in retrospect, the intense reaction should not have been a surprise.

One problem, said Maryann Napoli, the associate director of the Center for Medical Consumers in New York, is that mammography has become a big business in the United States, widely promoted by instrument makers, medical centers and the American Cancer Society as a way to ease the minds of women who have become terrified of breast cancer. As a consequence, few want to hear that its much-touted effectiveness may be in doubt for women under age 50.

"They've made us scared of the disease, and it's understandable that women want to believe that there's something they can do," Ms. Napoli said. "I feel the confusion stems from the fact that they sold women in their 40s on mammography before there was any evidence."

Cindy Pearson, the executive director of the National Women's Health Network, an advocacy group based in Washington, noted that the American Cancer Society, radiologists and medical centers had been advertising and otherwise pounding home the message that mammograms would find cancers early, when they can be snipped out, curing a woman of cancer that would otherwise kill her. "The message is that mammograms never miss," Ms. Pearson said.

As a result, Dr. Berry said, women are convinced that if they find cancer early, they will be saved. But he said it was clear that some cancers would kill women whether or not they were found on mammograms. Other cancers will not be deadly even if they are left untreated for years—even if they are left untreated until the women can feel the lumps.

Another "irrational bias," Dr. Berry said, is the widespread belief that women who had mammograms and survived cancer are alive today because of those mammograms. Nearly every woman knows someone who says her life was saved because she had a mammogram, he said, and mammograms are advertised with that message.

Of course, Dr. Berry added, there is no way of knowing whether a woman is alive because of, or in spite of, her mammogram. That is why it takes large clinical trials to search for benefits of the screening test.

The messages women have heard and endorsed have been "too reassuring" and "too simplistic," said Dr. Laufman, of Hematology Oncology Consultants. She had mammograms throughout her 40s "without questioning the advice," said Dr. Laufman, who just turned 50. She added, "I have recommended very many patients and family members to have mammograms over the years."

But after reviewing the evidence as a member of the panel, Dr. Laufman said, "I have a different opinion now."

She said she had confronted that question in her practice recently when she saw a cancer patient who was in her late 40s and who had come in for a checkup after a mastectomy and chemotherapy a year ago.

"She asked me, 'What should I tell my 29-year-old daughter?'" Dr. Laufman said. "I told her that I would tell her daughter what I would tell my own daughter: Start having mammograms when you're 50. And stay very, very tightly tuned to the research as it develops."

*January 28, 1997*

# Experts Decode Cancer Patient's Genes, Seeking Treatment Clues

## By DENISE GRADY

For the first time, researchers have decoded all the genes of a person with cancer and found a set of mutations that might have caused the disease or aided its progression.

Using cells donated by a woman in her 50s who died of leukemia, the scientists sequenced all the DNA from her cancer cells and compared it to the DNA from her own normal, healthy skin cells. Then they zeroed in on 10 mutations that occurred only in the cancer cells, apparently spurring abnormal growth, preventing the cells from suppressing that growth and enabling them to fight off chemotherapy.

The findings will not help patients immediately, but researchers say they could lead to new therapies and would almost certainly help doctors make better choices among existing treatments, based on a more detailed genetic picture of each patient's cancer. Though the research involved leukemia, the same techniques can also be used to study other cancers.

"This is the first of many of these whole cancer genomes to be sequenced," said Richard K. Wilson, director of the Genome Sequencing Center at Washington University in St. Louis and the senior author of the study. "They'll give us a whole bunch of clues about what's going on in the DNA when cancer starts to bloom."

The mutations—genetic mistakes—found in this research were not inborn, but developed later in life, like most mutations that cause cancer. (Only 5 percent to 10 percent of all cancers are thought to be hereditary.)

The new research, by looking at the entire genome—all the DNA—and aiming to find all the mutations involved in a particular cancer, differs markedly from earlier studies, which have searched fewer genes. The project, which took months and cost $1 million, was made possible by recent advances in technology that have made it easier and cheaper to analyze hundreds of millions of DNA snippets. The study is being published Thursday in the journal *Nature*.

Dr. Wilson said he hoped that in 5 to 20 years, decoding a patient's cancer genome would consist of dropping a spot of blood onto a chip that slides into a desktop computer and getting back a report that suggests which drugs will work best.

"That's personalized genomics, personalized medicine in a box," he said. "It's holy grail sort of stuff, but I think it's not out of the realm of possibility."

Until now, Dr. Wilson said, most work on cancer mutations has focused on just a few hundred genes already suspected of being involved in the disease, not the 20,000 or so genes that make up the full human genome.

The older approach is useful, Dr. Wilson said, "but if there are genes mutated that you don't know about or don't expect, you'll miss them."

Indeed, 8 of the 10 mutations his group discovered would not have been found with the more traditional approach.

A cancer expert not involved with the study, Dr. Stephen Nimer, chief of the hematology service at Memorial Sloan-Kettering Cancer Center, called the research a "tour de force" and the report "a wonderful paper." Dr. Nimer said the whole-genome approach seemed likely to yield important information about other types of cancer as well as leukemia.

"It is supporting evidence for the idea that you can't just go after the things you know about," Dr. Nimer said.

He added, "It would be nice to have this kind information on every patient we treat."

Dr. Nimer also predicted that oncologists would quickly want to start looking for these mutations in their patients or in stored samples from former patients, to see if they could help in predicting the course of the disease or selecting treatments.

Studying cancer genomes has become a major thrust of research. In the past few years the government has spent $100 million for genome studies in lung and ovarian cancers and glioblastoma multiforme, a type of brain tumor. The person who gave her cells for the study at Washington University became not only the first cancer patient, but also the first woman to have her entire genome decoded. Her information will be available only to scientists and not posted publicly, to protect her privacy and that of her family. The only other complete human genomes open to researchers so far have come from men, two scientists known for ego as well as intellect, who ran decoding projects and chose to bare their own DNA to the world: James D. Watson and J. Craig Venter. Their genomes are available for all to inspect.

The woman at Washington University had acute myelogenous leukemia, a fast-growing cancer that affects about 13,000 people a year in the United States and kills 8,800. Its cause is not well understood. Like most cancers, it is thought to begin in a single cell, with a mutation that is not present at birth but that occurs later for some unknown reason. Generally, one mutation is not enough to cause cancer; the disease does not develop until other mutations occur.

"Most of them are just these random events in the universe that add up to something horrible," said Dr. Timothy J. Ley, a hematologist at Washington University and the director of the study.

The researchers chose to study this disease because it is severe and the treatment has not improved in decades.

"It's one of the nastiest forms of leukemia," Dr. Wilson said. "It's very aggressive. It affects mostly adults, and there's really no good treatment for it. A very large fraction of the patients eventually will die from their disease."

Before starting treatment, the patient they studied had donated samples of bone marrow and skin, so the researchers could compare her normal skin cells to cancer cells from her bone marrow. Some of the patient's mutated genes appeared to promote cancer growth. One probably made the cancer drug-resistant by enabling the tumor cells to pump chemotherapy drugs right out of the cell before they could do their work. The other mutated genes seemed to be tumor suppressors, the body's natural defense against dangerous genetic mistakes.

"Their job is surveillance," Dr. Wilson said. "If cells start to do something out of control, these genes are there to shut it down. When we find three or four suppressors inactivated, it's almost like tumor has systematically started to knock out that surveillance mechanism. That makes it tougher to kill. It gets a little freaky. This is unscientific, but we say, gee, it looks like the tumor has a mind of its own, it knows what genes it has to take out to be successful. It's amazing."

Tests of 187 other patients with acute myelogenous leukemia found that none had the eight new mutations found in the first patient.

That finding suggests that many genetic detours can lead to the same awful destination, and that many more genomes must be studied, but it does not mean that every patient will need his or her own individual drug, Dr. Wilson said.

"Ultimately, one signal tells the cell to grow, grow, grow," he said. "There has to be something in common. It's that commonality we'll find that will tell us what treatment will be the most powerful."

*November 6, 2008*

CHAPTER 6

# Cloning—Stem Cells

# Scientist Reports First Cloning Ever of Adult Mammal

By GINA KOLATA

In a feat that may be the one bit of genetic engineering that has been anticipated and dreaded more than any other, researchers in Britain are reporting that they have cloned an adult mammal for the first time.

The group, led by Dr. Ian Wilmut, a 52-year-old embryologist at the Roslin Institute in Edinburgh, created a lamb using DNA from an adult sheep. The achievement shocked leading researchers who had said it could not be done. The researchers had assumed that the DNA of adult cells would not act like the DNA formed when a sperm's genes first mingle with those of an egg.

In theory, researchers said, such techniques could be used to take a cell from an adult human and use the DNA to create a genetically identical human—a time-delayed twin. That prospect raises the thorniest of ethical and philosophical questions.

Dr. Wilmut's experiment was simple, in retrospect. He took a mammary cell from an adult sheep and prepared its DNA so it would be accepted by an egg from another sheep. He then removed the egg's own DNA, replacing it with the DNA from the adult sheep by fusing the egg with the adult cell. The fused cells, carrying the adult DNA, began to grow and divide, just like a perfectly normal fertilized egg, to form an embryo.

Dr. Wilmut implanted the embryo into another ewe; in July, the ewe gave birth to a lamb, named Dolly. Though Dolly seems perfectly normal, DNA tests show that she is the clone of the adult ewe that supplied her DNA.

"What this will mostly be used for is to produce more health care products," Dr. Wilmut told the Press Association of Britain early today, the Reuters news agency reported.

"It will enable us to study genetic diseases for which there is presently no cure and track down the mechanisms that are involved. The next step is to use the cells in culture in the lab and target genetic changes into that culture."

Simple though it may be, the experiment, to be reported this coming Thursday in the British journal *Nature*, has startled biologists and ethicists. Dr. Wilmut said in a telephone interview last week that he planned to breed Dolly next fall to determine whether she was fertile. Dr. Wilmut said he was interested in the technique primarily as a tool in animal husbandry, but other scientists said it had opened doors to the unsettling prospect that humans could be cloned as well.

Dr. Lee Silver, a biology professor at Princeton University, said last week that the announcement had come just in time for him to revise his forthcoming book so the first chapter will no longer state that such cloning is impossible.

"It's unbelievable," Dr. Silver said. "It basically means that there are no limits. It means all of science fiction is true. They said it could never be done and now here it is, done before the year 2000."

Dr. Neal First, a professor of reproductive biology and animal biotechnology at the University of Wisconsin, who has been trying to clone cattle, said the ability to clone dairy cattle could have a bigger impact on the industry than the introduction of artificial insemination in the 1950s, a procedure that revolutionized dairy farming. Cloning could be used to make multiple copies of animals that are especially good at producing meat or milk or wool.

Although researchers have created genetically identical animals by dividing embryos very early in their development, Dr. Silver said, no one had cloned an animal from an adult until now. Earlier experiments, with frogs, have become a stock story in high school biology, but the experiments never produced cloned adult frogs. The frogs developed only to the tadpole stage before dying.

It was even worse with mammals. Researchers could swap DNA from one fertilized egg to another, but they could go no further. "They couldn't even put nuclei from late-stage mouse embryos into early mouse embryos," Dr. Silver said. The embryos failed to develop and died.

As a result, the researchers concluded that as cells developed, the proteins coating the DNA somehow masked all the important genes for embryo development. A skin cell may have all the genetic information that was present in the fertilized egg that produced the organism, for example, but almost all that information is pasted over. Now all the skin cell can do is be a skin cell.

Researchers could not even hope to strip off the proteins from an adult cell's DNA and replace them with proteins from an embryo's DNA. The DNA would shatter if anyone tried to strip it bare, Dr. Silver said.

Last year, Dr. Wilmut showed that he could clone DNA from sheep embryo cells, but even that was not taken as proof that the animal itself could be cloned. It could just be that the embryo cells had DNA that was unusually conducive to cloning, many thought.

Dr. Wilmut, however, hit on a clever strategy. He did not bother with the proteins that coat DNA, and instead focused on getting the DNA from an adult cell into a stage in its normal cycle of replication where it could take up residence in an egg.

DNA in growing cells goes through what is known as the cell cycle: it prepares itself to divide, then replicates itself and splits in two as the cell itself divides. The problem with earlier cloning attempts, Dr. Wilmut said, was that the DNA from the donor had been out of synchrony with that of the recipient cell. The solution, he discovered, was, in effect, to put the DNA from the adult cell to sleep, making it quiescent by depriving the adult cell of nutrients. When he then fused it with an egg cell from another sheep—after removing the egg cell's DNA—the donor DNA took over as though it belonged there.

Dr. Wilmut said in the telephone interview last week that the method could work for any animal and that he hoped to use it next to clone cattle. He said that he could use many types of cells from adults for cloning but that the easiest to use would be so-called stem cells, which give rise to a variety of other cells and are present throughout the body.

In his sheep experiment, he used mammary cells because a company that sponsored his work, PPL Therapeutics, is developing sheep that can be used to produce proteins that can be used as drugs in their milk, so it had sheep mammary cells readily available.

For Dr. Wilmut, the main interest of the experiment is to advance animal research. PPL, for example, wants to clone animals that can produce pharmacologically useful proteins, like the clotting factor needed by hemophiliacs. Scientists would grow cells in the laboratory, insert the genes for production of the desired protein, select those cells that most actively churned out the protein and use those cells to make cloned females. The cloned animals would produce immense amounts of the proteins in their milk, making the animals into living drug factories.

But that is only the beginning, Dr. Wilmut said. Researchers could use the same method to make animals with human diseases, like cystic fibrosis, and then test therapies on the cloned animals. Or they could use cloning to alter the proteins on the surfaces of pig organs, like the liver or heart, making the organs more like human organs. Then they could transplant those organs into humans.

Dr. First said the "exciting and astounding" cloning result could shake the dairy industry. It could allow the cloning of cows that are superproducers of milk, making 30,000 or even 40,000 pounds of milk a year. The average cow makes about 13,000 pounds of milk a year, he said.

"I think that if—and it's a very big if—cloning were highly efficient," Dr. First said last week, "then it could be a more significant revolution to the livestock industry than even artificial insemination."

Although Dr. Wilmut said he saw no intrinsic biological reason humans, too, could not be cloned, he dismissed the idea as being ethically unacceptable. Moreover, he said, it is illegal in Britain to clone people. "I would find it offensive" to clone a human being, Dr. Wilmut said, adding that he fervently hoped that no one would try it.

But others said that it was hard to imagine enforcing a ban on cloning people when cloning got more efficient. "I could see it going on surreptitiously," said Lori Andrews, a professor at Chicago-Kent College of Law who specializes in reproductive issues. For example, Professor Andrews said last week, in the early days of in vitro fertilization, Australia banned that practice. "So scientists moved to Singapore" and offered the procedure, she said. "I can imagine new crimes," she added.

People might be cloned without their knowledge or consent. After all, all that would be needed would be some cells. If there is a market for a sperm bank selling semen from Nobel laureates, how much better would it be to bear a child that would actually be a clone of a great thinker or, perhaps, a great beauty or great athlete?

"The genie is out of the bottle," said Dr. Ronald Munson, a medical ethicist at the University of Missouri in St. Louis. "This technology is not, in principle, policeable."

Dr. Munson called the possibilities incredible. For example, could researchers devise ways to add just the DNA of an adult cell, without fusing two living cells? If so, might it be possible to clone the dead?

"I had an idea for a story once," Dr. Munson said, in which a scientist obtains a spot of blood from the cross on which Jesus was crucified. He then uses it to clone a man who is Jesus Christ—or perhaps cannot be.

On a more practical note, Dr. Munson mused over the strange twist that science has taken.

"There's something ironic" about study, he said. "Here we have this incredible technical accomplishment, and what motivated it? The desire for more sheep milk of a certain type." It is, he said, "the theater of the absurd acted out by scientists."

In his interview with the Press Association, Britain's domestic news agency, Dr. Wilmut added early today: "We are aware that there is potential for misuse, and we have provided information to ethicists and the Human Embryology Authority. We believe that it is important that society decides how we want to use this technology and makes sure it prohibits what it wants to prohibit. It would be desperately sad if people started using this sort of technology with people."

*February 23, 1997*

# After Decades of Missteps, How Cloning Succeeded

By MICHAEL SPECTER WITH GINA KOLATA

Charles Darwin was so terrified when he discovered that mankind had not been specially separated from all other animals by God that it took him two decades to find the courage to publish the work that forever altered the way humans look at life on Earth. Albert Einstein, so outwardly serene, once said that after the theory of relativity stormed into his mind as a young man, it never again left him, not even for a minute.

But Dr. Ian Wilmut, the 52-year-old embryologist who astonished the world on Feb. 22 by announcing that he had created the first animal cloned from an adult—a lamb named Dolly—seems almost oblivious to the profound and disquieting implications of his work. Perhaps no achievement in modern biology promises to solve more problems than the possibility of regular, successful genetic manipulation. But certainly none carries a more ominous burden of fear and misunderstanding.

"I am not a fool," Dr. Wilmut said last week in his cluttered lab, during a long conversation in which he reviewed the fitful 25-year odyssey that led to his electrifying accomplishment and unwanted fame. "I know what is bothering people about all this. I understand why the world is suddenly at my door. But this is my work. It has always been my work, and it doesn't have anything to do with creating copies of human beings. I am not haunted by what I do, if that is what you want to know. I sleep very well at night."

Yet by scraping a few cells from the udder of a 6-year-old ewe, then fusing them into a specially altered egg cell from another sheep, Dr. Wilmut and his colleagues at the Roslin Institute here, seven miles from Edinburgh, have suddenly pried open one of the most forbidden—and tantalizing—doors of modern life.

People have been obsessed with the possibility of building humans for centuries, even before Mary Shelley wrote *Frankenstein* in 1818. Still, so few legitimate researchers actually thought it was possible to create an identical genetic copy of an adult animal that Dr. Wilmut may well have been the only man trying to do it, a contrast with the fiery competition that has become the hallmark of modern molecular biology.

Dr. Wilmut, a meek and affable researcher who lives in a village where sheep outnumber people, grew more disheveled and harried as the pressure-filled week wore on. A $60,000-a-year government employee at the institute, Scotland's leading animal research laboratory, Dr. Wilmut does not stand to earn more than $25,000 in royalties if his breakthrough is commercially successful.

"I give everything away," he said. "I want to understand things."

Dr. Wilmut has made no conscious effort to improve on science fiction in his work; he said, in fact, that he rarely read it. A quiet man whose wife is an elder in the Church of Scotland but who says he "does not have a belief in God," Dr. Wilmut is the least sensational of scientists. Asked the inevitable questions about cloning human beings, he patiently conceded that it might now become possible but added that he would "find it repugnant."

Dr. Wilmut's objectives have always been prosaic and direct: he has spent his life trying to make livestock healthy, more efficient and better able to serve humanity. In creating Dolly, his goal—like that of many other researchers around the world—was to turn animals into factories churning out proteins that can be used as drugs. Even though the work is early and tentative, and it needs many improvements before it can be used, no scientists have stepped forward to say that they doubt its authenticity.

Many scientists say they are certain that the day will eventually come when humans can also be cloned. Already, scientists in Oregon say they have cloned rhesus monkeys from very early embryo cells. That is not the same as cloning the more sophisticated cells of an adult animal, or even a developing fetus. But any kind of cloning in primates brings the work closer to human beings. That is why what has happened here has rapidly begun to resonate far beyond the tufted glens and heather hills of Scotland. In much the way that the Wright Brothers at Kitty Hawk freed humanity of a restriction once considered eternal, human existence suddenly seems to have taken on a dramatic new dimension.

The eventual impact of this particular experiment on business and science may not be known for years. But it will almost certainly cast important new light on basic biological science.

Already, even the simplest questions about the creation of Dolly provoke answers that demonstrate how profound and novel the research here has been. Asked if the lamb should be considered 7 months old, which is how long she has been alive, or 6 years old, since it is a genetic replica of a 6-year-old sheep, Dr. Wilmut's clear blue eyes clouded for a moment. "I can't answer that," he said. "We just don't know. There are many things here we will have to find out."

## The Goal: Aim Is Barnyard, Not Nursery

The Scots have an old tongue twister of an adage that says "many a mickle make a muckle," or, little things add up to big things. It is certainly true of the cloning of Dolly, who had her conceptual birth in a conversation in an Irish bar more than a decade ago and who was born after a series of painstaking experiments, years of doubt and several final all-night vigils—one bleating little lamb among nearly 300 abject failures.

While the world has become transfixed by the idea of creating identical copies from frozen cells, that was not the result that Dr. Wilmut, or any other scientists interviewed for this article, considers the most significant part of the research.

The true object of those years of labor was to find better ways to alter the genetic makeup of farm animals to create herds capable of providing better food or any chemical a consumer might want. In theory, genes could be altered so animals would produce better meat, eggs, wool or milk. Animals could be made more resistant to disease. Researchers here even talk about breeding cows that could deliver low-fat milk straight from the udder.

"The overall aim is actually not, primarily, to make copies," Dr. Wilmut said, interrupted constantly by the institute's feed mill as it noisily blew off steam. "It's to make precise genetic changes in cells."

Obscure as he may seem to those outside his field, Ian Wilmut has been quietly pushing the borders of reproductive science for decades. In 1973, having just completed his doctorate at Cambridge, he produced the first calf born from a frozen embryo. Cows give birth to no more than 5 or 10 calves in a lifetime. By taking frozen embryos produced by cows that provide the best meat and milk, thawing them and transferring them to surrogate mothers, Dr. Wilmut enabled cattle breeders to increase the quality of their herds immensely.

Since then, while always harboring at least some doubt that cloning was really possible, he has struggled to isolate and transfer genetic traits that would improve the utility of farm animals.

In 1986, while in Ireland for a scientific meeting, Dr. Wilmut heard something during a casual conversation in a bar that caught his attention and convinced him that cloning large farm animals was indeed possible. "It was just a bar-time story," he recalled this week, in the slight brogue he has acquired after living here for 25 years. "Not even straight from the horse's mouth."

What he heard was the rumor—true, it turned out—that another scientist had created a lamb clone from an already developing embryo. It was enough to push him in a direction that had already been abandoned by most of his colleagues.

By the early 1980s, many researchers had grown discouraged about the practicalities of cloning because of a hurdle that had come to seem insurmountable. Every cell in the body originates from a single fertilized egg, which contains in its DNA all the information needed to construct a whole organism. That fertilized egg cell grows and divides. The new cells slowly take on special properties, developing into skin, or blood or bones, for example. But each cell, however specialized, still carries in its nucleus a full complement of DNA, a complete blueprint for an organism.

The problem for scientists was stark and unavoidable: It was assumed that the nucleus of a mature cell, which has developed, or differentiated, so it could carry out a specific function in the body, simply could not be made to function like the nucleus of an embryo that had yet to begin the process of learning to play its special role. Even though the DNA, with all the necessary genes, was in the differentiated cell, the issue was how to turn it on so it would direct the process of growth that begins with the egg. The essential question for cloning researchers was whether the genes in an adult cell could still be used to create a new animal with the same genes.

The pivotal rumor Dr. Wilmut heard at the meeting in Ireland was that a Danish embryologist, Dr. Steen M. Willadsen, then working at Grenada Genetics in Texas, had managed to clone a sheep using a cell from an embryo that was already developing.

The story, which came from a veterinarian named Geoff Mahon, who worked at the same company, went beyond the research that Dr. Willadsen would publish later that year on cloning sheep from early embryos. Dr. Willadsen said in a telephone interview from his home in Florida that he had indeed done the more advanced work but had never published it.

What he did publish was the result of successfully cloning sheep from very early embryo cells: the first cloning of a mammal. Dr. Willadsen tried that experiment with three sheep eggs. In each case, he removed the egg's nucleus, with all its genetic information, and fused that egg, now bereft of instructions on how to grow, with a cell from a growing embryo. If the egg could use the other cell's genetic information to grow itself into a lamb, the experiment would be a success. It worked.

"The reality is that the very first experiment I did, which involved only three eggs, was successful," Dr. Willadsen said. "It gave me two lambs. They were dead on arrival, but the next one we got was alive." The paper was eventually published in *Nature,* the influential British science journal that last week published Dr. Wilmut's news of Dolly, and it created a sensation.

But it was the rumor of the unpublished work that captivated Dr. Wilmut. If it was possible to clone using an already differentiated embryonic cell, it was time to take another look at cloning an adult, Dr. Wilmut decided. "I thought if that story was true—and remember, it was just a bar-time story—if it was true, we could get those cells from farm animals," he said. And, he thought, he might even be able to make copies of animals from more mature embryos or eventually from an adult.

When Dr. Wilmut flew back to Scotland, he was already dreaming of Dolly. When he was flying back over the Irish Sea with a colleague, he said, "we were already making plans to try to get funds to start this work."

## The Quest: From Daydreams to Successes

Dr. Wilmut's dominance of the field grew from that day, almost by default. He was nearly alone, out on a limb. His tumultuous field seemed to have run out of steam. Many of its leaders and its students had departed, going to medical school and becoming doctors or accepting lucrative positions at in vitro fertilization centers, helping infertile couples have babies. Two of its stars published a famous paper concluding that cloning an adult animal was impossible, dashing cold water on their eager colleagues. Companies, formed in a flush of enthusiasm a decade earlier, folded by the early 1990s.

Most of the few cloning researchers left were focused on a much easier task. They were cloning cells from early embryos that had not yet specialized. And even though some had achieved stunning successes, none were about to try cloning an adult or even cells from mature embryos. It just did not seem possible.

The idea of cloning had tantalized scientists since 1938. When no one even knew what genetic material consisted of, the first modern embryologist, Dr. Hans Spemann of Germany, proposed what he called a "fantastical experiment": taking the nucleus out of an egg cell and replacing it with a nucleus from another cell. In short, he suggested that scientists try to clone.

But no one could do it, said Dr. Randall S. Prather, a cloning researcher at the University of Missouri in Columbia, because the technology was not advanced enough. It would be another 14 years before anyone could try to clone, and then they did it with frogs, whose eggs are enormous compared with those of mammals, making them far easier to manipulate. Dr. Spemann, who died in 1941, never saw his idea carried to fruition.

In fact, frogs were not successfully cloned until the 1970s. The work was done by Dr. John Gurdon, who now teaches at Cambridge University. Even though the frogs never reached adulthood, the technique used was a milestone. He replaced the nucleus of a frog egg, one large cell, with that of another cell from another frog.

It was the beginning of nuclear transfer experiments, which had the goal of getting the newly transplanted genes to direct the development of the embryo. But the frog studies seemed to indicate that cloning could go only so far. Although scientists could transfer nuclei from adult cells to egg cells, the frogs only developed to tadpoles, and they always died.

Most researchers at the time thought even that sort of limited cloning success depended on something special about frogs. "For years, it was thought that you could never do that in mammals," said Dr. Neal First of the University of Wisconsin, who has been Dr. Wilmut's most devoted competitor.

In 1981, after some rapid advances in technology, two investigators published a paper that galvanized the world. It seemed to say that mammals could be cloned—at least from embryo cells. But, in a crushing blow to those in the field, the research turned to be a fraud.

The investigators, Dr. Karl Illmensee of the University of Geneva and Dr. Peter Hoppe of the Jackson Laboratory in Bar Harbor, Me., claimed that they had transplanted the nuclei of mouse embryo cells into mouse eggs and produced three live mice that were clones of the embryos. Their mice were on the cover of the prestigious journal *Science*, and their work created a sensation.

"Everyone thought that article was right," said Dr. Brigid Hogan, a mouse embryologist at Vanderbilt University in Nashville. Dr. Illmensee, the senior author, "was getting enormous publicity and exposure, and accolades," Dr. Hogan said.

Two years later, however, two other scientists, Dr. James McGrath and Dr. Davor Solter, working at the Wistar Institute in Philadelphia, reported in *Science* that they could not repeat the mouse experiment. They concluded their paper with the disheartening statement that the "cloning of mammals by simple nuclear transfer is impossible." After a lengthy inquiry, it was discovered that Dr. Illmensee had faked his results.

Leaders in the field were shattered. Dr. McGrath gave up cloning, got an M.D. degree and is now a genetics professor at Yale University. Dr. Solter gave up cloning and is now the director of the Max Planck Institute in Freiburg, Germany. Most research centers abandoned the work completely.

"Man, it was depressing," said Dr. James M. Robl, a cloning researcher at the University of Massachusetts in Amherst. After the paper by Dr. Illmensee, "we all thought we would be cloning animals like crazy," Dr. Robl said. He had pursued research to try to clone cows and pigs. Suddenly, it seemed as though he was wasting his time.

"We had a famous scientist come through the lab," Dr. Robl said. "I showed him with all enthusiasm all the work I was doing. He looked at me with a very serious look on his face and said, 'Why are you doing this?'"

But not everyone was despondent. A few investigators forged on. One of them was Dr. Keith Campbell, a charismatic 42-year-old biologist at the institute here who specializes in studying the life cycle of the cell. Dr. Campbell, who joined the institute in 1991, said in an interview last week, "I always believed that if you could do this in a frog, you could do it in mammals." Dr. Campbell, who said he had enjoyed the cloning fantasy *The Boys From Brazil,* responded to questions about his earlier work on cloning in an interview last summer, saying "We're only accelerating what breeders have been doing for years."

Soon he had convinced his colleagues at the institute to try the experiments that eventually led to their success with Dolly. "But at that point, we still had much to learn," he said.

The most important step would be to find a way to grow clones from cells that had already developed beyond the very earliest embryonic stage. Whenever cloning had been tried with more specialized cells in the past, it had ended in failure. Until Dolly was born, nobody could be sure whether those failures were because older cells have switched off some of their genes for good or because nobody knew how to make them work properly in an egg.

Because no one knew whether cloning was even possible, it was hard to speculate about what the hurdles might be. But Dr. Campbell had what turned out to be the crucial insight. It could be, he realized, that an egg will not take up and use the genetic material from an adult cell because the cell cycles of the egg and the adult cell might be out of synchrony. All cells go through cycles in which they grow and divide, making a whole new set of chromosomes each time. In cloning, Dr. Campbell speculated, the problem might be that the egg was in one stage of its cycle while the adult cell was in another.

Dr. Campbell decided that rather than try to catch a cell at just the right moment, perhaps he could just slow down cellular activity, nearly stopping it. Then the cell might rest in just the state he wanted so it could join with an egg.

"It dawned on me that this could be a beneficial way of utilizing the cell cycle," he said, in what may turn out to be one of scientific history's great understatements.

What he decided to do was to force the donor cells into a sort of hibernating state, by starving them of some nutrients.

In Wisconsin, Dr. First had actually beaten the Scottish group to cloning a mammal from cells from an early embryo; that occurred when a staff member in the laboratory forgot to provide the nourishing serum, inadvertently starving the cells. The result, in 1994, was four calves. But even Dr. First and his colleagues did not realize the significance of how the animals had been created.

Two years later, Drs. Wilmut and Campbell tried the starvation technique on embryo cells to produce Megan and Morag, the world's first cloned sheep and, until now, the most famous sheep in history. Their creation really laid the foundation for what happened with Dolly, for Dr. Campbell succeeded in doing an end run around the problem of coordinating the cycles of the donor cell with the recipient egg.

Today, Megan and Morag munch contentedly in the same straw-covered pen with the new star of the Roslin Institute, angelic little Dolly. Megan and Morag seem completely normal, if slightly spoiled.

Megan is now expecting, and she got pregnant the old-fashioned way. "It will always be the preferred way of having children," Dr. Campbell said jokingly. "Why would anyone want to clone, anyway? It's far too expensive and a lot less fun than the original method."

When the scientists moved on to cloning a fully grown sheep, they decided to use udder, or mammary, cells, and that is how Dolly got her name. She was named after the country singer Dolly Parton, whose mammary cells, Dr. Wilmut said, are equally famous.

In the experiment that produced Dolly, Dr. Wilmut's team removed cells from the udder of a 6-year-old sheep. The cells were then preserved in test tubes so the investigators would have genetic material to use in DNA fingerprinting— required to prove that Dolly was indeed a clone. In fact, by the time Dolly was born, her progenitor had died.

The trick, Dr. Wilmut said, was the starvation of the adult cells. "You greatly reduce serum concentration for five days," Dr. Wilmut said. "That's the novel approach. That's what we submitted a patent for." And that is why the team was silent about the lamb's birth for months. Until the patent was applied for, nobody wanted the news to spread.

But success is a relative concept. Even Dr. Campbell's technique has failed far more often than it has succeeded. Dolly was the only lamb to survive from 277 eggs that had been fused with adult cells. Nobody knows, or can know, until the work is repeated, whether the researchers were lucky to get one lamb—whether in fact that one lamb was one in a million and not just one in 277 or whether the scientists will become more proficient with more refinement.

The cell fusion that produced Dolly was done in the last week of January 1996. When the resulting embryo reached the six-day stage, it was implanted in a ewe. Dolly's existence as a growing fetus was first discovered on March 20, the 48th day of her surrogate mother's pregnancy. After that, the ewe was scanned with ultrasound, first each month and then, as interest grew, every two weeks.

"Every time you scanned, you were always hoping you were going to get a heartbeat and a live fetus," said John Bracken, the researcher who monitored the pregnancy.

"You could see the head structure, the movement of the legs, the ribs," he said. "And when you actually identified a heart that was beating, there was a great sense of relief and satisfaction. It was as normal a pregnancy as you could have."

On July 5 at 4 p.m., Dolly was born in a shed down the road from the institute. Mr. Bracken, a few members of the farm staff and the local veterinarian attended. It was a normal birth, head and forelegs first. She weighed 6.6 kilograms, about 14½ pounds, and she was healthy.

Because it was summer, the few staff members present were very busy. There was no celebration.

"We phoned up the road to inform Ian Wilmut and Dr. Campbell," Mr. Bracken said.

But Dr. Wilmut does not remember the call. He does not even remember when he heard about Dolly's birth.

"I even asked my wife if she could recall me coming home doing cartwheels down the corridor, and she could not," he said.

## The Publicity: A Quiet Scientist in the Public Eye

As so often happens in science, the existence of the cloned lamb was a loosely kept secret. While Dr. Wilmut himself was close-mouthed because of the patent issue, hints of the astonishing news spread through the corridors of scientific meetings.

"I heard it through the grapevine," said Dr. Mark Westhusin, a cloning researcher at Texas A&M University in College Station. "You go to meetings, people are sitting around in the bar having a few beers," and the secret slips out, he said.

Dr. Robl said that he and Dr. Wilmut were good friends but that Dr. Wilmut was not about to confide in him. "I just talked to him three weeks ago at a meeting," he said. "We had dinner, and I did the best I could to extract his secrets."

But Dr. Robl added, "We have various strategies for getting secrets out." One of the best, he said, is to put the graduate students from different labs together.

To a person, these investigators say adamantly that they believe that Dr. Wilmut's result is real. Dr. Wilmut included scientific proof, like DNA fingerprinting, that Dolly is indeed a clone. In interviews here this week, Dr. Wilmut said he would be perfectly willing to let a legitimate researcher conduct an independent analysis of Dolly's blood or DNA.

Still, Dr. Wilmut said he was surprised by how many people had asked him whether he would open his research to the examination of others. In part, he is surprised because the Roslin scientists have impeccable credentials, and the validity or honesty of their research has never been in doubt.

The tiny center has been contending with the overwhelming and often hostile descent of the news media.

On Friday, as Dr. Wilmut looked deeply uncomfortable in a suit and tie, television crews from around the globe flung themselves at him as if he were an indicted government official. "Do you have any idea of the implications of this research?" a woman from German television shouted at him, becoming the thousandth person to do so. Dr. Wilmut squirmed, shrugged and simply said, "Yes."

One reporter from Greek television demanded permission to jump into the pen with Dolly, Megan and Morag so she could prove to the viewers at home that she was truly on the scene. She did not get it. Other reporters, ignoring completely the fact that this research is new and has been conducted only in sheep, pounded Dr. Wilmut relentlessly about the prospects for cloning human beings.

After all that, Dr. Wilmut now seems to understand that he is struggling with something beyond his control.

"People have sensationalized this in every way," he said, too tired of hearing the worries of everyone from the Vatican to President Clinton to muster any further outrage. He admitted dismay at learning that the leaders of the European Union had called for an investigation and that the British Government was considering cutting the highly respected institute's financing as a result of the work.

"People say that cloning means that if a child dies, you can get that child back," he said, tugging nervously at his neatly trimmed beard. "It's heart-wrenching. You could never get that child back. It would be something different. You need to understand the biology. People are not genes. They are so much more than that."

## The Hurdles: Thorny Problems Are Still Ahead

In the world of animal research, where breakthroughs are common and publicity is not, leading scientists applaud the work. But they are also clearly unhappy about how quickly people are drawing inaccurate conclusions about the utility and viability of cloning. No matter how frightening the prospect, however, cloning in humans is unlikely any time soon.

And it may prove difficult to repeat the experiment that has already been done in sheep. The hurdles are formidable: unless researchers can gain in efficiency and produce more than one lamb from hundreds of eggs, it would never be clinically useful. It is important to note that their work has not been reproduced elsewhere, that it has not yet been duplicated in a species other than sheep—which would be far less useful to science than cloned cattle—and that the experiment did not result in a genetically altered animal. Other than the manner of her conception, Dolly is a normal sheep.

"There is healthy skepticism whether you can accomplish this efficiently in another species," said Leonard Bell, president and chief executive of Alexion Pharmaceuticals, a New Haven–based company developing transgenic pigs to serve as organ donors. "They transferred a normal adult cell," he said. "The question is, Can you transfer a cell that you have genetically engineered? That is a very difference process, and you have to be able to accomplish that for most of the commercial potential here."

Dr. John Logan, executive vice president of Nextran, a Princeton-based unit of Baxter Healthcare also working on transgenic pigs as organ donors, drew a similar line between the impressive science and its practical applicability. He said: "Is this going to be a textbook reference, as in all future general biology textbooks? Absolutely." He added that "to show that you can generate an animal from an adult cell is truly significant," but he noted that the animal had not been genetically modified. "If that had been achieved, it would have been very exciting," he said.

## The Company: Private Enterprise Puts Up the Money

The development of the Roslin Institute clearly shows how, in the late 20th century, the needs and goals of basic science are often driven by and entwined with those of business.

Although the institute started in 1993, it grew from a predecessor created during World War II for a simple, urgent reason: German submarines were preventing ships from reaching Britain and the country was in danger of starving.

The Animal Breeding Research Organization, Roslin's predecessor, was assigned to use the emerging field of genetics to help produce more home-grown food.

"You can feel the pressure these days to cure AIDS and cancer," said Dr. A. John Clark, a molecular biologist at the institute. "It's hard to imagine now, but in the 40s, there was the same pressure to make food. The place was put here to make food."

In a way, they got too good at it. By the late 1960s, British agriculture was as efficient as any in the world. So the Animal Breeding Research Organization suddenly needed to find a new occupation. The researchers there chose to remake the place as a center of molecular biology and biotechnology.

Roslin is a government-financed organization, and its scientists make government salaries. Dr. Wilmut and his colleagues each earn roughly $60,000 a year. No matter how successful their work with Dolly proves to be, none will become rich from it because they do not own the patent.

Technically, the institute is run by a company, PPL Therapeutics P.L.C., which helps to finance it. But the workers at Roslin have almost no personal financial stake in PPL's success. The researchers had worried that their careers would be tainted by working for a for-profit company, so they refused to become executives or even to accept any shares in PPL when it was first formed.

The company is run by Ron James, a biochemist-turned-entrepreneur. Dr. James is an immaculately tailored man in his 50s with piercing blue eyes, white hair, a white beard and an accent and gruffness reminiscent of Sean Connery.

Dr. James was not particularly steeped in the intricacies of genetic engineering when he first showed up in Edinburgh. But he had an eye for business opportunities, and he had already developed a strong sense that there were possibilities of some sort in the area of breeding genetically engineered, or transgenic, animals.

"He is a very, very clever man," remarked Ian Leslie, assistant director of biotechnology projects at Scottish Enterprise, a government development agency that provided Dr. James with some early seed money.

"We came here because of the transgenic chickens," Dr. James said in an interview this week. "But once we got here, we found the sheep."

Three Roslin scientists had just produced the first genetically engineered sheep that secrete a human pharmaceutical protein in its milk, a protein called alpha-1 antitrypsin, or AAT, which could be helpful in relieving the symptoms of cystic fibrosis. And they had applied for a patent on the process they had used.

It was a major milestone, one that scientists at the University of Pennsylvania had been racing to achieve themselves. The technology was still rough, and the sheep could only produce a tiny amount of the drug. But the important point was that it had been done and that the same techniques could theoretically be used to produce many other invaluable human drugs.

Based in an office only a few hundred yards from Roslin's research site, Dr. James has created a curious partnership between academics and many entrepreneurs, one that seems almost quaintly puritanical by comparison with many of the big-money deals struck by some biotechnology researchers in the United States.

The British Ministry of Agriculture, which controlled the Roslin Institute, categorically prohibited either the institute or its scientists from acquiring an equity stake in the new company. "This was where a critical mistake was made," Dr. Clark said in an interview. "It's not so much us that lost out, it's the institute, which owns the patents and now won't be able to get nearly as much."

Ten years ago, however, Dr. Clark and his colleagues were just scrambling desperately to keep their jobs. Cloning research had fallen out of vogue, and few businesses showed any interest in starting such an enterprise.

"You would go to companies and tell them that we could make the drugs they wanted in sheep, and you would get a polite smile," Dr. Clark said. "But the message was clearly: Don't call us—we'll call you."

The only person who showed any serious interest was Dr. James. With seed capital and practical guidance from Scottish Enterprise, a government agency created to promote the formation of new companies, the institute licensed its key patent in 1987 to the new company, PPL Therapeutics. They set up an office right next door to the institute and spent the first several years simply overseeing research aimed at enhancing the initial breakthrough.

What the institute got was the promise of royalties if and when any of the technology generated revenues, a small portion of which would be shared with the individual scientists, as well as the promise that PPL would hire the institute for much of the research to extend the original sheep technology.

Dr. James raised only $400,000 at first, barely enough to get started.

"It was always difficult," Dr. James said. He was under constant pressure to raise more money, knowing that it would still be years before PPL generated meaningful sales of product.

After more than one false start, the company went public last June. Its initial price was 450 pence on the market. At first, it fell steadily. By the end of this week, however, PPL had closed at 512.5 pence.

"If we had only been able to invest properly in our own product, we would all be rich," said Dr. Campbell, again without any apparent regret. "Maybe next time."

## The Road Ahead Hopes and Fears for the Future

Six years ago, animal rights activists burned down two of Roslin's laboratories. It was the first time the public became aware that Dr. Wilmut and his colleagues were trying to do something momentous.

Even before that, cloning had already become a shorthand way to talk about all that many fear in science. It hardly matters that many of the tomatoes and apples sold in grocery stores are the products of genetic engineering or that advances in reproductive technology have brought new hope to millions of potential parents. To most people, the idea of cloning is frightening; it is evidence of technology speeding out of control, an Orwellian universe where the essence of humanity has been lost and the fact of it has been cheapened.

And the race to follow Dr. Wilmut's lead has now begun in earnest. In Wisconsin on Saturday, Dr. First—one of the United States' leading experts in the field—decided to try cloning a cow by the method Dr. Wilmut used.

When he called his technician to ask her to start starving some skin cells from a fetal calf to prepare them for cloning, the technician had already begun. She, too, had heard the news.

Dr. First said he doubted that his lab was alone. He suspects that all over the world, he said, people who know how to clone will "do like we did—grab whatever cells they have" growing in the laboratory and try to repeat Dr. Wilmut's work.

*March 3, 1997*

# Scientists Cultivate Cells at Root of Human Life

## By NICHOLAS WADE

Pushing the frontiers of biology closer to the central mystery of life, scientists have for the first time picked out and cultivated the primordial human cells from which an entire individual is created.

The cells, derived from fertilized human eggs just before they would have been implanted in the uterus, have the power to develop into many of the 210 types of cell in the body—and probably all of them. Because they can divide indefinitely when grown outside the body without signs of age that afflict other cells, biologists refer to them as immortal.

Eventually, researchers hope to use the cells to grow tissue for human transplants and introduce genes into the body to remedy inherited disease.

But there is a thicket of ethical and legal issues, as well as technical problems, to be tackled. The cells are obtained from embryos created at in vitro fertilization clinics and so far do not seem definably different from the handful of primordial cells from which an entire individual is created.

The scientists involved in the work, some of which was reported today in the journal *Science*, consider use of the cells justified because they come from embryos that would otherwise have been discarded. But others believe the cells have a special status in that they retain the potential to develop into an individual, and that the use of the cells may draw criticism if this status is not taken into account.

The new cells, known as human embryonic stem cells, have eluded capture until now because they exist in this state only fleetingly before turning into more specialized cells, and need special ingredients to be kept alive outside the body.

The cells have many possible uses, of which the most promising is to grow new tissue, of any kind, for transplant into a patient's body. The cells may also offer effective routes to human cloning, although both the researchers and their sponsor deny any interest in this application. Another likely use is in gene therapy, the insertion of new or modified genes into body tissue.

Two forms of human embryonic cells have been developed, one by a team under Dr. James A. Thomson of the University of Wisconsin in Madison, the other by Dr. John Gearhart and colleagues at the Johns Hopkins University School of Medicine in Baltimore, Md. Dr. Thomson's work is reported in *Science*. Dr. Gearhart's work will be described later this month in the *Proceedings of the National Academy of Sciences*.

Congress in 1995 banned Federal financing of research on fetal cells, including those derived from embryos, and the university researchers whose work was announced today were financed by the Geron Corporation of Menlo Park, Calif., a biotechnology company that specializes in anti-aging research.

The research "has potential health benefits which I think are extremely promising, and I am sorry that the law prevented us from supporting it," said Dr. Harold Varmus, director of the National Institutes of Health.

## Cells Are Specialized as They Develop

After an egg is fertilized, it divides several times and forms a blastocyst, a hollow sphere with a blob of 15 to 20 cells, known as the inner cell mass, piled up against one wall. It is from these cells that the embryo develops. Dr. Thomson grew his embryonic stem cells from the inner cell mass of blastocysts that had been left over from fertility treatments and were to be discarded. The donors of the blastocysts granted permission for them to be used in research.

As an embryo grows and develops, its cells become irreversibly committed to their fates as specialized components of the body's organs. A pocket of cells, known as embryonic germ cells, is protected from the commitment process so as to create the next generation of eggs and sperm. Dr. Gearhart's group has developed embryonic stem cells from the germ cells of aborted fetuses. The cells developed by the two groups may well be equivalent but this has yet to be proved.

If researchers are able to use the cells to grow new tissues, the work could alleviate the shortage of livers and other organs for transplant. Cultures of the cells in the laboratory could be nudged down different developmental pathways to become heart or bone marrow or pancreatic cells. Before reaching their final stages, the about-to-become heart cells, for example, could be injected into a patient's ailing heart. Guided then by the body's own internal regulatory signals, the cells would develop into new, young heart tissue, supplementing or replacing the heart cells already there.

The same approach should in principle work with any tissue of the body. Human embryonic stem cells would thus serve as a universal spare parts system. Because the cells grow and divide indefinitely in the laboratory, very few blastocysts would be needed.

Many technical problems remain to be resolved. The art of directing embryonic stem cells down specific pathways is in its infancy. But heart muscle cells have been grown from mouse embryonic stem cells and successfully integrated with the heart tissue of a living mouse. Dr. Thomson in 1995 isolated the embryonic stem cells of a monkey, and Geron intends to do pilot experiments in these cells.

Another problem lies in making grafted cells compatible with the patient's immune system. Dr. Thomas B. Okarma, Geron's vice president for research, said his company would explore several ways of doing this. One, the least preferred, would be to set up a bank with enough different human embryonic cells that most patients could be matched. Another would be to suppress the self-recognition genes that make the stem cells appear foreign to the patient's immune system or, more elegantly, to replace them with copies of the patient's own self-recognition genes.

A third approach would be to convert one of the patient's own body cells back to embryonic form by fusing it with a human embryonic stem cell whose own nucleus had been removed. Embryonic cells may have the power, not yet understood, to rescue an adult cell's nucleus from its specialized state by flicking all the switches on its DNA back to default mode. This reprogramming of DNA is presumably what happened when mice were cloned in July from adult cells.

## Concerns About Ethics Prevent Some Tests

The ethical status of the cells is also likely to be a matter of discussion. They cannot become a fetus, as their blastocyst no longer exists, yet they are very similar, if not identical, to the 20 or so primordial cells from which the embryo develops.

Both research groups refer to their cells as "pluripotent" because, when injected into a mouse with no immune system, the cells develop into many of the major tissues of the body. The tissues are disorganized and do not develop into a normal embryo.

The cells may also be "totipotent," meaning they can form every one of the body's cell types. The test for totipotency, developed with mouse embryonic stem cells, is to inject stem cells into another blastocyst. A normal mouse will usually develop, but it is composed of a patchwork of cells, some from the blastocyst and some from the injected embryonic stem cells, proving the stem cells retain all their powers.

It would be unethical to perform such an experiment on people, but if it could be done, it seems likely that the human embryonic cells cultured by the researchers would also be able to form each of the body's cell types. If so, they may be capable in principle of contributing to the generation of a new individual.

But ethicists say great care must be taken in work involving human embryonic cells. "Any time you take a cell off a blastocyst, that cell could be used itself to create a

145

human being, so some groups in our society believe in making it transplantable you have derailed it into becoming a kidney or some other tissue," said Dr. Lori Andrews, an expert on the laws governing reproductive technology at the Chicago-Kent College of Law.

"Some researchers say, 'It's just a bunch of cells, why should people care?' But that totally avoids the fact that some people do care, and I'm concerned that if the researchers don't take into consideration the variety of viewpoints about embryos, they might ultimately end up with more restrictive regulations," Dr. Andrews said.

Geron, which has exclusive licenses to use the cells, under patents held by the researchers' universities, says it regards them as qualitatively different from other cells used in research. "Because these cells are derived from human blastocysts there is a moral authority here, so we take these cells seriously," said Dr. Okarma, of Geron.

Dr. Okarma said he believed that use of the cells was justified because they were something less than a living embryo, and life-saving treatments might be derived from them. "We are not saying the ends justify the means, but that given that the moral authority of these cells is subordinate to that of the embryo, the work we contemplate with them is appropriate," he said.

But Dr. Gearhart said he did not consider the cells that he and Dr. Thomson have isolated to have a special moral status because "they cannot form a fetus—you cannot take one of these cells and form a being out of it."

Still, Dr. Gearhart said he would not argue with the view of Dr. Okarma that the cells had a different standing from ordinary cells. Dr. Johnson, too, said that they were "special cells."

Dr. Kevin T. Fitzgerald, a geneticist and Jesuit priest at Loyola University Medical School, said that if the human embryonic stem cells were able to make each of the body's cell types, "then you are disrupting the viability of life and we are back to the question of how to justify destroying life for the purposes of scientific advancement."

The new cells may well reawaken fears of human cloning, although many ethicists have now come around to believing that the public's fears, despite science fiction writers' portrayal of clonal armies of frenzied despots, are largely beside the point. Many experts now predict human cloning is more likely to end up as a rare treatment offered in fertility clinics, no different from others like in vitro fertilization and egg donation in that they were first bitterly denounced and are now regarded as routine.

"Human cloning will likely also be accepted once it becomes a reality. Most of today's ethical arguments against it were previously used against in-vitro fertilization and turned out to be false," writes Dorothy C. Wertz, a bioethicist at the Shriver Center, in the current issue of *Gene Letter.*

The availability of human embryonic stem cells suggests a quite different possibility to biologists, who are well aware of how mouse embryonic stem cells have long been used to generate genetically altered mice. The belief that humans can now be modified like the mouse "will be the knee-jerk reaction of the academic community," Dr. Thomson said.

He said human embryonic stem cells were unlikely to be used in this way because there were more promising approaches for gene therapy in people. For one thing, the mouse method requires the creation of many embryos in order to obtain the few in which new genes integrate in exactly the correct position, as well as the breeding of a male and female mouse that have been genetically altered. In its present form, the technique is evidently inapplicable to humans.

## Federal Law Shifts Research to Industry

The National Institutes of Health and the university scientists it finances often play a leading role in reviewing new biomedical technologies.

But because of the Federal financing ban, university scientists cannot get Government support to study human embryonic stem cells. But industry can do whatever research it pleases, without necessarily obtaining government approval. Academic biologists believe that this asymmetry is unfortunate and that the new technique would receive better and more detached review if the agency and its scientists could take part in the discussion.

Dr. Varmus said that an expert panel on human embryo research had recommended to the health institutes that attempts to derive stem cells from human embryos should be permitted, but Federal efforts along this line were thwarted in 1995, with the Congressional financing ban. Dr. Varmus said he believed the public "will see how important the benefits of this research might be."

A Senate bill to ban human cloning was defeated in February this year, the principal argument of its opponents being that its overly broad language would prohibit promising research on human embryonic stem cells.

In any event, any ultimate use of human embryonic stem cells may face legal hurdles in the nine states that have outright bans on research on human fetal tissues, Dr. Andrews said.

Some laws also prohibit payment for embryos, a restriction that might extend to cells and tissues derived from embryos.

## A Possibility of Eternal Cells

The technique reported today reaches to the central mysteries of life and death. As biologists have recently begun to understand, the body's cells are not inherently mortal. They become mortal only when committed to developing into one or another of the body's mature cell types. These specialized cells have mostly lost the ability to grow and divide, but a few, typically those of the skin and intestinal lining, can divide in culture about 50 times and then die.

In January this year, biologists at Geron learned how to manipulate the section of DNA that marks off the 50 or so permissible divisions. By reversing the changes in this section of DNA, called the telomere, they created lines of cells that divided well beyond the usual limit and are still going strong, while retaining their youthful vigor and appearance. Biologists refer to these cultured cells as immortal because they are expected to grow and divide indefinitely.

Embryonic stem cells are also immortal because, until they become committed to specialized fates, their telomeres are renewed each time they divide. Unlike ordinary cells, they grow indefinitely in culture.

In the lineage of living organisms, they cycle indefinitely from the embryo to the germ line to a new embryo, forever avoiding specialization into the mortal cell types that comprise the body.

Geron biologists believe they can manipulate the telomeres of the human embryonic stem cells so that the cells stay immortal even as they turn into specialized tissues. Can the mortal body therefore be repaired with new tissues that remain youthful indefinitely? "Exactly," Dr. Okarma said.

Critics have said it would be folly to tamper with the telomere division-counting system because it probably arose in evolution as the body's last-ditch defense against any runaway cell likely to become a cancer. Dr. Okarma said that new experiments had largely laid this concern to rest by showing that telomerised cells are no more likely to become malignant than are normal cells.

These grand schemes may or may not come to pass, but the techniques now at hand for manipulating human embryonic stem cells will at least allow them to be seriously attempted.

*November 6, 1998*

# Scientists Bypass Need for Embryo
# to Get Stem Cells

By GINA KOLATA

Two teams of scientists reported yesterday that they had turned human skin cells into what appear to be embryonic stem cells without having to make or destroy an embryo—a feat that could quell the ethical debate troubling the field.

All they had to do, the scientists said, was add four genes. The genes reprogrammed the chromosomes of the skin cells, making the cells into blank slates that should be able to turn into any of the 220 cell types of the human body, be it heart, brain, blood or bone. Until now, the only way to get such human universal cells was to pluck them from a human embryo several days after fertilization, destroying the embryo in the process.

The need to destroy embryos has made stem cell research one of the most divisive issues in American politics, pitting President Bush against prominent Republicans like Nancy Reagan, and patient advocates who hoped that stem cells could cure diseases like Alzheimer's. The new studies could defuse the issue as a presidential election nears.

The reprogrammed skin cells may yet prove to have subtle differences from embryonic stem cells that come directly from human embryos, and the new method includes potentially risky steps, like introducing a cancer gene. But stem cell researchers say they are confident that it will not take long to perfect the method and that today's drawbacks will prove to be temporary.

Researchers and ethicists not involved in the findings say the work, conducted by independent teams from Japan and Wisconsin, should reshape the stem cell field. At some time in the near future, they said, today's debate over whether it is morally acceptable to create and destroy human embryos to obtain stem cells should be moot.

"Everyone was waiting for this day to come," said the Rev. Tadeusz Pacholczyk, director of education at the National Catholic Bioethics Center. "You should have a solution here that will address the moral objections that have been percolating for years," he added.

The White House said that Mr. Bush was "very pleased" about the new findings, adding that "By avoiding techniques that destroy life, while vigorously supporting alternative approaches, President Bush is encouraging scientific advancement within ethical boundaries."

The new method sidesteps other ethical quandaries, creating stem cells that genetically match the donor without having to resort to cloning or the requisite donation of women's eggs. Genetically matched cells would not be rejected by the immune system if used as replacement tissues for patients. Even more important, scientists say, is that genetically matched cells from patients would enable them to study complex diseases, like Alzheimer's, in the laboratory.

Until now, the only way most scientists thought such patient-specific stem cells could be made would be to create embryos that were clones of that person and extract their stem cells. Just last week, scientists in Oregon reported that they did this with monkeys, but the prospect of doing such experiments in humans has been ethically fraught.

But with the new method, human cloning for stem cell research, like the creation of human embryos to extract stem cells, may be unnecessary. The new cells in theory might be turned into an embryo, but not by simply implanting them in a womb.

"It really is amazing," said Dr. Leonard Zon, director of the stem cell program at Children's Hospital Boston at Harvard Medical School.

And, said Dr. Douglas A. Melton, co-director of the Stem Cell Institute at Harvard University, it is "ethically uncomplicated."

For all the hopes invested in it over the last decade, embryonic stem cell research has moved slowly, with no cures or major therapeutic discoveries in sight.

The new work could allow the field to vault significant problems, including the shortage of human embryonic stem cells and restrictions on federal financing for such research. Even when scientists have other sources of financing, they report that it is expensive and difficult to find women who will provide eggs for such research.

The new discovery is being published online today in *Cell*, in a paper by Shinya Yamanaka of Kyoto University and the Gladstone Institute of Cardiovascular Disease in San Francisco, and in *Science*, in a paper by James A. Thomson and his colleagues at the University of Wisconsin. Dr. Thomson's work received some federal money.

While both groups used just four genes to reprogram human skin cells, two of the genes used differed from group to group. All the genes in question, though, act in a similar way—they are master regulator genes whose role is to turn other genes on or off.

The reprogrammed cells, the scientists report, appear to behave very much like human embryonic stem cells but were called "induced pluripotent stem cells," meaning cells that can change into many different types.

"By any means we test them they are the same as embryonic stem cells," Dr. Thomson says.

He and Dr. Yamanaka caution, though, that they still must confirm that the reprogrammed human skin cells really are the same as stem cells they get from embryos. And while those studies are under way, Dr. Thomson and others say, it would be premature to abandon research with stem cells taken from human embryos.

Another caveat is that, so far, scientists use a type of virus, a retrovirus, to insert the genes into the cells' chromosomes. Retroviruses slip genes into chromosomes at random, sometimes causing mutations that can make normal cells turn into cancers.

One gene used by the Japanese scientists actually is a cancer gene.

The cancer risk means that the resulting stem cells would not be suitable for replacement cells or tissues for patients with diseases, like diabetes, in which their own cells die. But they would be ideal for the sort of studies that many researchers say are the real promise of this endeavor—studying the causes and treatments of complex diseases.

For example, researchers could make stem cells from a person with a disease like Alzheimer's and turn the stem cells into nerve cells in a petri dish. Then they might learn what goes awry in the brain and how to prevent or treat the disease.

But even the retrovirus drawback may be temporary, scientists say. Dr. Yamanaka and several other researchers are trying to get the same effect by adding chemicals or using more benign viruses to get the genes into cells. They say they are starting to see success.

"Anyone who is going to suggest that this is just a sideshow and that it won't work is wrong," Dr. Melton predicted.

The new discovery was preceded by work in mice. Last year, Dr. Yamanaka published a paper showing that he could add four genes to mouse cells and turn them into mouse embryonic stem cells.

He even completed the ultimate test to show that the resulting stem cells could become any type of mouse cell. He used them to create new mice. Twenty percent of those mice, though, developed cancer, illustrating the risk of using retroviruses and a cancer gene to make cells for replacement parts.

Scientists were electrified by the reprogramming discovery, Dr. Melton said. "Once it worked, I hit my forehead and said, 'It's so obvious,'" he said. "But it's not obvious until it's done."

The work set off an international race to repeat the work with human cells.

"Dozens, if not hundreds of labs, have been attempting to do this," said Dr. George Daley, associate director of the stem cell program at Children's Hospital.

Ever since the birth of Dolly the sheep in 1996, scientists knew that adult cells could, in theory, turn into embryonic stem cells. But they had no idea how to do it without cloning, the way Dolly was created.

With cloning, researchers put an adult cell's chromosomes into an unfertilized egg whose genetic material was removed. The egg, by some mysterious process, then does all the work. It reprograms the adult cell's chromosomes, bringing them back to the state they were in just after the egg was fertilized. A few days later, a ball of stem cells emerges in the embryo, and every cell of the embryo, including its stem cells, is an exact genetic match of the adult.

The abiding questions, though, were: How did the egg reprogram the adult cell's chromosomes? Would it be possible to reprogram an adult cell without using an egg?

About four years ago, Dr. Yamanaka and Dr. Thomson independently hit upon the same idea. They would search for genes that are being used in an embryonic stem cell that are not being used in an adult cell. Then they would see if those genes would reprogram an adult cell.

Dr. Yamanaka worked with mouse cells, and Dr. Thomson worked with human cells from foreskins.

The researchers found more than 1,000 candidate genes. So both groups took educated guesses, trying to whittle down the genes to the few dozen they thought might be the crucial ones and then asking whether any combinations of those genes could turn a skin cell into a stem cell.

"The number of factors could have been 1 or 10 or 100 or more," Dr. Yamanaka said in a telephone interview from his laboratory in Japan.

If many genes had been required, the experiments would have failed, Dr. Thomson said, because it would have been impossible to test all the gene combinations.

As soon as Dr. Yamanaka saw that the mouse experiments succeeded, he began trying the same brute force method in human skin cells that he had ordered from a commercial laboratory. Some were face cells from a 36-year-old white woman and others were connective tissue cells from joints of a 69-year-old white man.

Dr. Yamanaka said he thought it would take a few years to find the right genes and the right conditions to make the human experiments work. Feeling the hot breath of competitors on his neck, he was in his laboratory every day for 12 to 14 hours a day, he said.

A few months later, he succeeded.

"We did work very hard," Dr. Yamanaka said. "But we were very surprised."

*November 21, 2007*

## CHAPTER 7

# Diabetes

# Diabetes Cure Confirmed by Treatment of 176 Cases

A great deal has been written and published in both the medical and lay press in recent years relative to the merits of the *Bacillus bulgaricus* as a therapeutic agent. Milk seems to be the normal habitat of this micro-organism. Remarkable instances of longevity among those European and Asiatic nations which, to use Kipling's expression, are the "most easterly of Western peoples and the most westerly of Eastern peoples," have been ascribed to the habitual and long-continued consumption of preparations of sour milk, under various names, which contain this non-pathogenic germ.

Some scientists "swear by" the *B. bulgaricus*. Prof. Elie Metchnikoff, the distinguished laboratory worker and medical investigator, is one of them. This harmless bacterium, if it had had its rights in times past and the science of bacteriology had been sufficiently developed, undoubtedly would have been incorporated in Brown-Séquard's "Elixir of Life"; if it had found a resting place in Ponce de León's spring and flourished there, that undiscoverable but highly desirable fountain of youth would be as well marked today, geographically speaking, as the Egyptian Sphinx and as consistently visited as Mecca itself.

## A Good Therapeutic Agent

The *Bacillus bulgaricus* is now a highly valued therapeutic agent, and after close observation and its employment as a remedial agent for more than a year it has been demonstrated that not only can severe cases of diabetes mellitus be checked and held in control by it, but that it will cure moderate cases. It is also believed by Dr. J. Wallace Beveridge of this city, who has contributed a comprehensive article on the treatment of this disease with cultures of the bacillus to the last two issues of the *New York Medical Journal*, that this common and dreaded ailment, which formerly was usually considered a fatal malady by the medical profession, can be prevented by the early use of the cultures in cases of intestinal putrefaction when this condition is recognized.

The first announcement in the lay press of the value of cultures of this bacillus in diabetes appeared in *The Times* last year and was based on information derived from Dr. Beveridge's observations. His present report is the result of treating 176 patients, who were suffering from well-defined diabetes, with cultures of this bacillus. In addition to giving exact statistical reports of several of his cases, Dr. Beveridge furnishes a number of facts concerning the cause of diabetes that are original, and also introduces for the first time in connection with the diagnosis of the ailment X-ray pictures indicating the intestinal conditions that are factors in the etiology of the disease.

The facts relating to faulty digestion and mechanical intestinal derangement as causative of diabetes, considered in conjunction with another set of facts brought out by another New York physician, Dr. I. L. Nascher, in an article on "Longevity and Rejuvenescence" printed in the New York Medical Journal on the same date that the first section of Dr. Beveridge's article appeared, constitute a startling arraignment of one of the apparently necessary contingents of modern civilization—cold-storage foods. Dr. Nascher says that cold-storage foods rapidly decompose in the stomach and intestines. Dr. Beveridge asserts that this rapid decomposition is largely responsible for diabetes. When asked about Dr. Nascher's declaration, Dr. Beveridge indorsed his views, and immediately declared that the present-day prevalence of diabetes— possibly one person in every fifteen more than 40 years old is attacked by it—was due undoubtedly to the enforced consumption of cold-storage foods in the larger centres of population. Neither physician, however, offers a solution of the cold-storage problem.

Dr. Nascher quotes from the report of the Field Secretary of the Provident Life Assurance Society of England to the effect that the death rate from diseases of the heart, kidneys, and circulatory system, including apoplexy, has increased 105 per cent, in the United States since 1880, while in England the increase in deaths from these diseases during this period was only 3 per cent. He attributes the increase in this country largely to the "strenuous life."

## Results Not Final

The distinguishing characteristic of diabetes mellitus is the presence of sugar in the secretion of the kidneys. This condition is known as glycosuria. The value of any therapeutic agent used in the treatment of diabetes is measured by its power to lower the sugar index. It is just a year ago since Dr. Beveridge said:

"In fact, in eleven cases so far treated that have been under constant care a sufficient length of time, and where the sugar index is now absent, the cure has been complete, and if the patients every now and then submit to an examination and, if necessary, resume medication for a short period, I believe that they will remain in the normal state regained through this new treatment."

"In presenting a new therapeutic measure for the treatment of diabetes," says Dr. Beveridge in the present report, "great caution should be maintained toward an optimistic viewpoint until a sufficient number of positive recoveries are noted, which would warrant an assertion that such a procedure as that herein recorded is of true value. The results in the 176 cases cited, and observations made by Dr. George P. Klemann and myself in this preliminary report, should in no way be considered as final."

The author gives a brief outline of the main etiological factors of the disease in order to sustain his argument, which theoretically indicates the employment of *B. bulgaricus* as the rational treatment. From this it appears that "the pancreas is the gland where secretion is known to have the most power in breaking down the carbohydrate group."

Carbohydrates are the sugars and starches, and are substances containing carbon, hydrogen, and oxygen, the two latter in the proportion to form water. When the carbohydrates are broken down by the internal secretions they split up into a variety of substances whose names are immaterial for the purposes of this article. As Dr. Beveridge explains, the most important carbohydrate as a food is starch, but, as such, is valueless, though easily broken down by the digestive ferments. The saliva and pancreatic juice contain a ferment which changes starch into maltose.

"During digestion," says the author, "the activity of the pancreatic secretion depends mostly upon the acidity in the duodenum and small intestine, this acidity causing a peripheral, local stimulating reflex action on the ganglionic cells scattered throughout the pancreas, while the reflexes of central origin remain inert.

## Results of Research

"Popielski, Wertheimer, and Le Page demonstrated that when an acid was introduced into the duodenum, pancreatic secretion was excited, and they were able to prove that pancreatic secretion could be induced by the injection of acid into the small intestine, the effect diminishing as the acid neared the lower end of the intestine. The name of the product formed inducing pancreatic activity is known as 'secretin.' Bayliss and Starling confirmed the results given above and justify the statement that 'when the acid gastric juice of digestion reaches the duodenum the prosecretin manufactured by the epithelial cells is converted into secretin, which is immediately absorbed into the blood stream, then carried to the cells of the pancreas, which at once are stimulated to secretory activity.'

"The process showing the power exerted through the stimulation of acid digestion in producing secretin, so necessary to the normal functionating of the pancreas, has never until now been brought forward as a factor in glycosuria. Hence, one can readily perceive that when chronic conditions arise to change the acidity of the gastric contents, a corresponding response will be noted in the production of secretin.

"According as a hyperacidity (increased acidity) or hypoacidity (lowered acidity) of the gastric chyle is apparent while passing through the duodenum and upper portion of the small intestine, the amount of secretin manufactured is either increased or diminished, and, reflexly, the pancreatic secretions will also be increased or diminished. Should this abnormal chemical reaction continue, whereby the pancreas receives inadequate stimulation during digestion, serious chemical and metabolic changes will in time manifest themselves, which may eventually combine and prevent complete carbohydrate metabolism.

"The other causes interfering with a normal production of secretin are intestinal putrefaction, ulcer of the duodenum or pylorus, and any lesion involving the mucosa of the duodenum and upper portion of the small intestine.

"The liver, next to the pancreas, furnishes the most important etiological factor, but in this paper a complete exposition of its action in digestion is impossible. Only a very brief indication of a few cardinal points will be undertaken. The power of the liver cell to change ammonia into urea is vital. When any abnormal cellular change manifests itself the urea content is lessened and the ammonia output increased.

"This fact is observed in all severe eases of diabetes, in anaemias, in some types of intestinal nephritis, in toxaemias, in hypertrophic and atrophic cirrhosis of the liver, in chronic inflammations of the gall duct, and in malignancy. A continued low urea output is an unfavorable sign in diabetes. Generally, we find that when the liver is unable to normally change ammonia into urea the secretion of the bile is affected, the production is lessened, and the bactericidal action diminished.

"The intestinal tract also plays a most important part in carbohydrate metabolism. In more than 90 per cent of the cases under observation there was intestinal putrefaction, usually traced to chronic constipation, intestinal stasis, or lack of proper bodily care. The normal action of digestion is dependent upon the daily intestinal elimination and non-absorption of the waste products; otherwise interference with oxidation, as a result of auto-intoxication, will co-ordinately affect the entire internal secreting glandular system, and, should such a chronic state ensue, cellular changes in the thyroid, pituitary, and pancreas ofttimes begin. Of course, constipation is the main cause of all intestinal disturbances, and to-day we can be reasonably certain whether a chemical or mechanical derangement is paramount.

"The chemical faults may be ascribed primarily to improper food, such as food of poor quality, food badly prepared, or unbalanced food consisting either of carbohydrates or proteids in excess; interference with the chemical activating agents of peristalsis, i.e. bile &c., and the noxious chemical products of intestinal putrefaction, come under this heading.

"The mechanical faults are demonstrated by the radiograph, briefly indicated from observations made by Dr. A. J. Quimby, Professor of Radiography at the New York Polyclinic Medical School, on some 350 patients and upon cases submitted by me, in which the patient's stomach and intestines have been radiographed following a test meal of bismuth. In this series the mechanical defects portrayed were frequently marked, and the data obtained through this accurate determination of the stomach and intestines have proved most valuable, especially in the prognosis and treatment."

Dr. Beveridge then describes the different mechanical faults that interfere with normal digestive processes, as revealed by the X-ray plates, and continues:

"The preceding facts readily demonstrate why glycosuria often follows a grave cellular change in the pancreas, liver, or small intestine; so that we now know that a chemical fault or a mechanical one, or both combined, is always necessary for a diabetic state to manifest itself."

This interesting information concerning the discovery of the *Bacillus bulgaricus* is recorded:

## Who Deserves Credit?

"Much controversy has arisen, since the international employment of the *Bacillus bulgaricus* culture for intestinal putrefaction, as to whom the credit should belong for first isolating this organism. It seems that Prof. Kern, in 1881, first published an article describing the micro-organisms found in Russian kefir. At this early period the bacteriological technique was perhaps untrustworthy for accurate information, and judgment should therefore be withheld on the question whether the true *Bacillus bulgaricus* of to-day was isolated at that time. Beijerinck unquestionably was the first to positively demonstrate the isolation of the *Bacillus caucasicus*, which belongs to the *bulgaricus* group.

"Two distinct classes of this organism have been demonstrated, and the first investigators to prove this fact were Rist and Khoury. A true bacillus isolated from the Bulgarian yoghurt by Grigoroff, a member of Prof. Massol's laboratory staff, and first described by him as the *Bacillus bulgaricus,* is the organism now used as a therapeutic agent.

"A further point of interest is the report by Heinemann and Hefferan that they were able to isolate this bacillus from many sources, asserting they found a bacillus identical to that of the *bulgaricus* in a great variety of sour and aromatic foods, in the human saliva, in the normal gastric juice, and in the gastric juice when hydrochloric acid is absent in the fermented milk and ordinary sweet milk. Cohendy devised the present media for active growth."

The writer goes on to describe the morphological characteristics of the bacillus, the methods of cultivation, and the microscopic appearance of the cultures of both classes. Experimentation has shown that these cultures act on the carbohydrates in a manner similar to the ferments of normal digestive activity.

"The *Bacillus bulgaricus,*" Dr. Beveridge continues, "is non-pathogenic to man or the usual laboratory animals. No untoward effects have been observed following the ingestion of large amounts of this culture.

"The cultures of the *Bacillus bulgaricus* employed by me are grown upon a modified Cohendy medium, which from time to time I have had examined in reference to the purity and viability of the organism by the Gram positive method, the average count being 285,000,000+ positive per cubic centimeter, with an acid activity of from 1 to 3.6 per cent, in twenty-four hours upon sweet milk.

"In the preceding description of the *Bacillus bulgaricus* its action upon sugar, with the formation of lactic acid, is indicated. In diabetes the carbohydrate radicle is attacked in the intestinal tract by this bacillus and converted into lactic acid. The necessity for starch as a food is well known, and if digestion is unable to break down the molecules of starch, in glycosurias it is harmful. But by this action of the *Bacillus bulgaricus* this much needed carbohydrate may be taken with little, if any, excess of sugar appearing.

## An Important Reaction

"This chemical reaction is of great importance when the normal combustion of sugar in the alimentary tract is at fault, and if we are able to continue the use of an active culture aid is given the pancreas, and liver to complete the carbohydrate digestion. When the pancreas receives weak stimulation by the lack of a normal quantity of secretin forming, as a result of a low gastric acidity, the potency of this bacillus to make lactic acid is of value in further stimulating the duodenum and upper portion of the small intestine.

"The antiseptic and corrective power of the bacillus, by overcoming auto-intoxication and all conditions of intestinal putrefaction, is very marked. Its distinct action in attacking the hosts of intestinal flora and the chemical action of the lactic acid upon the waste products such as indol, skatol, zanthin, and hyper-zanthin, may possess, according to Prof. Belonowsky, a still greater cleansing influence by an active product created during the proliferation of the bacillus. He positively asserts that this substance continues exercising a protective influence against reabsorption. The action of this culture is never manifested unless the micro-organisms are viable when administered."

Dr. Beveridge goes on to give the histories of a dozen patients treated, together with detailed tables of the laboratory findings in each case. Some of these patients were discharged as cured, while others improved.

Continuing, the author says:

"The patients under observation might be divided into two great classes: the glycosurias without acidosis, and the glycosurias with acidosis. (Acidosis is a condition in which an excess of acid products is excreted.)

"Glycosuria without Acidosis (First Class). During the early period or onset there may be a total absence of any classical sign which would direct either the patient's or the physician's attention to a beginning of glycosuria, unless, perhaps, discovered by an insurance examination. These cases may go for a considerable length of time without noticing any untoward symptoms, possibly complain a little of constipation, heartburn, or indigestion after eating. Then, as the disease progresses, a severe shock, such as worry, exposure, overindulgence or a rheumatic attack, will cause the first unpleasant symptoms to appear, which are generally described as weakness in the legs, cramps in the calves and knees, loss of weight, polyuria of varying intensity, constipation, indigestion, headache, impaired vision and hearing, dryness of the skin, with brittleness of the finger nails and falling out of the hair. These symptoms may gradually increase in severity, while in others the tolerance for considerable quantities of sugar is acquired with the subsequent abatement in many of the unpleasant physiological reactions. The patients who do poorly are the ones which lose weight rapidly, and the sugar index conditions above 5 per cent. Such cases should he placed under strict observation, and a special effort made to prevent the loss of weight and the continued excessive production of sugar; otherwise, at any moment, a severe acidosis with coma may involve the patient.

## The Second Class

"Glycosuria with Acidosis (Second Class) should be classified, for convenience, into three stages, those with acetone, those with a trace of acetone and diacetic acid, and those with marked acetone and diacetic acid, a condition always accompanied by the production of beta oxybutyric acid. The symptoms in this class are similar to glycosuria with acidosis, but the increasing weakness and malaise are more pronounced. One symptom always present is drowsiness, while vertigo and headache, if accompanied by other indications of digestive disturbance, such as vomiting, obstinate constipation and severe heartburn, or by acute gastritis, are always forerunners of grave sequalae which often end in coma. If seen before the disease has advanced to a degree in which the involvement and systemic changes have become so great that nothing can be done, patients will, as a rule, readily improve under treatment. The cases observed range from 9 to 74 years in age, and include glycosurias from those with very small amounts of sugar up to the most severe types of acidosis with dropsical effusion.

"The treatment of diabetes requires more time and consideration on the part of the physician than most diseases that come under his care. The difficulty of keeping the patient upon a strict diet and making him understand the necessity for following any good therapeutic procedure is almost insurmountable, because the moment diabetic patients begin to feel an improvement or notice the symptoms disappearing, the desire to eat forbidden food and do things that are inadvisable seems to overcome their better judgment, and they submit to these inordinate desires.

"The cases under observation are divided, as already indicated, into two classes. The first class presents the widest field for scientific work, especially by preventing this disease from a progressive development. Chronic constipation with intestinal putrefaction is the major difficulty encountered requiring correction, and a systematic examination should be undertaken to determine whether the intestinal tract, through a mechanical fault or a chemical derangement during digestion, is responsible for the condition.

"Knowing the fault causing intestinal putrefaction, our efforts are then directed toward giving relief. Should this condition be due to gastric or liver inactivity, the usual, accepted drugs are given, with from four to six tubes (equal to twelve or eighteen centimeters) of the *bulgaricus* culture each day. The action by this culture, as shown, begins at once to stop intestinal putrefaction. The culture is continued until an indican-tree secretion has persisted for five weeks, then the culture is gradually diminished until one tube (three cubic centimeters) every other day suffices. Not until every trace of sugar has been absent for a period of three months do we entirely discontinue using the culture.

"The mechanical defects, unless very serious, may be greatly aided by abdominal exercises, daily massage, and the galvanic treatment.

"It is necessary to ascertain in the very beginning what the carbohydrate tolerance of each patient may be, and then, by a gradual increase of starch in the daily diet we find exactly what the capacity for the daily production of sugar during the twenty-four-hour elimination is. If the carbohydrate tolerance is fairly high, and the percentage of sugar indicated in the urine analysis moderate, a liberal diet is permitted."

The author outlines the diabetic diet, but space does not permit its repetition here.

"Those patients," he continues, "whose pancreas, liver, or small intestine is not seriously damaged by a chronic lesion will recover. Every case, in this series, of glycosuria without acidosis has responded to the treatment described, and all the symptoms of discomfort have permanently subsided."

If the patient has a secondary anaemia, sodium cacodylate is given every third day by subcutaneous injection.

"When acetone bodies form as a complication to glycosuria," the report continues, "the beginning of a more serious condition is indicated, and our efforts should be directed toward overcoming this evil chemical derangement. If the patient is under control and follows suggestions made, acidosis is preventable. The abolishing of carbohydrates from the diet is one of the principal factors in the cause of acidosis. We may be able to greatly diminish the percentage of sugar, but by so doing the changed metabolism of the cell, owing to the absence of carbohydrates, increases the possibility of acidosis. Should acidosis be present we place the patient upon a fluid diet, insisting on milk, clear broths, and fruit juice, suggesting that he remain in bed during this interval for about three weeks. A culture of *Bacillus bulgaricus* is given up to 24 cubic centimeters per day."

The administration of other therapeutic agents is described but must be omitted here, with the exception of mention of the fact that glandular extracts are given to patients inclined toward obesity. The cases treated as indicated above responded favorably, losing all signs of acidosis, unless the disease had advanced to such an extent that there was marked emaciation and changes in the viscera. In these cases, medication was without avail.

"In cases of the first class," says the report, "the symptoms entirely subsided during treatment. Only seven still have traces of sugar, and if they are kept under observation from time to time, I believe will remain in a fairly normal state."

## His Conclusions

"In cases of the second class, the results have not been so marked, although all the patients have shown considerable improvement, with most of the major symptoms disappearing. The gain in weight has averaged from three to eighteen and a half pounds. The proportion of recoveries, however, is very small, and out of seventy-nine cases of acidosis we would say that five have recovered, twenty-seven have apparently been greatly benefited; the rest, with the exception of two, remaining about the same as when first observed. These two patients, both under 15 years of age, have since passed away."

These are the author's conclusions:

"1. The efficacy of this culture in diabetes is undoubtedly due to its power to prevent intestinal putrefaction.

"2. The stimulating effect upon the pancreas by its acidity is potent.

"3. Its power to convert starch into lactic acid is an important factor.

"4. By relieving auto-intoxication many of the symptoms in diabetes are stopped.

"5. The use of the X-ray in diagnosis is most valuable.

"6. The necessary analysis of the gastric contents should be made, so that a consistent method may be followed in treatment.

"7. The routine examination of the blood, not only for acetone, but sugar, is advisable.

"8. The prevention of this disease and the overcoming of its progress is unquestionably possible, and I believe by systematic, thorough care of all glycosurias in the first class a permanent recovery will be the reward.

"9. Glycosurias of the second class do not apparently respond, although their condition seems to be greatly benefited.

"10. The use of this culture in diabetes is far superior to that of opium, and offers the only rational internal therapy really of value."

*July 20, 1913*

# Diabetes Discovery Not a Positive Cure

An announcement from Cleveland, printed here yesterday, that a cure for diabetes had been discovered at the Rockefeller Institute for Medical Research, and that it had been tried successfully at the Lakeside Hospital in Cleveland, aroused much interest in medical circles yesterday. It was learned that the new treatment for the disease had been tried at the Presbyterian Hospital here with excellent results.

The discovery is at present only a new treatment, according to the New York physicians familiar with it, and cannot be called a cure, at least until there has been sufficient time to ascertain whether the disease will return after the patient has been discharged from a hospital.

The treatment was developed by Dr. Allen of the Rockefeller Institute, and before it was tried on patients he got good results with experiments on animals. It is remarkably simple, and consists almost entirely of starving out the disease. In this it is only a development of the treatment that has long been used. The most generally adopted treatment consists of eliminating carbohydrates, or foods containing starch, from the patient's diet, and allowing the patient practically a normal supply of fats and proteins. Dr. Allen's method eliminates the carbohydrates, but also reduces all other diet as much as the patient can stand.

The treatment calls for absolute fasting of the patient at stipulated periods. In some cases alcohol is given during the early stages. This is a new feature, though the alcohol is given to stimulate the patient and make up for the lack of food at first to some extent.

The policy of giving the patient bicarbonate of sodium to neutralize the effect of acids is adhered to in the new treatment, one of the physicians said yesterday, though it is considered questionable whether this has much to do with the results obtained. Bicarbonate of sodium has been administered in cases of diabetes for nearly thirty years. It is given in cases where there is sufficient poisoning in the system to cause nervous disorders, such as coma and fainting.

Despite its simplicity the new treatment has been producing results considered almost remarkable by the medical profession. It has been tried at the Cleveland Hospital, Johns Hopkins in Baltimore, and the Presbyterian Hospital here, and is still in use at all three institutions. It was first tried at the Presbyterian Hospital early in the year.

"Excellent results have been obtained at this hospital with the new treatment," said Dr. J. Eliot Overlander, the Assistant Superintendent of the hospital. "All of the patients treated by the method have improved rapidly."

It was learned that between fifteen and twenty patients had been treated by the new method at the hospital, and that all but one had been discharged. On leaving the hospital they said that they felt better than they had at any time before since contracting the disease. They were instructed to continue on a somewhat reduced diet after being discharged, but were allowed to eat a small amount of foods containing starch.

*October 11, 1915*

# Serum Proves Boon in Fighting Diabetes

Experiments in the treatment of diabetes, hitherto regarded as practically incurable, have met with remarkable success, according to reports officials of the Carnegie Corporation, which has made an appropriation toy research work at the Potter Metabolic Laboratory and Clinic in California. The treatment that is being administered has given relief in practically all the cases under observation.

The ravages of the disease have been checked by application of a serum discovered by Canadian physicians working under Dr. J. J. R. Macleod of the University of Toronto. This serum has been used at the Potter laboratory. Thus far relief has been dependent upon constant application of the serum. It is too early, physicians say, to describe the treatment as a "sure cure" for diabetes, for the experiments at the Potter laboratory have been going on for only about eighteen months.

Dr. Henry S. Pritchett, President of the Carnegie Corporation, who recently visited the Potter clinic and observed the experiments there, has made a report on the study and treatment there of diabetes, for incorporation in the annual report of the corporation.

## Dr. Potter First Started Work

Dr. Potter's metabolic research began at the French Hospital here. He removed to Santa Barbara, Cal., where a metabolic clinic and laboratory was built by public-spirited Californians. The Carnegie Corporation has aided the work by an annual appropriation. Dr. Potter died in 1919, and since then the work has been carried on under the direction of W. D. Sansum.

Intensive studies on the internal secretion of the pancreas had been carried on in the meantime under Dr. Macleod in Canada. It has long been known that some pathology of the pancreas is responsible for diabetes. Dr. F. G. Banting, working under Dr. Macleod, carried on intensive experiments to extract a substance from pancreatic tissues. This substance was first injected into dogs suffering with diabetes. The diabetic symptoms disappeared with the application of the serum, which is known as insulin. Convincing results of the efficacy of the serum were obtained by Dr. Banting in the cases of humans suffering with the disease.

"On account of the admirable facilities in the Potter Metabolic Clinic in Santa Barbara and the opportunity afforded by the close association of laboratory and hospital," Dr. Pritchett's report says, "Dr. Macleod and his associates most generously and kindly communicated to Dr. Sansum and his staff in Santa Barbara such full information as they had and because of the urgent need for such an extract of the pancreas urged their immediate co-operation. With the information thus generously given through Dr. Macleod, the staff of the Potter Metabolic Clinic began strenuous efforts in the insolation of the internal secretion of the pancreas now known as insulin. They were immediately successful and within two months had been able to secure a sufficient amount of insulin to use on nine severe cases of diabetes.

## Success of Treatment Established

The results have been so convincing that there can be no doubt of the great value of this substance in the treatment of diabetes and it is quite within the possibilities that the discovery may result in the relief and cure of great numbers of people from this scourge. The following cases will illustrate the extraordinary sort of results which have been obtained:

"A patient of 53 years of age was sent to the clinic on the verge of diabetic coma, apparently death within a few days awaited him. Following the administration of insulin he became immediately free from sugar, his diet could be increased to normal and he is rapidly gaining in strength and weight.

"A boy of 12 in extreme illness through diabetes became free from sugar after twenty-four hours of treatment with insulin [and] has remained free although his diet has been increased to practically normal. This boy is gaining weight at the rate of half a pound a day and is leading the type of life that any normal active child would lead. By the older dietary methods partial starvation would have been necessary even to prolong life, to say nothing of restoration to health. The results in the other cases have been equally astonishing."

## Expense of Serum Is Very Great

"The problem is of course still in its infancy. Insulin is prepared at present at very great expense. Cheaper methods of production must be devised. A study of the intricate chemistry of the product will undoubtedly add materially to our knowledge of the oxidative processes going on in the body about which practically nothing is known at present. But the great gains seem to be that patients with the use of this new agent will not only be able to be sugar free, but will be able to have normal diets with the strength and health which can come alone from the use of such food.

"The brilliant success which has come from this study and the still more brilliant prospects of the future which it holds out form a source of the greatest encouragement to the trustees of the corporation that their gifts may, if given with discretion, advance the cause of medical knowledge and thereby increase human happiness and usefulness in the most desirable fashion. Mr. Carnegie had always in mind the desire to 'find the efficient man and enable him to do his work.' Not every research can show the brilliant results which have come out of these investigations, but all patient, long-continued study adds, little by little, to the sum of knowledge, enriches life, and helps to turn away misfortune.

"Not the least pleasing feature of this investigation lies in the generous and admirable attitude in which two sets of investigators, each of whom has revived modest help from the Carnegie Corporation, have co-operated toward their common end. It was a graceful and generous act on the part of Dr. Macleod and his colleagues to put at the service of the Potter Metabolic Clinic the full results of their important researches, but this action is in entire consonance with the spirit and the purpose of true scientific research."

*October 8, 1922*

# Virus Link Is Found in Diabetes Patient

By HAROLD M. SCHMECK JR.

In the first thoroughly documented instance of its kind, a virus has been linked to a fatal case of diabetes under circumstances that make it almost certain that the virus caused the disease.

A report of the case has been published in the current issue of the *New England Journal of Medicine*, together with an editorial that described the new evidence as "highly important."

The case and research related to it provide strong evidence that virus infection is among the causes of the most serious form of diabetes, known as juvenile-onset diabetes. How common this kind of link may be is unknown. Juvenile-onset diabetes is distinct in many respects from the more common adult-onset diabetes and tends to be more severe.

A Government announcement described the case as the first in which a virus had been recovered from the pancreas of a juvenile diabetes patient.

## Classic Requirements for Proof

For almost a century scientists have tried, but always failed, to prove that some juvenile diabetes is caused by virus infection. The new research seems to fulfill all the classic requirements for proof. The new evidence also indicates that heredity is a factor in susceptibility to virus-caused damage to the pancreas.

The editorial said the new findings offered "challenges for future research" and "cause for optimism" concerning the understanding and treatment of this serious illness. The editorial suggested the possibility of a vaccine for some persons who might be at high risk of developing diabetes and use of anti-inflammatory or immunosuppressive treatment for some diabetics to minimize damage to the pancreas, the gland where insulin is produced.

The possibility of such a vaccine, however, is conjectural and perhaps far in the future. The concept is complicated by the fact that the virus involved in this case and other viruses suspected of possible links to some juvenile diabetes cases are widespread in the human population while the disease is much less common.

The new report was by scientists of the National Institute of Dental Research and the National Naval Medical Center in Bethesda, Md. They described the case of a 10-year-old boy who had no previous evidence of diabetes but developed a serious form of that disease two days after what appeared to be a mild flu-like illness.

The boy was hospitalized because of severe lethargy and abdominal cramps. He also showed some of the common symptoms of diabetes, including excessive thirst and urination. Doctors soon found that he had the biochemical derangements typical of serious diabetes. Even though he was given insulin and other treatment, he died about a week after the illness began.

## Recovered the Virus

Scientists recovered a virus called Coxsackie B4 from the boy's pancreas. They grew this in tissue culture and then injected it into mice, some of which developed the same serious form of diabetes with destruction of the insulin-producing cells of the pancreas.

Thus, the team of scientists fulfilled all of the classic conditions required for proof that a given virus or bacterium is the cause of a specific illness.

They took elaborate care to rule out the possibility that the virus was a laboratory contaminant. The fact that some strains of laboratory mice developed diabetes while others did not suggests that heredity influences the risk that virus infection will cause the disease. Persons of certain identifiable tissue types are known to be more likely than others to develop diabetes. Furthermore the boy had relatives who were diabetics.

An announcement yesterday from the dental research institute said the case was the first documented instance of recovery of a virus from the pancreas of a patient with juvenile diabetes. The institute is a unit of the National Institutes of Health.

The combined evidence of the research and the highly unusual case in a young boy has suggested to the scientists that hereditary susceptibility, virus infection and a situation in which the body assaults its own tissues may be responsible for some cases of juvenile diabetes.

## Circumstantial Evidence

Although they have no indication of how common virus-linked diabetes may be, the scientists note in their report that there has been much circumstantial evidence over the years linking it to various virus infections. This is not believed to be true of adult-onset diabetes, a more common condition that some scientists believe to be essentially a different disease from the serious so-called juvenile form.

Authors of the report in the medical journal were Drs. Ji-Won Yoon, Marshall Austin, Takashi Onodera and Abner Louis Notkins. Dr. Austin is a pathologist and virus specialist of the Naval Medical Center, where the boy's pancreas was studied. The others are scientists of the dental research institute who have long been interested in possible virus links to diabetes.

In earlier research, the team led by Dr. Notkins produced the equivalent of diabetes in mice by infecting them with certain strains of Coxsackie virus and another variety called Reo virus type 3. Strains of both viruses are far more widespread in the human population than is juvenile diabetes.

Coxsackie virus, named for a community in upstate New York where it was discovered several decades ago, is known to produce flu-like infections. It has also been suspected of contributing to some cases of diabetes, because of the laboratory research on mice.

In an interview, Dr. Notkins said it was clear that diabetes was not a common result of infection with Coxsackie virus because at least 50 percent of Americans have been infected with it at some time, while less than one-tenth of 1 percent of Americans ever develop juvenile diabetes. The scientist said the virus-diabetes situation might be somewhat analogous to that of polio virus infections, only a few of which actually produce paralysis.

*May 24, 1979*

CHAPTER 8

# Diagnostics

# Prof. Röntgen's X-Rays

The preliminary communication of Prof. Wilhelm Conrad Röntgen to the Würzberg Physico-Medical Society of his discovery of a new form of radiant energy appears this week translated in full in several of the English papers. As the chief interest of men of science is centred in the question of the nature of the rays, those portions of Prof. Röntgen's paper which deal with this aspect of the subject are here reproduced in full.

The name given by Prof. Röntgen to the newly discovered form of radiant energy is X-rays. The translation appended was made by Arthur Stanton, and appears in the current number of *Nature*. After describing his experiments in making shadow photographs of various substances, Prof. Röntgen says:

"7. After my experiments on the transparency of increasing thicknesses of different media, I proceeded to investigate whether the X-rays could be deflected by a prism. Investigations with water and carbon bisulphide in mica prisms of 30° showed no deviation either on the photographic or the fluorescent plate. For comparison, light rays were allowed to fall on the prism as the apparatus was set up for the experiment. They were deviated 10 mm. and 20 mm. respectively in the case of the two prisms.

"With prisms of ebonite and aluminium I have obtained images on the photographic plate which point to a passible deviation. It is, however, uncertain, and at most would point to a refractive index 1.05. No deviation can be observed by means of the fluorescent screen. Investigations with the heavier metals have not as yet led to any result, because of their small transparency and the consequent enfeebling of the transmitted rays.

"On account of the importance of the question it is desirable to try in other ways whether the X-rays are susceptible of refraction. Finely powdered bodies allow in thick layers but little of the incident light to pass through, in consequence of refraction and reflection. In the case of the X-rays, however, such layers of powder are for equal masses of substance equally transparent with the coherent solid itself. Hence we cannot conclude any regular reflection or refraction of the X-rays. The research was conducted by the aid of finely powdered rock salt, fine electrolytic silver powder, and zinc dust already many times employed in chemical work. In all these cases the result, whether by the fluorescent screen or the photographic method, indicated no difference in transparency between the powder and the coherent solid.

"It is, hence, obvious that lenses cannot be looked upon as capable of concentrating the X-rays; in effect, both an ebonite and a glass lens of large size prove to be without action. The shadow photograph of a round rod is darker in the middle than at the edge; the image of a cylinder filled with a body more transparent than its walls exhibits the middle brighter than the edge.

"8. The preceding experiments and others which I pass over point to the rays being incapable of regular reflection. It is, however, well to detail an observation which at first sight seemed to lead to an opposite conclusion.

"I exposed a plate, protected by a black paper sheath, to the X-rays, so that the glass side lay next to the vacuum tube. The sensitive film was partly covered with star-shaped pieces of platinum, lead, zinc, and aluminium. On the developed negative the star-shaped impression showed dark under platinum, lead, and more markedly under zinc; the aluminium gave no image. It seems, therefore, that these three metals can reflect the X-rays; as, however, another explanation is possible, I repeated the experiment with this only difference, that a film of thin aluminium foil was interposed between the sensitive film and the metal stars. Such an aluminium plate is opaque to ultra-violet rays, but transparent to X-rays. In the result the images appeared as before, this pointing still to the existence of reflection at metal surfaces.

"If one considers this observation in connection with others—namely, on the transparency of powders, and on the state of the surface not being effective in altering the passage of the X-rays through a body—it leads to the probable conclusion that regular reflection does not exist, but that bodies behave to the X-rays as turbid media to light.

"Since I have obtained no evidence of refraction at the surface of different media, it seems probable that the X-rays move with the same velocity in all bodies, and in a medium which penetrates everything, and in which the molecules of bodies are imbedded. The molecules obstruct the X-rays, the more effectively as the density of the body concerned is greater.

"9. It seemed possible that the geometrical arrangement of the molecules might affect the action of a body upon the X-rays, so that, for example, Iceland spar might exhibit different phenomena according to the relation of the surface of the plate to the axis of the crystal. Experiments with quartz and Iceland spar on this point lead to a negative result.

"10. It is known that Lenard, in his investigations on kathode rays, has shown that they belong to the ether, and can pass through all bodies. Concerning the X-rays the same may be said.

"In his latest work, Lenard has investigated the absorption coefficients of various bodies for the kathode rays, including air at atmospheric pressure, which gives 4.10, 3.40, 3.10 for 1 cm., according to the degree of exhaustion of the gas in the discharge tube. To judge from the nature of the discharge, I have worked at about the same pressure, but occasionally at greater or smaller pressures. I find, using a Weber photometer, that the intensity of the fluorescent light varies nearly as the inverse square of the distance between screen and discharge tube. This result is obtained from three very consistent sets of observations at distances of 100 and 200 mm. Hence, air absorbs the X-rays much less than the kathode rays. This result is in complete agreement with the previously described result, that the fluorescence of the screen can be still observed at two metres from the vacuum tube. In general, other bodies behave like air; they are more transparent for the X-rays than for the kathode rays.

"11. A further distinction, and a noteworthy one, results from the action of a magnet. I have not succeeded in observing any deviation of the X-rays even in very strong magnetic fields.

"The deviation of kathode rays by the magnet is one of their peculiar characteristics; it has been observed by Hertz and Lenard that several kinds of kathode rays exist, which differ by their power of exciting phosphorescence, their susceptibility of absorption, and their deviation by the magnet; but a notable deviation has been observed in all cases which have yet been investigated, and I think that such deviation affords a characteristic not to be set aside lightly.

"12. As a result of many researches, it appears that the place of most brilliant phosphorescence of the walls of the discharge tube is the chief seat whence the X-rays originate and spread in all directions; that is, the X-rays proceed from the front where the kathode rays strike the glass. If one deviates the kathode rays within the tube by means of a magnet, it is seen that the X-rays proceed from a new point—i.e., again from the end of the kathode rays.

"Also for this reason the X-rays, which are not deflected by a magnet, cannot be regarded as kathode rays which have passed through the glass, for that passage cannot, according to Lenard, be the cause of the different deflection of the rays. Hence I conclude that the X-rays are not identical with the kathode rays, but are produced from the kathode rays at the glass surface of the tube.

"13. The rays are generated not only in glass. I have obtained them in an apparatus closed by an aluminium plate 2 mm. thick. I purpose later to investigate the behavior of other substances.

"14. The justification of the term "rays," applied to the phenomena, lies partly in the regular shadow pictures produced by the interposition of a more or less permeable body between the source and a photographic plate or fluorescent screen.

"I have observed and photographed many such shadow pictures. Thus I have an outline of part of a door covered with lead paint; the image was produced by placing the discharge tube on one side of the door, and the sensitive plate on the other. I have also a shadow of the bones of the hand, of a wire wound upon a bobbin, of a set of weights in a box, of a compass card and needle completely inclosed in a metal case, of a piece of metal where the X-rays show the want of homogeneity, and of other things.

"For the rectilinear propagation of the rays I have a pinhole photograph of the discharge apparatus, covered with black paper. It is faint, but unmistakable.

"16. Researches to investigate whether electrostative forces act on the X-rays are begun, but not yet concluded.

"17. If one asks, what then are these X-rays; since they are not kathode rays, one might suppose, from their power of exciting fluorescence and chemical action, them to be due to ultra-violet light. In opposition to this view, a weighty set of considerations presents itself. If X-rays be, indeed, ultra-violet light, then that light must possess the following properties:

"(a) It is not refracted in passing from air into water, carbon bisulphide, aluminium, rock salt, glass, or zinc. (b) It is incapable of regular reflection at the surfaces of the above bodies. (c) It cannot be polarized by any ordinary polarizing media. (d) The absorption by various bodies must depend chiefly on their density.

"That is to say, these ultra-violet rays must behave quite differently from the visible, infrared, and hitherto-known ultra-violet rays.

"These things appear so unlikely that I have sought for another hypothesis.

"A kind of relationship between the new rays and light rays appears to exist; at least the formation of shadows, fluorescence, and the production of chemical action point in this direction. Now, it has been known for a long time that, besides the transverse vibrations which account for the phenomena of light, it is possible that longitudinal vibrations should exist in the ether, and, according to the view of some physicists, must exist. It is granted that their existence has not yet been made clear, and their properties are not experimentally demonstrated. Should not the new rays be ascribed to longitudinal waves in the ether?

"I must confess that I have in the course of this research made myself more and more familiar with this thought, and venture to put the opinion forward, while I am quite conscious that the hypothesis advanced still requires a more solid foundation."

The *London Electrician*, in its last number, points out briefly the similarity and difference between the Röntgen rays and the Lenard, or true kathode rays, as follows:

"It may not be without interest at the present moment to recall the main points of difference and of similarity between Röntgen rays and Lenard rays—to use two brief and convenient expressions. Röntgen rays are not deflected by a magnet; Lenard rays are. Röntgen rays suffer far less absorption and diffusion than Lenard rays. Lenard found that his kathode rays failed to pass through anything but the thinnest soap films, glass, and aluminium foil, &c; the Röntgen variety will traverse several centimeters of wood and several millimeters of metal or glass. Röntgen was able to take 'shadowgraphs' and detect fluorescence 200 cm. away from the discharge tube; 6cm. or 8cm. were enough to wipe out Lenard rays in air at atmospheric pressure, and even in hydrogen gas at only 0.0164mm. pressure, the 'radiation length' for kathode rays was only 130cm.; hydrogen at atmospheric pressure behaving as a decidedly turbid medium. These are, however, rather differences in degree than in kind. Lenard rays emanate, of course, from the kathode itself, but Röntgen rays, according to their discoverer, start from the luminescent spot on the glass wall of the discharge tube, at which the kathode rays terminate.

"The points of similarity between Röntgen and Lenard rays are their photographic activity, their rectilinear propagation (as evidenced by the sharp shadows cast), and the fact that in both cases it would seem the total mass of molecules contained in unit volume of any substance practically determines its transparency. All things tend to show that we are on the verge of a great scientific discovery, which may oblige us, nolens volens, to 'rearrange our ideas.'"

Even the *Lancet* has succumbed to the photographic evidence presented to it, and says in an editorial paragraph in its current issue:

The application of this remarkable phenomenon to the discovery of bullets and abnormalities in the structure of bone has already been made, with very promising results. It is reported already from Vienna, for instance, that photographic pictures taken by this means showed with the greatest clearness and precision the injuries caused by a revolver shot in the hand of a man and the position of the bullet. In another case, that of a girl, the position and nature of a malformation in the left foot were ascertained. As the conditions of these experiments become perfected with regard to the source of the radiations, there is no doubt that the result will be even more brilliant."

An abstruse extract taken from Lord Kelvin's Baltimore lectures, delivered at Johns Hopkins University in 1884, which is quoted in *Nature*, seems to show that he anticipated some discovery which would prove that ether was compressible like ordinary forms of matter. The point is to show that the new energy behaves more like sound than like light. It is worthy of note that Prof. Sylvanus Thompson has already termed the new form of energy "ultra-violet sound."

*February 5, 1896*

# 3-Dimensional X-Ray Is Tested for New View of Body

## By JANE E. BRODY

ROCHESTER, MINN.—"Take a deep breath and hold it, sir," the technician told the patient stretched out in what looked like a guillotine about to slice through his abdomen. But rather than a knife, this "guillotine" would use X-rays to produce a radically new view of the human body.

The ring of instruments encircling the man's body began to rotate, whirring and clicking for 20 seconds until it had made a half circle around him. The technician said, "Breathe now, sir," and in a few minutes a picture appeared on a television screen showing the patient's kidneys, pancreas and other internal organs as if he had been sliced in half crosswise.

The moment was historic. The man, who has an abdominal cancer, was the first patient at the Mayo Clinic here to be examined by an experimental machine that could either revolutionize diagnosis of many internal ailments or turn out to be a half-million-dollar dud.

Mayo is one of two dozen institutions in the United States that are now cautiously and systematically testing this new generation of medical equipment, called a body scanner, to find out just what it can and cannot do for diagnosis. In a few months, as the machines proliferate, several dozen other medical centers will join in the search.

The body scanner uses a technique called computed axial tomography, or CAT. Unlike conventional X-ray machines, which send a broad X-ray beam over a large area—say, from the shoulders to the diaphragm—CAT scanners direct a pencil-point-thin line of X-ray photons through a narrow cross section, or slice, of the body.

As the beam moves around the body in the same plane, a minicomputer analyzes how much of the X-rays were absorbed as they passed through the various internal organs and structures. Up to eight "slices," one centimeter apart, may be taken at a time, with the total radiation dose comparable to that of a single ordinary X-ray exposure.

Ordinary X-rays take a "flat" view, superimposing organs in the front of the body on organs in the back—a two-dimensional picture of a three-dimensional object. They also give poor pictures of soft tissues.

## Sensitive to Tissues

The scanner also produces a two-dimensional picture but mainly of the third "depth" dimension that is missed on regular X-rays. And by taking serial slices through the patient and flipping the pictures rapidly on the television screen, the impression of a three-dimensional object—the body—can be recreated.

The scanning X-ray is also far more sensitive to differences between tissues than an ordinary X-ray beam and is therefore theoretically able to show structures or abnormalities that would otherwise be missed.

CAT scanners have already created an undisputed revolution in diagnosing brain disorders, heretofore inaccessible to ordinary flat X-rays because the bony skull absorbs most of the X-ray beam and obscures the view of what lies within it.

The special techniques, such as injecting dyes and air into the brain, used to overcome these limitations are painful and dangerous and involve costly hospitalization. A brain scan does the job in half an hour on an outpatient basis and without endangering the patient. At Toronto General Hospital, one brain scanner resulted in a saving of $2 million in patient costs in one year.

## Future Is Cloudy

Brain scans have enabled doctors to diagnose blood clots, cysts, tumors, hemorrhages and other physical brain abnormalities safely and rapidly. In the scores of institutions where brain scanners are in use, they have largely replaced the more hazardous X-ray techniques and enabled doctors to diagnose some conditions that were previously impossible to detect without surgically exploring the brain, an approach avoided in all but the most extreme or obvious cases.

But whether the new whole body scanners will set off a similar revolution for the rest of the human organism remains to be seen. Most observers familiar with the devices are betting on something, but they do not yet know what.

"You need the imagination of a Jules Verne to see what this technology will mean to the rest of the body in years to come," observed Dr. Eugene Gedgaudas, head of radiology at the University of Minnesota, where an instrument similar to Mayo's has been in use since June.

"There are incredible possibilities, but there are also limitations," Dr. Gedgaudas continued. "There are so many hurdles that it will be some time before this can be added to existing radiographic techniques."

He said that the results of body scanning must be compared to ultrasound, X-ray examinations using radioactive materials and other established procedures "to see where it fits—what it adds, what it will replace, what new things it will allow."

At Mayo, radiologists are excited about the seemingly endless possibilities but are similarly cautious.

"If the scanner only makes pictures, it will be a very expensive way to see slices of bodies," Dr. Hillier Baker, Mayo radiologist, remarked.

## Issue of Differentiation

Among the possibilities under study are the following:

- Can the scanner distinguish between an abscess, a cyst and a tumor, or between a benign and a malignant tumor?

- Can it spot an early cancer before it could be found by other means? Similarly, can it detect hidden metastases?

- Could it be used to monitor the results of cancer therapy, guiding the therapist on where and how much to treat?

- Could it detect such postoperative complications as a hemorrhage or abscess?

Other possibilities include detecting early stages of bone demineralization, finding gallstones without injecting a dye, diagnosing an aortic aneurysm—a blowout in the body's main artery—without further endangering the patient's life, and quantifying the amount of iodine in the thyroid gland.

While what may be in the future for body scanners is in doubt, that they will have a future of some kind is virtually guaranteed by the fact that 18 electronics companies in the United States and in Europe are racing to develop the fastest, most accurate and economical body scanner.

## 3 Companies Producing

Three companies are producing commercial instruments: EMI Ltd., a British-based company that pioneered in the field by developing the first brain scanner; Pfizer

Medical Systems, Inc., which is manufacturing an ACT-Scanner developed by Dr. Robert Ledley of Georgetown University in Washington, and Ohio Nuclear, Inc. of Cleveland, which produces the Delta-Scanner.

The three machines differ mainly in price and scan time, the EMI-Scanner, which the Mayo Clinic has, being the fastest and most expensive. Speed is important because patient motion, including the movements of breathing, can distort the image projected by the computer.

Thus far, the EMI, with a 20-second scan time, is the only machine fast enough to permit the patient to hold his breath. But several companies are working on a ten-second and even a five-second machine, and biophysicists at Mayo are experimenting with a prototype unit that may one day be incorporated into a device that scans in one one-hundredth of a second—fast enough to "stop" the motion of a beating heart.

Most of the body scanners in use are being applied mainly to brain studies, where the extraordinary value of CAT-scanning has been well established. Experimental scans of the rest of the body, funded by research grants, are being squeezed in during off hours—at the University of Minnesota, at nights and on weekends.

The first published report on the results of 119 body scans, prepared by researchers at Georgetown University in the current issue of the *Journal of the American Medical Association,* is notable mainly in that it did not pinpoint any unique usefulness for the device in the first year of tests.

Dr. Laura Knight, a radiologist at the University of Minnesota, pointed out that the brain was so precisely organized that any deviation could be regarded as abnormal.

"But in the body you can have a lot of displacement of organs and still be within normal bounds. Such things as fluid, gas, food and feces can affect the shape, position and densities of organs, making it harder to learn what's what," Dr. Knight said.

Dr. Gedgaudas is distressed by what he regards as premature proliferation of body scanners, some of which are being bought by places that never used a brain scanner and have no notion of the body scanner's probable limitations.

"We shouldn't be piling on machines until their place in medicine is clearly established," he remarked. "We shouldn't be adding to medical costs until we know we are adding something truly valuable."

*October 22, 1975*

**CHAPTER 9**

# Diet and Obesity

# Nutritive Value of Food

In order to ascertain the customs and methods of persons of different stations in life regarding the purchase and use of their food a series of investigations are being conducted by the Department of Agriculture. These inquiries are of a distinctly practical character, and they are made with the co-operation of a number of experiment stations, colleges, and other organizations, as well as of private individuals, in different parts of the country. The general scope of the investigations includes the determination of the amounts and nutritive value of the food consumed by a given number of persons during a certain number of days, and the deducting of the quantities per man per day.

It is believed that such information, coupled with that derived from the study of the composition, digestibility, and nutritive value of food materials in common use on the one hand, and with that which comes from research into the laws of nutrition on the other hand, will gradually make it possible to judge what are the more common dietary errors and how improvements may be made to the advantage of health, purse, and home life. A variety of digestion experiments have already been made, and others are in progress, under Governmental supervision. Accounts of studies of dietaries of families, boarding houses, and clubs are from time to time made the subject of official reports.

## How Experiments Are Made

In these studies account is taken of the amounts, composition, and cost of all food materials of nutritive value in the house at the beginning, purchased during and remaining at the end of each experiment, and of all the kitchen and table wastes. Such accessories as baking powder, essences, salt, condiments, tea, coffee, &c., although of interest from a pecuniary standpoint, are of no practical value as regards nutriments. The sum of the different food materials on hand at the beginning and those received during the experiment is taken, and from this sum the quantities remaining at the end are subtracted, thus giving the amount of each material actually used. From the amount thus obtained and the composition of each material, as shown by analysis, the amounts of the nutritive ingredients are estimated. From these are subtracted the amounts of nutrients in the waste, and thus the amounts of nutrients actually eaten are learned. In all of these experimental inquiries account is kept of the meals taken by the different members of the family and by visitors.

The number of meals for one man, to which the total number of actual meals taken is equivalent, is estimated upon the basis of the potential energy. These energy equivalents are somewhat arbitrary, and it is acknowledged that they will require revision in the light of accumulating information.

Following is a table of estimated relative quantities of potential energy in nutrients required by persons of different classes:

| | |
|---|---|
| Man at moderate work | 1.0 |
| Woman at moderate work | .8 |
| Boy between 14 and 16, inclusive | .8 |
| Girl between 14 and 16, inclusive | .7 |
| Child between 10 and 13, inclusive | .6 |
| Child between 6 and 9, inclusive | .5 |
| Child between 2 and 5, inclusive | .4 |
| Child under 2 | .3 |

## Where Studies Have Been Made

The dietary studies already made include a boarding house, a blacksmith's family, a jeweler's family, a chemist's family, an infant nine months old, a college students' eating club, a Swedish laborer's family, a female college students' club, farmer's family, a camping party in Maine, a poor widow's family, a man in the Adirondacks under treatment for consumption, and a mason's family. As a general thing, the figures used for the percentages of nutrients in each food material are taken from the averages given for like food materials in *Bulletin No. 28* of the Office of Experiment Stations of the Department of Agriculture. The figures in that bulletin represent the results of a compilation of analyses made previous to Jan. 1, 1895. In estimating the fuel values of the nutritive ingredients, the proteine and carbohydrates are assumed to contain 4.1 and the fats 9.3 calories of potential energy per gram. These correspond to 1,860 calories for one pound of proteine, or carbohydrates, and 4,220 calories for one pound of fats.

## Fuel Values of Bacon, Turkey and Cod

Bacon has a very large percentage of fuel value. The latest official analysis shows that a portion of bacon, with the inedible parts discarded, contains 17.8 parts water, 9.8 parts of proteine, 68 parts fat, and 4.4 parts ash, and has a fuel value of 3,050 calories per pound. By the same analysis, the edible portion of a turkey is found to contain 55.5 parts water, 20.6 parts proteine, 22.9 parts fat, and 1 part ash, with a fuel value of 1,350 calories per pound. Codfish (edible portion) contains 82.0 parts water, 15.8 parts proteine, .4 part fat, and 1.2 parts ash, and has a fuel value of 310 calories per pound.

In each of the dietary studies reported the data regarding the kinds and amounts of food material, the persons by whom they were eaten, and the number of days and meals were sent to the Government Experiment Station at Middletown, Conn., where the necessary computations were made. For the sake of simplicity and convenience, the computed quantities for one man for ten days are given, instead of the actual quantities consumed, or the quantities for one man for one day. If the quantities were stated as actually consumed in the period of each dietary, it would not be easy to compare the quantities in different dietaries. By putting the quantities for all of the dietaries on one basis, however, the relative amounts of the different kinds of food materials, as meats, milk, bread, and the like in the different dietaries are readily compared. If the quantities were given per man per day, some would be too small for printing without the use of an inconvenient number of decimal places.

## What a Laborer's Family Ate

A fourteen days' study was given to the dietary of a laborer's family in Hartford, Conn. The family consisted of man and wife, three girls, aged respectively four, six, and eleven years; a boy, two and a half years old, and an infant. The father was a laborer in a coal yard, earning $8 per week. The mother had worked as a servant before her marriage and did her own cooking. The food materials bought by this family consisted of beef, veal, mutton, pork, salt codfish, eggs, butter, milk, rice, flour, rolled oats, bread, beans, sugar, potatoes, onions, and raisins. The consumption of food, calculated for one man ten days, was: 13.2 pounds of animal food, 9.6 pounds of cereals and sugars, 11.1 pounds of vegetables, and 2 pounds of fruit, a total of 34.1 pounds. This total quantity cost $1.53, and it contained 2.41 pounds of proteine, 2.24 pounds of fat, and X.XX pounds of carbohydrates, the aggregate fuel value being 31,760 calories per pound. The following table shows the nutrients and potential energy in the food purchased, rejected, and eaten by this entire family during the period of fourteen days:

### For Family, 14 Days—Food Purchased

#### Nutrients

| Food Materials | cost | Proteine grams | Fat grams | Carbohydrates grams | Fuel Value calories |
|---|---|---|---|---|---|
| Animal | $5.62 | 3,312 | 5,239 | 1,076 | 66,710 |
| Vegetable | $3.51 | 2,816 | 444 | 23,519 | 112,100 |
| Total | $9.13 | 6,128 | 5,683 | 24,595 | 178,810 |
| Total Waste | | 38 | 99 | 98 | 1,480 |
| Total Food Actually Eaten | $9.13 | 6,090 | 5,584 | 24,497 | 177,330 |

#### Per Man Per Day—Food Purchased

| | | | | | |
|---|---|---|---|---|---|
| Animal | $0.10 | 59 | 94 | 15 | 1,175 |
| Vegetable | $0.06 | 50 | 8 | 420 | 2,000 |
| Total | $0.16 | 109 | 102 | 435 | 3,175 |
| Total Waste | | 1 | 2 | 2 | 30 |
| Total Food Actually Eaten | $0.16 | 108 | 100 | 433 | 3,165 |

## What a Camping Party Required

In the Summer of 1895, four young men, from nineteen to twenty-two years of age, spent some time canoeing and camping on the Allagash River, in Maine. As they took their journey leisurely, they may be considered as being engaged in light work. The whole time included in the dietary study of this party is estimated as equivalent to 115 days for one man. The following table shows the nutrients and potential energy in the food purchased, rejected, and eaten by this camping party:

## Food Materials

### Nutrients

| | Proteine | Fat | Carbohydrates | Fuel Value for Party |
|---|---|---|---|---|
| | **grams** | **grams** | **grams** | **calories** |
| **Food Purchased** | | | | |
| Animal | 12,169 | 27,396 | 2,331 | 314,230 |
| Vegetable | 7,616 | 2,625 | 59,018 | 297,610 |
| Total | 19,785 | 30,021 | 61,349 | 611,840 |
| **Per Man Per Day—Food Purchased** | | | | |
| Animal | 106 | 238 | 20 | 2,730 |
| Vegetable | 66 | 23 | 513 | 2,590 |
| Total | 172 | 261 | 533 | 5,320 |

The average of thirty-eight dietaries recorded by the Government officials make the following interesting showing:

## Dietaries

### Nutrients

| | Proteine | Fat | Carbohydrates | Fuel Value |
|---|---|---|---|---|
| | **grams** | **grams** | **grams** | **calories** |
| Food purchased | 111 | 140 | 447 | 3,595 |
| Food waste | 7 | 11 | 13 | 185 |
| Food eaten | 104 | 129 | 434 | 3,410 |
| Estimated digestible nutrients in food eaten | 96 | 124 | 423 | 3,235 |

## Character of Sandow's Food

About a year ago, during an engagement of Eugene Sandow, the "strong man," in Washington, an attempt was made to determine the character and amount of the food he consumed. Mr. Sandow claims to be the strongest man in the world, and at the time of the investigation he had the appearance of being in perfect health. He did not then follow any prescribed diet, but ate whatever he desired, always being careful, as is his custom, to eat less than he craved. He always ate very slowly. He smoked a great deal and drank beer and other beverages. Below is the result of a study of Sandow's dietary for one day:

| | **Nutrients** | | | |
|---|---|---|---|---|
| Food Consumed *(Quantities in Ounces)* | Proteine | Fat | Carbohydrates | Potential Energy |
| | **Lb.** | **Lb.** | **Lb.** | **calories** |
| **Dinner, Jan. 10** <br> 2 oysters, 10 soup, <br> 1 celery, 3 fish, 1 potatoes, <br> 2 oyster plant, 1 green peas, <br> 1 tomatoes, 2 bread, 2 roast beef, <br> 2½ chicken, 4 ice cream, <br> 3 orange sherbet, ½ cakes, <br> 1 butter, 11 wine (Burgundy) | .17 | 14 | .34 | |
| **Supper** <br> 8 roast beef, <br> 7½ rye bread, <br> 3½ Camembert cheese, <br> 2 water biscuit, <br> 3½ cakes, 4.4 lb. beer | .26 | .14 . | 61 | |
| **Breakfast, Jan. 11** <br> 9 vegetable soup, 2 potatoes, <br> 3 veal (breaded chop), <br> ½ green peas, 2 roast beef, <br> 4½ bread pudding, <br> ½ cakes, 14 beer | .14 | .05 | .06 | |
| **Total in pounds** | .67 | .33 | 1.11 | 4,462 |
| **Total in grams** | 304 | 151 | 502 | |

It was noted that Sandow rejected all of the visible fat of the meat served him, and in his case it was shown that while the amount of carbo-hydrates and fat consumed did not differ very greatly from the standard for a man at muscular work, the amount of proteine (albumen) was very large. The fact that so much proteine was consumed by Sandow sustains the theory advanced by scientific experimenters that the energy which is used in the production of severe muscular labor is furnished by the combustion of proteine.

Official experiments regarding the digestibility of food by healthy men are now in progress. It has been demonstrated that 98 per cent of the proteine and 97 per cent of the fat in animal foods is readily digested; also that 85 per cent of the proteine and 90 per cent of the fat in cereals and sugars, and 80 per cent of the proteine and 90 per cent of the fat in vegetables and fruits is readily digested.

*June 6, 1897*

# Insurance Study Finds Close Correlation Between Weights and Mortality Rates

By WILLIAM L. LAURENCE

The Society of Actuaries, most of whose members are in the field of life insurance, published last week a report on its twenty-year study of body build and blood pressure. The survey, described by the Institute of Life Insurance as "by far the most extensive statistical investigation ever undertaken in the health field," is based on vital statistics provided by several million insured individuals.

The policy holders, studied over a period dating back to 1935, provide a picture of mortality in relation to weight and blood pressure for comparison with previous figures, some dating back to the turn of the century.

According to the institute, the findings "make obsolete" the figures on average weights now shown on weighing machines and used by physicians throughout the country. These figures are based on an actuarial study of thirty years ago.

The study of the variations in mortality according to weight included nearly 5,000,000 insured persons and covered a period of twenty years. In addition, the study covers mortality rates according to variation in blood pressure among nearly 4,000,000 insured individuals.

## Women Weigh Less

Women were found to weigh less than they did a generation ago, while men tend to be heavier. The weights of women in their twenties average at least five pounds less than those of three to four decades ago, and, in fact, women of all ages now tip the scales several pounds less. This, it was stated, is partly due to lighter clothing (they were clothed when weighed) but reflects mainly the established vogue of slenderness.

In contrast, the average weights of short and medium-height men in their twenties and thirties are now five pounds higher. The increase in men's weights at other ages and for tall men has been generally smaller.

Average weights for both men and women increase with age through the fifties. However, the pattern of the increase is different in the two sexes. Men start putting on weight in the twenties and level off in the forties, while women stay slim into the thirties and do not usually begin putting on weight until after the mid-thirties.

The study shows a correlation between overweight and higher mortality rates. Men weighing twenty pounds above the average have a 10 per cent higher mortality rate; those weighing 25 pounds above the average have an excess mortality of 25 per cent, while a weight of fifty pounds above the average is associated with a death rate as much as 50 to 70 per cent higher. Women were found to stand added weight better than men.

The study shows that overweight is accompanied by markedly increased mortality from diabetes and some digestive diseases, such as those of the gall bladder. With greater increases in weight, the death rate from heart disease rises sharply.

## Below Average

In both sexes, the lowest mortality at ages over thirty is found among those 15 to 20 per cent below average weight. In the teens, a slightly above average weight shows a small advantage. Edward A. Lew, statistician for Metropolitan Life and chairman of the committee that made the study, commented that the data show the average American to be about twenty pounds overweight.

The study showed that reducing adds years to life. The mortality rate dropped to normal in a group that was overweight when insured but later got standard insurance by showing sustained weight reduction.

The most striking revelation was that even a small increase in blood pressure above the average, the level at which most physicians tell you not to worry, may significantly shorten the lifespan. Among men, the study showed, a systolic blood pressure (the pressure when the heart contracts) of 150 or a diastolic blood pressure (when the heart relaxes) of 100 are associated with excess mortality of 75 to 125 percent. Women were found to withstand high blood pressure much better than men.

The lowest mortality among both men and women was found among those with below average blood pressures.

## Blood Pressure

Overweight in combination with elevated blood pressure is found to be a warning of increased danger. Where the two conditions occur together, the rise in death rate is much greater than is accounted for by the two conditions considered separately. Dr. John J. Hutchinson, Medical Director of the New York Life Insurance Company, said he could "offer no obvious explanation of the mechanism whereby moderate overweight in combination with blood pressure of only the slightest departure from the normal produces a mortality experience nearly twice the expected."

Individuals with high blood pressure or overweight in combination with albumin in the urine are similarly subject to significantly higher mortality than that associated with each of these conditions alone. A history of two or more cases of early cardiovascular (heart and blood vessel) kidney disease in the family is also associated with markedly higher mortality, particularly from heart disease, the new data show.

*October 25, 1959*

# Federal Heart Panel Asks Public to Eat Fewer Fats

By JANE E. BRODY

A national commission of medical experts recommended in a report released yesterday that Americans make "safe and reasonable" changes in their diets to lower blood cholesterol levels in the hope of stemming the current "epidemic" of heart disease.

At the same time, the commission urged the immediate adoption of a national policy committed to the primary prevention of premature atherosclerosis and its attendant cardiovascular diseases.

Of the 600,000 American deaths attributed to heart disease each year, 165,000 are "premature" deaths occurring in persons under the age of 65. Men are three times more likely than women to be the victims of premature coronary death.

The dietary changes recommended yesterday included a halving of the current average daily consumption of cholesterol and saturated fats and a substantial reduction in total fat intake.

To achieve this, the commission advised Americans to cut down on egg yolks, butter fat, fatty meats, organ meats, shellfish and fat-rich baked goods and candies and to substitute wherever possible products prepared with unsaturated fats. Most vegetable oils are unsaturated.

The commission's recommendation was based on a large body of data gathered from both animals and man that suggest that changes in the typical fat-rich American diet can help prevent or at least delay cardiovascular diseases.

Noting that definitive evidence linking dietary fats and cholesterol to human heart disease is not available, the commission called for large-scale, long-term, Government sponsored studies to determine once and for all the effect that changes in diet and other factors may have on the nation's slowly rising coronary mortality rate.

Such a study would involve perhaps 100,000 persons followed for five to 10 years at an estimated cost of $50 million to $100 million.

The commission said that it was recommending a change in diet despite the lack of definitive evidence because "the American public would probably have to wait at least 10 years for the results of these studies [and] at times urgent public health decisions must be made on the basis of incomplete evidence."

## Other "Risk Factors"

In addition to diet and its effect on blood fat levels, the commission singled out high blood pressure and cigarette smoking as the major "risk factors" leading to premature heart disease and coronary deaths. Accordingly, the report recommended an "orderly phasing out" of the cigarette industry with strict restraints on the sale and advertising of cigarettes and a major national effort to detect and treat victims of high blood pressure.

The commission, called the Intersociety Commission for Heart Disease Resources, consists of 115 leading American medical and nursing personnel. It was set up under the Regional Medical Programs, sponsored by the Federal Government, to formulate policy guidelines to prevent premature heart disease and improve care of coronary patients.

Under the chairmanship of Dr. Irving Wright, professor emeritus at Cornell University, and the direction of Dr. Donald T. Fredrickson, the commission will produce a series of reports in the coming months on other aspects of coronary care.

The current report, considered the commission's major effort, was discussed at a news conference at the Biltmore Hotel here yesterday. The full report will be published in this month's issue of the journal *Circulation*.

Dr. Fredrickson summarized the commission's dietary recommendations as follows:

The current American diet, which draws about 40 per cent of its calories from fat, should be cut down to include no more than 35 per cent fats; the saturated fat level, currently at 16 to 20 percent, should be cut in half, and the cholesterol level, currently at 600 to 750 milligrams a day, should be no more than 300 milligrams daily.

Foods high in cholesterol include egg yolks and dairy and animal fats.

At the same time, Dr. Fredrickson said, intake of polyunsaturated fats (the oils of corn, peanuts, soybeans and the like), which currently averages 7 per cent of calories, should not exceed 10 per cent. The remaining dietary fats should come from monounsaturated fats like olive oil.

## Change in Standards

According to Dr. Frederick H. Epstein, epidemiologist at the University of Michigan, such a dietary change "can lower serum cholesterol by 10 to 15 per cent."

"At a conservative estimate," he said, "such an effect on serum cholesterol might lower the incidence of coronary heart disease by as much as 30 per cent."

To help Americans achieve this dietary change, the commission urged that Federal food standards be changed to permit the sale of processed meats and dairy products in which unsaturated fats substitute for saturated fats. Under current standards, for example, milk that has part or all of its butter fat replaced by vegetable oil must be called "imitation milk."

The commission also called upon the Food and Drug Administration to change its labeling laws to permit manufacturers to list the exact fat contents of their products so that Americans would have a better idea of what they were eating in the way of fats and cholesterol.

Other risk factors that the commission linked to premature heart disease were diabetes, obesity, sedentary living, a family history of heart disease and possibly "psychological tensions."

*December 16, 1970*

# Atkins Diet: A "Revolution" That Has Medical Society Up in Arms

By JANE E. BRODY

The Medical Society of the County of New York yesterday denounced Dr. Robert C. Atkins's "revolutionary" no-carbohydrate diet as "unscientific," "unbalanced" and "potentially dangerous," especially to persons prone to kidney disease, heart disease and gout.

At a news conference called by its Committee on Public Health, the society said that the side effects of the kind of diet Dr. Atkins promotes in his best-selling book may include weakness, apathy, dehydration, loss of calcium, nausea, lack of stamina and a tendency to fainting.

The Atkins diet is basically a high-protein, high-fat, no- to very-low-carbohydrate diet in which, it is claimed, the dieter can eat all he wants of the permitted foods and still lose weight.

The society's criticisms, which echo those made last week by the Council of Foods and Nutrition of the American Medical Association, were generally denied by Dr. Atkins, who said that neither group had reviewed his yet-unpublished records nor studied a group of patients who had faithfully followed his diet.

The seven doctors who participated in yesterday's news conference said that more serious effects of the diet might include kidney failure in persons with kidney disease, disturbances in normal heart rhythm, too much uric acid in the blood (a precursor to gout) and too much blood fats (a precursor to heart disease).

And if followed by pregnant women, as recommended in Dr. Atkins's book, Dr. Karlis Adamsons of Mount Sinai Medical Center said that the diet could impair the intellectual development of the unborn child.

## Below Normal Amount

The first week of the Atkins diet cuts out carbohydrates altogether. That means fruits, juices and nearly all vegetables as well as the traditional diet no-no's—cake, ice cream, candy, etc.

As the diet progresses, the dieter is permitted to add tiny amounts of very-low-carbohydrate foods—some vegetables and fruits—but at most, the maintenance

Atkins diet still contains only about one-sixth the amount of carbohydrates present in the ordinary American diet.

A variation on the old "calories don't count" theme, the Atkins diet is designed to cause a condition called ketosis, which is at the heart of many of the medical society's objections.

Ketosis is the presence of large amounts of chemicals called "ketone bodies" that spill over into the blood and urine as a result of the incomplete metabolism of fats.

## Warns of Problems

Dr. Robert Kark, professor of medicine at Rush College of Medicine in Chicago, told the news conference that in otherwise normal healthy persons ketosis can cause nausea, vomiting, apathy, fatigue and low blood pressure, and in persons with kidney disease, it can produce kidney failure. Several participants said they had seen or heard of such symptoms developing in adherents to the Atkins diet.

Dr. Atkins, interviewed at his office here, said that "the scientific basis of the medical society's allegations are in total disagreement with my findings, which are based on careful clinical observation of 10,000 obese subjects studied for nine years."

He added that the A.M.A. had declined his invitation to look over his data. He said he is now tabulating the data in computer form for detailed analysis.

"I can tell you on the basis of a preliminary hand tabulation that renal [kidney] shutdown has never happened among my patients, and complaints of nausea, fatigue and apathy occur less often than on a balanced low-calorie diet—in fact, about one-tenth as often," Dr. Atkins said.

## Discusses Cholesterol

As to whether his diet will contribute further to the nation's already out-of-hand epidemic of heart disease, Dr. Atkins said that on the average blood cholesterol and triglyceride levels fall in people following his diet, even though it contains large amount of cholesterol and saturated fats.

He said that about 8 or 9 per cent of Atkins dieters respond with rises in blood cholesterol and that these patients "may have an increased risk," but that about 40 per cent experience "a significant reduction" in cholesterol levels.

With regard to pregnancy, Dr. Atkins now says that his diet "has not been tried sufficiently in pregnant women to recommend its use at this time." Dr. Adamsons said that, all other things being equal, children have an I.Q. 10 points lower on the average if their mothers experienced ketosis during pregnancy.

It remains to be seen what the criticisms will mean to the hundred of thousands of Americans who are now following Dr. Atkins's dietary regimen (his book, *Dr. Atkins' Diet Revolution,* is a runaway best-seller with more than 600,000 copies sold within five months of publication).

## Some Express Misgivings

Some of the Atkins faithful reported yesterday that they already feel a little nervous about continuing on the diet. But, as a 46-year-old 300-pounder said, "I ate more stupidly than this when I was not on the diet. At this point, I'm willing to take my chances about heart disease. After the way I've eaten all these years, anything is an improvement."

The man said the "diet is the first he has ever tried—"and believe me, I've tried everything, including doctors' diets with and without pills"—on which he could lose weight and not be hungry.

"For the first time in my life, I can turn things down without willpower, which I've never had," he said, "And I feel great, psyched up, almost like I was taking amphetamines."

He outlined a typical day's diet: A cheese omelet with two eggs and a glass of seltzer for breakfast; two cheeseburgers without bread, a small wedge of lettuce with oil and vinegar and two glasses of water for lunch, a serving of broiled fish, and other wedge of lettuce and low-calorie gelatin pudding for dinner, and a couple of chunks of cheese for a bedtime snack.

## "I Don't Get Hungry"

When told that the reporter weighs one-third what he does and eats more than that, the man conceded that he was indeed consuming many fewer calories than he ordinarily did, but that "it's easy to do it because I really don't get hungry."

The medical society panel questioned the long-run success of such a diet as Dr. Atkins proposes. It called such a diet "unbalanced."

Dr. Roger Lerner of the Columbia University College of Physicians and Surgeons said that "losing weight is a learning experience—the patient has to learn the caloric and nutritional values of foods. There are no panaceas. A low-calorie diet with a balance of protein, fat and carbohydrate is the most successful in the long run."

Dr. Jules Hirsch of Rockefeller University, whose studies have shown that fat people have more and larger fat cells in their bodies than thin people, predicted that the Atkins diet fad would flourish and fade just like its dozens of predecessors, "among them the drinking man's diet, the grapefruit diet, the hard-boiled egg diet, the Stillman diet, the Air Force diet—there are almost as many passé diets as there are calories in a piece of chocolate layer cake."

Despite them all, Dr. Hirsch said, about a third of the nation continues to suffer from unwanted, excess body fat.

But it was Dr. Ethan Allan Sims, obesity expert from the University of Vermont Medical Center, who cited one of the most inhibiting aspects of the Atkins diet.

"It's a Jet Set diet—poor people couldn't afford to live on proteins and fats," he said. "Besides America is already living off the top of the food chain—its resources couldn't support the consumption of more animal proteins."

*March 14, 1973*

# Metabolism Found to Adjust for a Body's Natural Weight

### By GINA KOLATA

In a new study that helps explain one of the givens of obesity—that the body has a weight that it naturally gravitates to—researchers have found that all people, fat or thin, adjust their metabolism to maintain that weight.

The body burns calories more slowly than normal after weight is lost, and faster than normal when weight is gained, the study found. This means it is harder both to lose and, perhaps surprising to some, to gain weight than to maintain the same level. In the study, researchers found that in volunteers who gained weight, metabolism was speeded up by 10 percent to 15 percent, and in those who lost weight, metabolism was 10 percent to 15 percent slower than normal. The volunteers, both female and male, ranged in age from their 20s to their 40s, but the effect on metabolism was independent of age and sex.

The researchers also found that the way the body adjusts its metabolism is by making muscles more or less efficient in burning calories. Their findings mean that a 140-pound woman, for example, who has lost 15 pounds to achieve that weight will burn about 10 percent to 15 percent fewer calories when she exercises than a woman who maintains that weight effortlessly. Conversely, if a 140-pound woman gains 15 pounds, she will burn about 10 percent to 15 percent more calories when she exercises than a woman who had always weighed 155 pounds.

The study, conducted by researchers at Rockefeller University in an unusually rigorous manner, was published today in the *New England Journal of Medicine*. Dr. Jules Hirsch, physician in chief at Rockefeller and the senior author of the study, said the findings showed that obesity, rather than being an eating disorder, is "an eating order." Obese people, he said, eat to maintain the weight that puts their energy metabolism precisely on target for their height and body composition.

One myth the study demolishes is that excessive dieting deranges the metabolism. The study showed equally perturbed metabolisms in those who gained and lost weight, whether they had ever dieted and whether they were fat or lean.

Another myth the study debunks is that obese people have unusually slow metabolisms. The only people in the study who showed sluggish metabolisms were those who were trying to maintain a body weight that was lower than their natural weight.

The researchers suggest that the best way to help dieters in the future might be to understand what makes the muscles more or less efficient with weight gain or loss, rather than focusing on diets and psychological counseling.

"I'd say this is a landmark investigation," said Dr. Albert Stunkard, a psychiatrist and weight-loss expert at the University of Pennsylvania School of Medicine. Calling the work "first rate," he said the group's data were so carefully gathered and the study so thorough that "what they are proposing is almost certainly right."

Dr. William Ira Bennett, a psychiatrist at Cambridge Hospital in Cambridge, Mass., who wrote an editorial accompanying the paper, praised the work, saying "what it shows is very very interesting" particularly because it was done on humans, not laboratory animals on which so much of the work on obesity and metabolism has been done.

Weight control is an obsession for many Americans and a big business in this country, but Dr. Rudolph L. Leibel, an author of the study, said what was surprising was how little weight people actually gain. Data from the Framingham Heart Study, an ongoing study of more than 10,000 people in Massachusetts, showed that adults increased their weight, on average, by just 10 percent over 20 years.

For a man to gain 20 pounds over 30 years, he would have had to consume about 60,000 calories more than he needed, Dr. Leibel said. But, he pointed out, those extra 60,000 calories are a minuscule fraction of the 300 million the man had to consume just to maintain his weight. "It's frightening how fine that control is," Dr. Leibel said.

Most people find it easier to gain weight than to lose it. Although it is easy to eat just an extra 200 or so calories a day, resulting in added pounds, it is much harder to subtract 200 or so calories. "It's painful; it hurts to be in negative energy balance," Dr. Leibel said.

Dr. Leibel said he and his colleagues, Dr. Hirsch and Dr. Michael Rosenbaum, began their study because they wanted to understand why it was that the hardest part of dieting was keeping the weight off.

The group recruited 18 people who were obese and 23 who had never been overweight. They were required to live at the clinical center at Rockefeller while their diet and activities were carefully controlled.

For the first four to six weeks, the volunteers ate only a liquid diet that kept their weights absolutely stable. The researchers knew each subject's energy intake and knew that their body weight was not changing, which meant that the subjects were expending the same amount of calories they were taking in.

Then the volunteers purposely gained weight by eating 5,000 to 6,000 additional calories a day until they were 10 percent above their normal weights. Gaining weight was difficult for everyone.

"Some people might imagine that an obese person, given free rein to eat as much as they want, would have a field day," Dr. Leibel said. "But that was absolutely not the case. If anything, the obese subjects had a harder time gaining the extra 10 percent and were more uncomfortable with it."

After the subjects had added 10 percent to their body weight, they were fed liquid formula for four to six weeks with enough calories to keep their weight stable. The researchers repeated the metabolic studies and found increased metabolism.

Then the volunteers lost weight, by consuming 800 calories a day. When they were 10 percent below their normal weights, the researchers maintained them there for four to six weeks with a liquid formula and repeated the metabolic studies, which this time showed a decreased metabolic rate.

The normal-weight volunteers, who were mostly students, received $40 a day for participating, Dr. Leibel said. The obese volunteers were not paid but were promised that at the end of the study, the researchers would keep them on a special diet at the clinical center until they no longer were fat. Some spent a year there after the end of the study, Dr. Leibel said. Most reduced to within 20 percent to 30 percent of the recommended weight for their height and build, and some got down to that weight, but none were able to maintain the weight loss. Inexorably, their weight crept up again.

"This tells you why the recidivism rate to obesity is so enormous," Dr. Leibel said. "Even at a weight loss of 10 percent, the body starts to compensate."

The investigators also studied what the body does to change its metabolism. They found that about 65 percent to 70 percent of calories burned each day are used to keep up the routine body functions—the pumping heart, the working kidneys, the metabolizing liver. About 10 percent to 15 percent are spent eating and assimilating food. And the rest, about 15 percent to 25 percent, are spent by the muscles' exercising.

Now, Dr. Leibel said, "we need to figure out what the heck is going on in muscle."

One possibility is that the muscle fibers themselves may change their composition slightly. The red muscles, which are used for long-distance walking or running, for example, use fewer calories to do their work. The white muscles, used for sudden bursts of energy in activities like lifting weights or sprinting, burn more calories. When a person's weight is 10 percent or more above his or her natural weight, Dr. Leibel speculated, that person "may shift from predominantly red to predominantly white fibers, or have enzymes that do that."

But, Dr. Bennett said, the answer for dieters is not in the immediate offing. "Over and over again, people have been told there's an answer, and it's a terrible betrayal to have people think we are close," he said.

For now, Dr. Bennett added, "the key thing is to use the muscles." He added: "I'm speaking from personal experience. I bought a car five years ago and gained 30 pounds.

*March 9, 1995*

# Some Extra Heft May Be Helpful, New Study Says

## By GINA KOLATA

People who are overweight but not obese have a lower risk of death than those of normal weight, federal researchers are reporting today.

The researchers—statisticians and epidemiologists from the National Cancer Institute and the Centers for Disease Control and Prevention—also found that increased risk of death from obesity was seen for the most part in the extremely obese, a group constituting only 8 percent of Americans.

And being very thin, even though the thinness was longstanding and unlikely to stem from disease, was correlated with a slight increase in the risk of death, the researchers said.

The new study, considered by many independent scientists to be the most rigorous yet on the effects of weight, controlled for factors like smoking, age, race and alcohol consumption in a sophisticated analysis derived from a well-known method that has been used to predict cancer risk.

It also used the federal government's own weight categories, which define fatness and thinness according to a "body mass index" correlating weight to height, regardless of sex. For example, 5-foot-8 people weighing less than 122 pounds are underweight. If they weighed 122 to 164 pounds, their weight would be normal. They would be overweight at 165 to 196, obese at 197 to 229, and extremely obese at 230 or over.

Researchers had a full gamut of responses to the unexpected findings, being reported today in the *Journal of the American Medical Association.*

Some saw the report as a long-needed reality check on what they consider the nation's near-hysteria over fat.

"I love it," said Dr. Steven Blair, president and chief executive of the Cooper Institute, a research and educational organization in Dallas that focuses on preventive medicine.

"There are people who have made up their minds that obesity and overweight are the biggest public health problem that we have to face," Dr. Blair said. "These numbers show that maybe it's not that big."

Others simply did not believe the findings.

Dr. JoAnn Manson, chief of preventive medicine at Brigham and Women's Hospital in Boston, which is affiliated with Harvard, pointed to the university's own study of nurses that found mortality risks in being overweight and even greater risks in being obese. (That study involved mostly white women and used statistical methods different from those in the newly reported research.)

"We can't afford to be complacent about the epidemic of obesity," Dr. Manson said.

In fact, the new study addressed the risk only of death and not of disability or disease. There has long been conclusive evidence that as people move from overweight to obese to extremely obese, they are more and more likely to have diabetes, high blood pressure and high cholesterol levels.

But the investigators said it was possible that being fat was less of a health risk than it used to be. They mentioned a paper, also being published today in the journal, in which researchers including Dr. Edward W. Gregg and Dr. David F. Williamson, both of the C.D.C., report that high blood pressure and high cholesterol levels are less prevalent now than they were 30 or 40 years ago, largely because of breakthroughs in medication.

As for whether there is truly a mortality risk in being underweight, Dr. Mark Mattson, a rail-thin researcher at the National Institute on Aging who is an expert on caloric restriction as a means of prolonging life, said it was not clear that eating fewer calories meant weighing so little, since some people eat very little and never get so thin. In any event, while caloric restriction may extend life, Dr. Mattson said, "there's certainly a point where you can overdo it with caloric restriction, and we don't know what that point is."

Some statisticians and epidemiologists said that the study's methods and data were exemplary and that the authors—Dr. Williamson and Dr. Katherine M. Flegal of the disease control centers, and Dr. Barry I. Graubard and Dr. Mitchell H. Gail of the cancer institute—were experienced and highly regarded scientists.

"This is a well-known group, and I thought their analysis and their statistical approaches were very good," said Dr. Barbara Hulka, an emerita professor of epidemiology at the University of North Carolina.

The study did not explain why overweight appeared best as far as mortality was concerned. But Dr. Williamson said the reason might be that most people die when they are over 70. Having a bit of extra fat in old age appears to be protective, he said, giving rise to more muscle and more bone.

"It's called the obesity paradox," Dr. Williamson said. But, he said, while the paradox is real, the reasons are speculative. "It's raw conjecture," he said.

The new study comes just 13 months after different researchers from the disease control centers published a paper warning that obesity and overweight were causing an extra 400,000 deaths a year and were poised to overtake smoking as the nation's leading preventable cause of premature death.

That conclusion caused an uproar, and scientists, particularly those who examine the consequences of smoking, questioned the study's methods. In January, the agency's researchers corrected calculation errors and published a revised estimate of 365,000 deaths.

Now the new study says that obesity and extreme obesity are causing about 112,000 extra deaths but that overweight is preventing about 86,000, leaving a net toll of some 26,000 deaths in all three categories combined, compared with the 34,000 extra deaths found in those who are underweight.

Dr. Donna Stroup, director of the Coordinating Center for Health Promotion at the C.D.C., noted that the previous study had used different data and different methods of analysis.

"Counting deaths is not an exact science," Dr. Stroup said.

For now, said Dr. Dixie Snider, the disease control centers' chief science officer, the agency will not take a position on what is the true number of deaths from obesity and overweight. "We're too early in the science," Dr. Snider said.

Dr. Stroup said of the new findings, "From a scientific point of view, they are a step forward." But she added that the agency considered illness that is linked to obesity to be just as important as the number of deaths.

"Mortality really only represents the tip of the iceberg of the magnitude of the problem," she said.

Estimating deaths due to overweight or obesity is a statistical challenge, the study's investigators said. The idea is to determine, for each person in the population, what would be the risk of dying if that person's weight were normal.

For people whose weight is already in that range, there would be no change in the risk, of course. But what happens to the risk for people whose weight is above or below the normal range? The idea is to control for factors like age, smoking and gender, and ask what would happen if only the weight were changed.

Now that the researchers have done their analysis, Dr. Williamson said, the message, as he sees it, is that perhaps people should take other factors into consideration when deciding whether to worry about the health risks of their weight.

Dr. Williamson, who is overweight, said that "if I had a family history—a father who had a heart attack at 52 or a brother who developed diabetes—I would actively lose weight."

But "if my father died at 94 and my mother at 97 and I had no family history of chronic disease," he said, "maybe I wouldn't be as concerned."

Dr. Barry Glassner, a sociology professor at the University of Southern California, had another perspective.

"The take-home message from this study, it seems to me, is unambiguous," Dr. Glassner said. "What is officially deemed overweight these days is actually the optimal weight."

*April 20, 2005*

CHAPTER 10

# Ethics

# Nazi Medical Horrors Revealed at New Trials

By DANA ADAMS SCHMIDT

Following close upon the exposure of the cosmic crimes of the war lords and politicians tried before the International Military Tribunal, an American Military Government Tribunal at Nuremberg is now ferreting out details of crimes committed by a part of the German medical profession so hideous that the Nazis bent every effort to keep them secret.

The trial of twenty doctors and scientists and three laymen, now nearing its end, has exposed ghoulish experiments on living men and women and a program of extermination by gassing, lethal injection and sterilization conducted in remote clinics, asylums and concentration camps.

Specifically, the case has become a trial of the Nazi racial doctrine. For the victims of experiments and extermination were drawn from "inferior peoples"—Russians, Poles and other Slavs, and Jews and gypsies. The experiments were pretended to further military medical science, but were really to devise new methods of inconspicuous mass killing, of "inferior, useless or undesirable people." This is what Brig. Gen. Telford Taylor in his opening address called the science of thanatology. To it certain German medical men, abandoning the Hippocratic oath and all codes of ethics, devoted themselves. Some of the men who bore top administrative responsibility for this activity, such as Dr. Leonard Conti, chief of civilian medical services, committed suicide at the end of the war. The others today blame orders imposed by Hitler and Himmler.

## Fields Explored

Gerhardt Rome, an expert in tropical medicine with an international reputation, is professionally the most "distinguished." Today he professes to despise the unscientific and barbarous activities of the others in the dock but he provided fly eggs for malaria experiment on inmates of the Dachau concentration camp, causing 300 or 400 deaths.

Lesser administrators and doctors performed the gruesome tasks. In addition to those mentioned the subjects of their experiments included the effects of high altitude and freezing, poisoning induced by bullets and woodshavings or ground glass rubbed into wounds, spotted fever, bone and muscle transplanting, uses of sulphanilamide, and effects of mustard gas and incendiary bombs.

In a report on one of the high altitude experiments at Dachau defendants Siegfried Ruff and Hans Romberg described as follows the reactions of a Jewish delicatessen clerk who, deprived of an oxygen mask, had been raised to an atmospheric elevation of 47,000 feet inside a low pressure chamber:

"Spasmodic convulsions, arms stretched stiffly forward, sits up like a dog, legs spread stiffly apart, agonal convulsive breathing, convulsions and groaning, yells aloud, convulses arms and legs, grimaces, bites his tongue, does not respond to speech, gives the impression of someone who is completely out of his mind."

## Victims Frozen to Death

Also at Dachau defendants under the direction of an arch fiend named Sigmund Rascher, now believed dead, exposed victims to freezing temperatures for fourteen hours or immersed them in near-freezing water for three hours. Herta Oberheuser, the lone woman on trial, was charged with having selected young and healthy inmates of the Ravensbruck women's camp for experiments. Karl Gebhardt, surgical adviser to the Waffen SS, is charged with having gone to Ravensbruck to perform sterilizations and of having removed a bone from the shoulder of a healthy Polish woman to transplant it on the shoulder of an ailing friend. Victor Brack, who handled the administrative details of the euthanasia program, wrote recommendations that Russians and others should be sterilized by X-ray emanating from a counter before which they would be required to pass, ostensibly to fill out forms.

Equally horrifying practices have come to light in the trials of forty-three members of the staffs of the Eighberg Kaimenof and Hadamar medical institutions before a German court in Frankfort on the Main. At Hadamar, naked men and women were driven into a "shower" room where they were gassed and later cremated until the ceaseless smoke from the crematorium induced the Bishop of Limburg to protest to Hitler.

## Defense Denies Race Theory

None of the defendants before the United States or German courts has dared to invoke the Nazi motive for his act. This was that the victims were physically, mentally or racially inferior and must be eliminated to make way for the pure-bred master race. Instead they refer to a higher authority that they dared not oppose.

They maintain, also, that they thought the victims of the experiments were volunteers, condemned criminals who had received a promise of pardon if they survived or that the mass killings were merciful euthanasia.

All this has been faithfully reported to the German public. Two dozen German correspondents are in attendance in Nuremberg, including representatives of the German news agencies of all four zones. The United States zone radio network broadcasts three fifteen-minute commentaries on the trials. One this week was devoted to the Strasbourg University skeleton collection, for which eighty-six representative Jewish types were selected and slaughtered.

Nearly 100 German spectators observe the Nuremberg medical trials daily. They are checked only for criminal records before admission and many erstwhile Nazis are known to attend. Frequently groups of medical students ask for passes.

The German public at large, however, has heard these or similar stories over and over during the long series of trials.

## Germans Satiated

Today Germans are satiated with horror. Many a German wearily switches off the radio when talk on the concentration camp atrocities begins. With satiation appear to have come these reactions:

1. Almost all Germans will admit today that these things happened—that they are not mere propaganda.

2. They will hasten to add they knew nothing of such horrors at the time and were certainly in no way responsible. They knew there were concentration camps but this, never.

3. While there is no sign of any feeling of collective guilt, there is a widespread feeling of revulsion against the acts committed by some leading Nazis.

Few observers would risk the opinion that German reaction goes much beyond revulsion at present. But it is the higher purpose of the trials, as laid down by General Taylor, to lead the Germans to the broader conclusions that such crimes epitomize the Nazi way of life and that they and other disasters followed inevitably when the Germans allowed their individual reason and conscience to be swept away by a dictator with an irrational and immoral doctrine of racial superiority.

In the long run it will be up to German writers, politicians and leaders in all fields to make this an integral part of German thought.

The initial impulse is in the hands of United States judges and attorneys in charge of the trials. Among them are Justice Walter B. Beals, former Chief Justice of the Supreme Court of the State of Washington; H. L. Sebring, judge of the Supreme Court of Florida, and Johnson T. Crawford, on the bench of the Oklahoma District Court for twenty-two years. An alternate is Lieut. Col. V. C. Swearinger, former assistant attorney general of Michigan, who served as a combat intelligence officer during the war.

The prosecuting attorney is James M. McHaney of Little Rock, Ark., formerly of the New York law firm of Cabin, Gordon, Salhry & Reindal. His deputy is Alexander G. Hardy of Boston, Mass., veteran of three years' service with the Navy.

*March 2, 1947*

# Many Scientific Experts Condemn Ethics of Cancer Injection

By JOHN A. OSMUNDSEN

Medical research circles are buzzing over the disclosure last week of experiments in which persons were injected with living cancer cells without their knowledge.

Discussion centers less on the legality of the experiments than on the ethics and morality of them. Opinion is varied, but it leans heavily toward condemnation of the failure to inform the subjects of the research about exactly what was being done to them.

Varied reactions were expressed in interviews with several scientists active in clinical research and other authorities who have studied the ethics and morality of human experimentation.

Judgment ranged from the opinion that the experiments were "completely indefensible" on ethical grounds, and should not have been conducted at all, to the view that the experimenters were justified in the way they did their research. Both extremes were minority opinions.

The majority expressed the view that the studies were important and productive and should have been done, but that it was unethical not to tell the subjects that they were receiving living cancer cells instead of just "cells," as the experimenters had described the tests to the patients.

## Scientists Disagree

The scientists who did this work, on the other hand, insisted that to tell many of the patients who took part in the research that they were receiving cancer cells would have been unethical.

The reason they gave for this was that a person who has cancer and will not admit it to himself—or has not been told of it—would be forced into the realization of his condition and that this would be psychologically harmful to him.

The problem came to light last Monday when it was disclosed that 22 patients at Brooklyn's Jewish Chronic Disease Hospital had been injected with living cancer cells with their consent but without their knowing what the injections really consisted of.

It came out subsequently that nearly 300 other patients at the Sloan-Kettering

215

Institute for Cancer Research and Memorial Hospital for Cancer and Allied Diseases had also participated in this work and that many of them had, similarly, not been told that the injections contained living cancer cells.

A third group, inmates of the Ohio State Penitentiary in Columbus, Ohio, volunteered for the tests, knowing that the injections consisted of cancer cells.

The research, under the direction of Dr. Chester M. Southam of Sloan-Kettering, has been going on for 10 years. It is aimed at studying the nature of the body's defense mechanisms—the immune reactions—in healthy persons, cancer patients and persons suffering from chronic diseases other than cancer.

The important outcome of the study so far is that a cancer patient's immune mechanisms are deficient, compared with those of the two other groups. The nature of the deficiency is now being studied.

Possible fruits of the work include the knowledge of how to help cancer patients fight their own tumors with immune reactions, how to manipulate the reaction so that grafts of foreign tissues would be practicable, and how to transfer immunity to disease from one person to another.

## Value Not Questioned

Thus, there has never been any question of the potential value of the research.

Neither has there been much doubt about the safety of experiments. Sufficient experience with the injection of cancer cells in animals and in humans—many of them scientists, or volunteers who were told what they were getting—has shown that the risk of, say, causing cancer by the injections was considered to be very low.

Nor has there been any question of the competence and high standards of Dr. Southam, who is recognized as one of the world's leading authorities in this field.

Two supporters of the manner in which the work was done, in fact, declared that if the same procedure had been followed by almost any scientist other than Dr. Southam they would have thought it unethical, their regard for him was so high.

Rather, the question of ethics has been raised over the matter of whether the scientists usurped the rights of the subjects to make their own decisions about taking part in the experiments.

It was pointed out by several critics of the work that these experiments were distinctly different from the sort of clinical research that is aimed at evaluating the efficacy of a new drug or vaccine or other therapeutic procedure.

Such studies, they pointed out, are of direct potential benefit to the individual being tested. By contrast, the possibility of immediate benefit to the subject was not a consideration of the Sloan-Kettering project.

Moreover, the critics said, because a physical act on the person of the subject was involved in the research, a finite—though small—risk was involved. They asserted that this called for the complete disclosure to the subject of the nature of the injection.

In this respect, Dr. Southam said in an interview:

"It is not necessary to present [the subject] with what you feel are inconsequential data and [it is] unethical to ram down his throat information which is detrimental to his condition."

Asked whether it would not be possible to use as subjects cancer sufferers who knew of their condition and so would not suffer from the revelation, Dr. Southam replied:

"You just don't know what the patient really knows or has accepted by himself."

Dr. Southam was asked why the subjects at Jewish Chronic Disease Hospital who did not have cancer were similarly deprived of the knowledge that the injections contained living malignant cells.

He replied that the preparation of the patients and acquisition of their consent was left up to Jewish Hospital officials, who had decided simply to follow procedures that had been used for so long by the Sloan-Kettering team.

The controversy gains significance because of the growing amount of human experimentation. The ethics and morality of such experimentation have been discussed in medical journals in this country and abroad and by panels in medical schools.

## Code Adopted

An ethical code has been adopted by some institutions in this country and elsewhere: the Nuremberg Code for Permissible Human Experiments.

The first article of that code states:

"The voluntary consent of the human subject is absolutely essential. This means that the person involved should have legal capacity to give consent; should be so situated as to be able to exercise free choice, without the intervention of any element of force, fraud, deceit, duress, overreaching, or other ulterior form of constraint or coercion; and should have sufficient knowledge and comprehension of the elements of the subject matter involved as to enable him to make an understanding and enlightened decision."

State health officials are reported to be studying whether a stricter code of ethics for clinical research would be needed or justified.

The board now has no regulations about what kind of consent, written or oral, is required from patients in scientific experiments.

Although many hospitals "do not go in for 'paper,'" as one authority phrased the attitude toward written consent, some experts believe that this is the only ethical form of agreement and that vocal consent is not enough.

*January 26, 1964*

# Physician Scores Tests on Humans

By JOHN A. OSMUNDSEN

AUGUSTA, MICH.—A noted medical researcher assailed today what he said "seem to be breaches of ethical conduct in experimentation" on humans.

The critic was Dr. Henry K. Beecher, Henry I. Dorr Professor of Research in Anesthesia at Harvard University and chief anesthetist at Massachusetts General Hospital.

He attacked experiments performed on persons without their informed consent that "cannot by any stretch of the imagination be construed as for [their] benefit."

Dr. Beecher cited cases in which 23 charity patients died in 1963 because they were deprived of the standard treatment for typhoid fever. He also mentioned 25 United States servicemen who were "crippled for life" in 1956 because they were denied treatment that would have prevented the development of rheumatic fever.

Instances of such practice, the scientist said, "are by no means rare but are almost, one fears, universal" and are increasing as the amount of experimentation on man grows.

## Dr. Beecher Countered

"Dr. Beecher's views came under immediate attack from other medical scientists who attended a two-day symposium on clinical research given by the Upjohn Company here.

One called the criticism "a gross and irresponsible exaggeration" and another declared that the charges would do serious damage to medical research in this country.

Dr. Beecher emphasized that he was not referring to the clinical testing of new drugs or of new procedures that are done for the patient's good. He indicated that obtaining the "informed consent" of the patient in such instances was not required because "the necessary consent is understood in the presentation of the patient to the physician for treatment."

Dr. Beecher was concerned about the use of hospitalized patients, military personnel, convicts, medical students and laboratory personnel for experiments in which the subjects are not asked for their permission nor told what is being done and what the risks might be.

The Boston physician asserted that such cases of clinical research "are easy to find." A British colleague has compiled a list of 500 examples, he said.

In his paper "Ethics and the Explosion of Human Experimentation," Dr. Beecher cited 50 examples of clinical experiments that he thought were ethically questionable.

These are some of the examples Dr. Beecher described.

Last year, 18 children ranging in age from 3½ months to 18 years old were selected from a group about to undergo surgery for congenital heart disease. Of that number, 11 were to have their thymus glands removed, the remaining seven to serve as controls, retaining that gland in their chests. In addition, the skin from an unrelated adult was grafted to the chest wall of each child. The experiment was described as "part of a long-range study of the growth and development of these children over the years."

## Heart Experiment Cited

In another case in 1960, seven patients were put under general anaesthesia and a double needle was thrust through their chest so that one part entered a chamber on the right side of the heart and the other a chamber on the left.

"No indication is given as to the source of the patients or the relevancy of this test to their required medical care," Dr. Beecher said. He observed that the experimenters who did the work believed that their method "may be valuable clinically as soon as safety has been confirmed by additional work."

Another study in 1962 of the effect of a drug on liver function was performed on 50 inmates of a children's center who included mental defectives and juvenile delinquents. None had a disease worse than acne, Dr. Beecher said, yet some were given repeated doses of the drug, which caused abnormal liver function for as long as five weeks.

In disagreement with Dr. Beecher were Dr. Thomas Chalmers, professor of medicine at Tufts University, and Dr. David Rutstein, professor of preventive medicine at Harvard Medical School.

Neither, however, disagreed with Dr. Beecher's contention that humans should not be subjected without their knowledge and consent to experiments that could not benefit them.

Dr. Beecher said that informed, paid volunteers were about the only type of acceptable subjects for such experimentation.

*March 24, 1965*

# Willowbrook Doctor Is Striving to End 2 Snake Pits

## By HOMER BIGART

At Willowbrook State School for the mentally retarded, two locked wards merit the term snake pits.

Wards A and C in Building 9 of the Staten Island institution each contain 75 profoundly retarded and severely disturbed men. Kept docile by massive doses of tranquillizers, they represent the total negation of human dignity and hope.

"With proper facilities and adequate staff, something could be done to improve the condition of these men," said Dr. Jack Hammond, director of the school, as he unlocked the door to Ward C for a visitor late Friday. "But there is nothing I can do now."

The door swung open. A staff assistant had prepared the visitor for shock: "You'll be lucky if you don't see a patient drinking from a lavatory."

The dayroom, a few steps beyond the toilets, was crowded with nude, shapeless male bodies.

## Slumped, Dozing, Staring

Some of the men, slouched against the drab walls, were standing in puddles of their own urine. Others shambled about, muttering incoherent sounds. There were heavy benches in the center of the room, and these were filled with slumping men, dozing or staring vacantly at the floor.

There was a violent stench. The men were bathed twice a day, Dr. Hammond said, but were always fouling themselves.

The ward attendant was a woman. In her white uniform, looking as placid as though she were in a well-ordered hospital, the attendant was surrounded by milling, grunting men.

Dr. Hammond said it was very difficult to get male attendants to work in this ward. Actually, the woman attendant was quite safe from sexual assault, he said, because these patients lacked the psycho-sexual development to be interested in heterosexual acts.

This was the ward that had prompted Senator Robert F. Kennedy to describe the institution as "filthy" and "zoo-like." It was the ward where, two months ago, one man slugged another in the neck, fracturing his larynx so that the man died quickly of suffocation.

Wards A and C are "disgraceful," Dr. Hammond said, so crowded that it is quite impossible to prevent assaults, even homicides. There have been five violent deaths in the institution—two of them homicides—in the 14 months of Dr. Hammond's tenure.

All could have been avoided with adequate staffing, Dr. Hammond said in a voice cold with anger.

Instead of herding 75 severely disturbed men in one ward, Dr. Hammond would put them in groups of no more than 15 each and give them therapeutic programs. But at the moment there aren't even enough attendants to toilet-train these men.

"They are being de-humanized," Dr. Hammond said. "Nobody talks to them."

The other wards, even the wards for children, were also desperately understaffed. And although conditions there seemed tolerable, Dr. Hammond warned that unless the children received more training, attention and human contact, many might become as profoundly retarded and disturbed as the men in Building 9.

In one of the children's wards, two attendants were trying to feed 40 children.

## An Occasional Whimper

A stillness, unusual in children's wards, was broken only by an occasional whimper. Several mongoloid children were in the room and there were a few others who were afflicted with hydrocephalus, a condition caused by the accumulation of fluid within the head.

On a wheelchair sat a startling figure. Irene, a 6-year-old girl with hydrocephalus, looked at first like a doll whose maker had attached a head grotesquely large to the image of a normal child's torso.

Irene's head rocked slowly back and forth, rhythmic as the pendulum of a clock, but she was in no pain and she gave a sweet smile while Dr. Hammond spoke to her.

Turning to the visitor, Dr. Hammond said: "If these retarded children were in the community and able to live at home, they'd be attending special classes in public schools; they'd be in school from 9 a.m. to 3 p.m., and there would be one teacher for every 15 children.

"Here," and his voice became indignant, "only about 15 of 186 children in this building are exposed to a teacher for one and one-half hours a day."

Dr. Hammond began a fight for more facilities and more staff soon after taking office in July, 1964. He reported a "most deplorable condition" at Willowbrook to his chief, the late Dr. Paul Hoch, Commissioner of the New York State Department of Mental Hygiene.

## Shut-off Urged

At that time the institution was even more crowded than now, with more than 6,000 patients squeezed into buildings designed for little more than 4,000.

Dr. Hammond urged the shut-off of all new admissions except for children under 5. Dr. Hoch approved the recommendation and ordered admissions closed for a 90-day period, after which they were reopened on a selective basis and only to those buildings where a vacancy occurred within the allowed capacities.

There have been no vacancies except in buildings for children under 5, and for which there is a waiting list of almost 400. For those over 5, there is now a waiting list of nearly 500 names.

When he came to Willowbrook, Dr. Hammond discovered to his "utter amazement" that patients were hastily screened on the day of admission and immediately assigned to buildings. This had resulted in the mixing of dangerous and aggressive persons with patients who were docile and only moderately retarded.

With Dr. Hoch's approval, Dr. Hammond instituted a preadmission evaluation of each patient and established a diagnostic and counseling center for the careful screening of applicants for admission.

There are still "about three or four" dangerous individuals at Willowbrook. Dr. Hammond has asked the State Supreme Court for authority to transfer three of them to the Eastern Correctional Institution at Napanoch. The necessary papers were filed several months ago, but the patients are still in Willowbrook.

One, with a history of arson, has set two fires within the institution, Dr. Hammond said. In July, 1964, the court sent back the papers, suggesting they be submitted through the District Attorney's office. This was done, but there has been no further action.

## Plans Outlined

In his report to Dr. Hoch a year ago, Dr. Hammond also outlined some long-range plans for increasing the therapeutic and training services.

He said he received prompt and complete backing from both Dr. Hoch and the present Acting Commissioner, Dr. Christopher F. Terrance. And Governor Rockefeller always supported the department's budget recommendations, he added.

But getting the money out of the Legislature was not easy. The Governor asked for a $100 million increase in the current budget for the department, which had spent $280 million last year. The Legislature allowed only a $30 million increase.

What Senator Kennedy said about Willowbrook was true enough, Dr. Hammond said yesterday, but he wished that the Senator had added a few kind words about his overworked staff and the fact that some happy developments were taking place there.

## Research Sought

These included a research program by the New York University School of Medicine, which is trying to develop a measles vaccine (a mother afflicted with German measles in pregnancy can give birth to a mentally defective child), and the construction of a $7 million Institute for Basic Research in Mental Retardation at the east end of the campus.

There is also some hope for getting adequate custodial help.

Dr. Hammond has been authorized five additional physicians (there are now 29), 182 more attendants, an additional psychologist and two social service workers.

But there is no immediate prospect of relieving the overcrowding, and this unpleasant condition is the main reason for the excessive turnover in employees.

Nearly one out of every four new employees quits after only two months at Willowbrook.

*September 13, 1965*

# U.S. Issues Rules on Human Testing

By HAROLD M. SCHMECK JR.

The Department of Health, Education and Welfare published today regulations codifying its policies for protecting the rights of human subjects of research.

A cardinal principle of the code is a regulation that require review committees at every institution doing research with support from the department if the research involves human subjects.

Another basic principle is that the subjects of the research be informed of the risks and potential benefits and that they voluntarily consent to take part, with the understanding that they can withdraw at any time.

The regulations also specify that the research must offer potential benefits to patients or to scientific knowledge sufficient to justify the risks and discomforts the studies might involve.

The Secretary of Health, Education and Welfare is given broad discretion to rule on the adequacy of the committees and to restrict the use of specific research procedures and the types of individual taking part as subjects of research.

While the specifics addressed in the new regulations are aimed largely at problems of medical research, the language appears to be broad enough to include also research in education, sociology and even such items as experiments in income maintenance for welfare patients. Some persons familiar with the regulations say this aspect raises potential problems. For example, would informed consent be necessary before a teacher could introduce an innovation in teaching arithmetic to elementary school pupils?

## Some Untouched Areas

The new regulations do not contain specific guidelines for such controversial subjects as psychosurgery, research on the human fetus or research involving prisoners. Proposed regulations concerning these areas are to be publicized this summer.

In general, an official involved in drafting the regulations said today, the statement published in the *Federal Register* amplifies and codifies policies that have been developed in the department over the last decade.

Review committees and informed consent, for example, have long been required. The new regulations give specifics such as the requirement that membership in a review committee must not be limited to employees of the institution where the research is done or to professional groups such as physicians, psychologists or sociologists.

The research subject's informed consent is defined in terms of the Nuremberg code: "The knowing consent of an individual or his legally authorized representative, so situated as to be able to exercise free power of choice without undue inducement or any element of force, fraud, deceit, duress or other form of constraint or coercion."

The Nuremberg code, covering the ethics of medical research, was drawn up in connection with the trials of war criminals after World War II.

The health department's regulation concerning the subject's right to withdraw from a research project specifies that this shall be "without prejudice."

*May 31, 1974*

# U.S. Apologizes for Syphilis Tests in Guatemala

By DONALD G. MCNEIL JR.

From 1946 to 1948, American public health doctors deliberately infected nearly 700 Guatemalans—prison inmates, mental patients and soldiers—with venereal diseases in what was meant as an effort to test the effectiveness of penicillin.

American tax dollars, through the National Institutes of Health, even paid for syphilis-infected prostitutes to sleep with prisoners, since Guatemalan prisons allowed such visits. When the prostitutes did not succeed in infecting the men, some prisoners had the bacteria poured onto scrapes made on their penises, faces or arms, and in some cases it was injected by spinal puncture.

If the subjects contracted the disease, they were given antibiotics.

"However, whether everyone was then cured is not clear," said Susan M. Reverby, the professor at Wellesley College who brought the experiments to light in a research paper that prompted American health officials to investigate.

The revelations were made public on Friday, when Secretary of State Hillary Rodham Clinton and Health and Human Services Secretary Kathleen Sebelius apologized to the government of Guatemala and the survivors and descendants of those infected. They called the experiments "clearly unethical."

"Although these events occurred more than 64 years ago, we are outraged that such reprehensible research could have occurred under the guise of public health," the secretaries said in a statement. "We deeply regret that it happened, and we apologize to all the individuals who were affected by such abhorrent research practices."

In a twist to the revelation, the public health doctor who led the experiment, John C. Cutler, would later have an important role in the Tuskegee study in which black American men with syphilis were deliberately left untreated for decades. Late in his own life, Dr. Cutler continued to defend the Tuskegee work.

His unpublished Guatemala work was unearthed recently in the archives of the University of Pittsburgh by Professor Reverby, a medical historian who has written two books about Tuskegee.

President Álvaro Colom of Guatemala, who first learned of the experiments on Thursday in a phone call from Mrs. Clinton, called them "hair-raising" and "crimes against humanity." His government said it would cooperate with the American investigation and do its own.

The experiments are "a dark chapter in the history of medicine," said Dr. Francis S. Collins, director of the National Institutes of Health. Modern rules for federally financed research "absolutely prohibit" infecting people without their informed consent, Dr. Collins said.

Professor Reverby presented her findings about the Guatemalan experiments at a conference in January, but nobody took notice, she said in a telephone interview Friday. In June, she sent a draft of an article she was preparing for the January 2011 issue of the *Journal of Policy History* to Dr. David J. Sencer, a former director of the Centers for Disease Control. He prodded the government to investigate.

In the 1940s, Professor Reverby said, the United States Public Health Service "was deeply interested in whether penicillin could be used to prevent, not just cure, early syphilis infection, whether better blood tests for the disease could be established, what dosages of penicillin actually cured infection, and to understand the process of re-infection after cures."

It had difficulties growing syphilis in the laboratory, and its tests on rabbits and chimpanzees told it little about how penicillin worked in humans.

In 1944, it injected prison "volunteers" at the Terre Haute Federal Penitentiary in Indiana with lab-grown gonorrhea, but found it hard to infect people that way.

In 1946, Dr. Cutler was asked to lead the Guatemala mission, which ended two years later, partly because of medical "gossip" about the work, Professor Reverby said, and partly because he was using so much penicillin, which was costly and in short supply.

Dr. Cutler would later join the study in Tuskegee, Ala., which had begun relatively innocuously in 1932 as an observation of how syphilis progressed in black male sharecroppers. In 1972, it was revealed that, even when early antibiotics were invented, doctors hid that fact from the men in order to keep studying them. Dr. Cutler, who died in 2003, defended the Tuskegee experiment in a 1993 documentary.

Deception was also used in Guatemala, Professor Reverby said. Dr. Thomas Parran, the former surgeon general who oversaw the start of Tuskegee, acknowledged that the Guatemala work could not be done domestically, and details were hidden from Guatemalan officials.

Professor Reverby said she found some of Dr. Cutler's papers at the University of Pittsburgh, where he taught until 1985, while she was researching Dr. Parran.

"I'm sifting through them, and I find 'Guatemala . . . inoculation . . .' and I think 'What the heck is this?' And then it was 'Oh my god, oh my god, oh my god.' My partner was with me, and I told him, 'You aren't going to believe this.'"

Fernando de la Cerda, minister counselor at the Guatemalan Embassy in Washington, said that Mrs. Clinton apologized to President Colom in her Thursday phone call. "We thank the United States for its transparency in telling us the facts," he said.

Asked about the possibility of reparations for survivors or descendants, Mr. de la Cerda said that was still unclear.

The public response on the Web sites of Guatemalan news outlets was furious. One commenter, Cesar Duran, on the site of *Prensa Libre* wrote: "APOLOGIES ... please ... this is what has come to light, but what is still hidden? They should pay an indemnity to the state of Guatemala, not just apologize."

Dr. Mark Siegler, director of the Maclean Center for Clinical Medical Ethics at the University of Chicago's medical school, said he was stunned. "This is shocking," Dr. Siegler said. "This is much worse than Tuskegee—at least those men were infected by natural means."

He added: "It's ironic—no, it's worse than that, it's appalling—that, at the same time as the United States was prosecuting Nazi doctors for crimes against humanity, the U.S. government was supporting research that placed human subjects at enormous risk."

The Nuremberg trials of Nazi doctors who experimented on concentration camp inmates and prisoners led to a code of ethics, though it had no force of law. In the 1964 Helsinki Declaration, the medical associations of many countries adopted a code.

The Tuskegee scandal and the hearings into it conducted by Senator Edward M. Kennedy became the basis for the 1981 American laws governing research on human subjects, Dr. Siegler said.

It was preceded by other domestic scandals. From 1963 to 1966, researchers at the Willowbrook State School on Staten Island infected retarded children with hepatitis to test gamma globulin against it. And in 1963, elderly patients at the Brooklyn Jewish Chronic Disease Hospital were injected with live cancer cells to see if they caused tumors.

Elisabeth Malkin contributed reporting from Mexico City.

*October 1, 2010*

CHAPTER 11

# The Flu

# Spanish Influenza Here, Ship Men Say

A disease, which the officers of a Norwegian steamship which arrived here yesterday insisted was the Spanish influenza, caused the death of four persons on the voyage. When the vessel reached this port yesterday ten men and women severely ill and exhibiting all the symptoms of the disease which caused the death of the other four were taken ashore for treatment. One of these patients, Mrs. Jensine Olsen, who lived in Flint, Mich., and was on her way to join her husband, died in the Norwegian Hospital soon after she reached that institution.

Whether the disease was the true Spanish influenza was not officially determined yesterday, but Dr. Edward G. Cornwell of 1218 Jackson Avenue, Brooklyn, who treated the patients from the ship, said yesterday that the immediate cause of Mrs. Olsen's death was bronchial pneumonia. As far as he could determine, he added, no symptoms of Spanish influenza had been evident in any of the cases, and he was treating them on a diagnosis of pneumonia.

At the hospital it was learned that the patients had not been isolated, and, it was asserted, they would not have passed quarantine had they been suffering from true Spanish influenza. One of them is Arvid Sundstrom, 17 years old, whose father makes his home at the Hotel Lorraine.

## 200 Passengers Ill at One Time

Late last night it was said that all the cases with one exception were diagnosed as pneumonia and that the exception was a child afflicted with bronchial pneumonia. It was also said, however, that some of the passengers on board asserted that during the voyage 200 passengers had been sick at one time, the illness lasting several days.

When asked whether the illness might not have been seasickness the passengers said that the illness was accompanied by high fever. One of the patients in the Norwegian Hospital, an educated woman with two children, told the hospital physician she was sure that the illness was not seasickness. Her children, she said, were taken with it and they both had high fever. The physician in charge at the hospital said that evidently there had been some kind of an epidemic on board, but he was unable to tell the exact nature of it because he did not have the history of the patients.

The officers of the ship said yesterday that the disease was brought on board at Bergen by a woman passenger in the third class, who came from Finland. After the first victim died four days out from the port one of the crew, an assistant cook, who looked after the third-class passengers, contracted the disease and also died, and was buried at sea. The Spanish influenza, which was said to have really started among the Russian armies on the eastern frontier in the Winter of 1915, commenced with pains followed by fever and delirium generally lasting four days, and left the patients so weak that it took two weeks or more to recover.

The victims of the disease on the Norwegian steamship, it was asserted, had pneumonia after the fever, which was the cause of death in 33 per cent of the cases. The death of the cook was followed by two of the women in the third class, which occurred just before the steamship put into Halifax, and they were buried at sea.

## Health Officer Passed Ship

The cases of mysterious illness were reported to the health officer by the surgeon when the steamship arrived at the quarantine station yesterday, and he did not regard the disease as contagious for healthy persons evidently because he had permitted the vessel to go to her pier. With the exception of the case of the assistant cook all the patients on the ship were passengers in the third class, and it had not affected those who were well fed before they came on board the ship. Every effort would be made, the agents of the line said yesterday, to fumigate the vessel and eradicate any germs that might remain in the third-class cabins, dining rooms and hospitals before she goes to sea again.

C. Stanley King, who arrived here yesterday from England, after being abroad doing war work since last December, contracted the Spanish influenza in England and lost nearly forty pounds in weight.

"The Spanish flue, as it is called in England for short," Mr. King said, "has spread all over the country, and caused schools, factories, and even shipyards to suspend work on account of the great number of pupils and workmen that have been laid up by it. The last reports I heard from France in official circles before leaving London was that the German Army was almost incapacitated by the Spanish flue in certain sectors, and the French, British, Canadian, and Australian soldiers were also great sufferers from it. The American soldiers have not yet been affected by the disease very much, which the medical experts put down to the fact that their physical condition was so good they were able to throw the germs off.

"The general impression, so far as I could ascertain, was that the spread of the Spanish flue to such a great extent was chiefly due to the people in

Europe having to live upon bad bread, which poisoned all around the gums and undermined the public health. The disease has gone all through Europe from Constantinople to Caithness, and I do not think there is any doubt that it will come to the United States.

"I had a bad attack myself just before sailing, commencing with fever and delirium, and then the weakness which left me helpless. I was not able to leave my cabin after we sailed from England ten days ago, and had a submarine attack taken place I should have been unable to move."

*August 14, 1918*

# Drastic Steps Taken to Fight Influenza Here

In order to prevent the complete shutdown of industry and amusement in this city to check the spread of Spanish influenza, Health Commissioner Copeland, by proclamation, yesterday ordered a change in the hours for opening stores, theatres and other places of business.

The Department is of the opinion that the greatest sources of spread of the disease are crowded subway and elevated trains and cars on the surface lines and the purpose of the order is to diminish the "peak" load in the evenings and mornings on these lines by distributing the travelers over a greater space of time. This will reduce crowding to a minimum.

Dr. Copeland's action was taken after a statement made by Surgeon General Blue, Chief of the Public Health Service in Washington, was called to his attention, in which Dr. Blue advocated the closing of churches, schools, theatres and public institutions in every community where the epidemic has developed. Dr. Blue said:

"There is no way to put a nationwide closing order into effect, as this is a matter which is up to the individual communities. In some States the State Board of Health has this power, but in many others it is a matter of municipal regulation. I hope that those having the proper authority will close all public gathering places if their community is threatened with the epidemic. This will do much toward checking the spread of the disease."

## 1,695 New Cases Here

There were reported in the twenty-four hours ending at 10 o'clock yesterday morning 1,695 new cases of influenza and 188 of pneumonia. The influenza cases were thus distributed: Manhattan, 615; Bronx, 367; Brooklyn, 421; Queens, 97; Richmond, 195.

In the same period the deaths were 42 from influenza, and 84 from pneumonia. The influenza deaths were thus distributed: Manhattan, 11; Bronx, 5; Brooklyn, 24; Richmond, 2.

The decision to issue a proclamation changing the hours of work and the opening and closing of amusement places was arrived at after a series of conferences in the Department of Health offices in Centre Street that lasted nearly all day. Dr. Copeland met first the heads of the various departments, and afterward he conferred with the departmental staff of nurses and the Medical Inspectors of every district.

Business interests were represented at the afternoon meeting. At that conference there were present:

Charles Bulkley Hubbell, Chairman of the Public Service Commission; E. A. Maher Jr., Vice President of the Third Avenue lines; W. Leon Pepperman, Assistant to the President of the Interborough and the New York Railways Companies; John R. Young, representing the Merchants' Association; Dr. W. L. Ettinger, Superintendent of Schools; Dr. Melville A. Hays, representing the State Labor Department; E. W. Estes, Secretary of the Broadway Association; J. E. Roach, representing the American Federation of Labor; William G. Lipsey; Superintendent of Bloomingdale Brothers, and these representing the theatrical and moving picture interests: Marc Klaw, Alf Hayman, J. J. Shubert, V. Kiraly, Patrick Casey, David Bernstein, J. J. Maloney, Edward Mallon, and A. Toxen Worm.

One of the decisions reached is to close all stores other than those dealing exclusively in food or drugs at 4 o'clock in the afternoon. To prevent evasions of this rule Dr. Copeland made it plain that department stores which carry either food or drugs as a department would have to close and not keep open on the ground that they were dealers in either food or drugs.

All moving picture houses and theatres outside of a certain district are considered community houses and are held to draw their patronage from within walking distance. There was debate on the proposition to close the schools and churches and other places of assemblage, but it was decided against at this time.

## Has Power to Close Up City

As to the legal right of the Health Department to put the order into effect, the Commissioner said that it was a question of obeying the order now or having the city closed up. The department has the power to do the latter, but it does not want to do it. Those at the conference understand the position taken by the department, and Dr. Copeland looks for the heartiest support of all.

The proclamation, with orders for the changes in opening and closing hours, which go into effect today and are to continue until further notice, is as follows:

"At a meeting of the Board of Health of the Department of Health, City of New York, held Oct. 4, 1918, the following resolution was adopted:

"Whereas, the epidemic of so-called Spanish influenza and pneumonia, while not alarming at the present moment, necessitates care on the part of the citizens of the City of New York, and

"Whereas, the particular things to be avoided, in order to escape contagion is to prohibit crowding and congestion, particularly in places of public assemblage, and

"Whereas, one of the chief places of crowding is in the subway, surface cars, elevated trains, steam railways and other public conveyances used for the transportation of passengers, and

"Whereas, the opening and closing of the vast majority of mercantile, manufacturing and business establishments take place at the same hours in the morning and afternoon or evening and are the principal factor in causing such overcrowded conditions of the subway and other public conveyances during the peak hours of travel, and

"Whereas, the conditions hereinbefore set forth constitute, in the opinion of the Board of Health, a condition prejudicial to health of the persons using such public conveyances and frequenting other places of public assemblage, therefore be it

"Resolved. That the Board of Health hereby declares the conditions hereinbefore set forth to be prejudicial to health, and hereby orders:

"1. That the institutions and buildings used in commerce, manufacture, trade, industry and labor, transportation, and recreation shall maintain hours of opening and closing in accordance with the following schedule:

"(a) All stores, except retail food and drug stores, shall open at 8 a.m. and close at 4 p.m.

"(b) All wholesale and jobbing establishments shall open at 8:15 a.m. and close at 4:15 p.m.

"(c) All offices shall open at 8:30 a.m. and close at 4:30 p.m.

"(d) All textile manufacturing establishments shall open at 9 a.m. and close at 5 p.m.

"(e) All nontextile manufacturing establishments shall open at 9:30 a.m. and close at 5:30 p.m.

"(f) All establishments formerly opening before 8 a.m. and closing later than 6 p.m. shall not be disturbed. The particular purpose of this exemption is to prevent any interference with munition factories or war industries."

## Theatre Opening Hours

"(g) Theatres and places of amusement shall open in accordance with the following schedule:

"7 p.m.—Rivoli, Rialto, Strand, Broadway, New York, and other leading moving picture houses situated between Fourteenth and Fifty-ninth Streets, must arrange for their night shows to begin at this hour.

"8 p.m.—Lexington Opera House, Hippodrome, Palace, Columbia, and all two-a-day vaudeville houses.

"8:15 p.m.—Winter Garden, Century, Broadhurst, Casino, Park, Harris, New Amsterdam, Cohan, Globe, Cort, Liberty, Shubert, Majestic. (Brooklyn.)

"8:80 p.m.—Lyric, Plymouth, Astor, Comedy, Morosco, Lyceum, Criterion, Knickerbocker, Montauk. (Brooklyn.)

"8:45 p.m.—Manhattan, Central, Selwyn, Booth, Belmont, Hudson, Gaiety

"9:00 p.m.—Longacre, Bijou, Forty-eighth Street, Playhouse, Maxine Elliott, Republic, Eltinge, Empire, Cohan & Harris, Belasco, Punch and Judy.

"By order of the Board of Health.

"ROYAL S. COPELAND,

"Commissioner.

"We have not closed up New York City largely because this community is not stricken with the epidemic," said Dr. Copeland. "The increase reported today has, however, caused us some serious hours. I had a conference this morning with the department nurses and the medical inspectors. These nurses and inspectors go into the schools and their testimony is that there are few sick school children in this city. "I had a conference with the Superintendent of Schools, Dr. Ettinger, and he has had a survey of the schools made and he found there were few sick there. He agrees with the department that the schools should be left open. We feel this way because New York is a great, cosmopolitan city and in some homes there is careless disregard of modern sanitation. From these homes, however, thousands of children are carefully washed up and their teeth scrubbed before they are sent to school. In the schools the children are under the constant guardianship of the medical inspectors.

"This work is part of our system of disease control. If the schools were closed at least 1,000,000 children would be sent to their homes and become 1,000,000 possibilities for the disease. Furthermore, there would be nobody to take special notice of their condition."

## Conditions Different Here

"I don't want to be in the position of giving an interview that would appear antagonistic to what Surgeon General Blue has said. He is dealing with the nation. He finds a variety of conditions while we face only one here. For instance, in Oswego, with 23,000 persons, there were found 3,500 cases today. Now, if we had one-sixth of the population here affected with Spanish influenza we would have 1,000,000 cases. We would have to close everything up. We have had about 6,000 cases here, while Philadelphia has had 20,000 and Boston 100,000. One half of the 6,000 cases here are in 600 homes.

"It has been the position of the Department of Health from the first that no individual is in danger if he or she escapes the mouth or nasal secretion of some other person who has it. We believe it is proper to keep the theatres and churches open if we can eliminate the sneezers, coughers, and spitters. We pointed out to the theatre managers the importance of making the public who go to their places know that these things are prohibited. Today we ordered these managers to instruct their ushers and attendants to escort from their theatres those who violate the Department rules and to use force if necessary. We will back them up.

"In this city the chief danger of spread of the disease lies in the subways—and the other lines to a lesser extent. The crowds carried at the morning and evening peak of the load must be diminished. For years there has been talk of establishing a relay system of travel or a zone system so that persons would go to and from work at different hours. This plan, we have established.

"The plan means general inconvenience. That is granted, but its purpose is to prevent the spread of disease, and we expect our big public to take to it as patriotically as they have obeyed the mandates of this Federal Government in measures affecting the war.

"The Department of Health was faced with the problem of either doing this or closing the subways, and we have worked out this plan with as little hindrance to business and amusement as possible. We have given orders to the public utilities companies to keep the car windows open and the fans going in the subway. This means warm clothing and so it is again put up to the public to do its part."

## To Permit Fires Earlier

Dr. Copeland said also that State Fuel Administrator Cooke has promised that he will issue a statement permitting fires in the homes and the heating twice a day of places in which persons are engaged in sedentary occupations.

It was reported that a quarantine had been established on Blackwell's Island, but no order was issued by the Health Department. There have been several cases among the prisoners, but no deaths, and the prison authorities decided yesterday to revoke all pass privileges of visitors.

Twenty persons were summoned to Yorkville Court yesterday for violation of the Sanitary Code in not providing properly cleansed glasses for the serving of drinks. Some were fined and some released on their promise to use more care. One hundred and twenty-five men were summoned to Jefferson Market Court for spitting in the public thoroughfares. Each was fined $1 and warned.

Ten spitters were arraigned in Yorkville Court and nine in the Tombs Court. In Yorkville Court most of the prisoners were fined $3 each, but those arraigned in the Tombs Court were held in $200 bail for trial in Special Sessions. Twenty-two spitters paid small fines in Harlem Court, and three in the West Side Court.

A call for the mobilization of all nurses and women with elementary training in the care of the sick was sent out yesterday from the headquarters of the Atlantic Division of the Red Cross to the 223 nursing committees in New York, New Jersey, and Connecticut. They are wanted to help combat the Spanish influenza epidemic. The call, Ethan Allen, manager of the division, explained, was a preparatory measure.

A large number of nurses from the Atlantic Division, in response to a special call last week, are now serving in Massachusetts, but in the future the work will be organized so that the resources of the Red Cross will be distributed systematically. Miss Clara D. Noyes, Director of the Bureau of Field Nursing at national headquarters in Washington, is making arrangements to coordinate the work. It is planned that groups of ten and fifteen nurses in each community will form the nucleus for a complete mobilization of all nursing personnel.

As fast as nurses are enrolled by the various nursing committees, the records will be forwarded to the division headquarters.

Demands for nurses are being received hourly at division headquarters, Mr. Allen said, and the present supply is far below the demand. He urges every woman who is capable and can spare the time to communicate at once with the local headquarters of the nearest chapter.

The Red Cross gives a course of instruction at the New York Chapter, Teaching School, 453 Madison Avenue. Fifteen lessons, one and a half hours each, covering three weeks, and seventy-two hours in a hospital, are required to qualify for service under ordinary conditions. At present, however, the pupils are taking their hospital training with their instruction, going directly from the classrooms to the wards.

The Board of Freeholders of Burlington County, New Jersey, yesterday were requested by State Commissioner of Charities and Corrections Burdette G. Lewis to authorize the use of Burlington County Hospital for the Insane at New Lisbon for the care and treatment of the present and future cases of Spanish influenza in Camp Dix.

*October 5, 1918*

# Swine Flu Program Suspended in Nation; Disease Link Feared

## By LAWRENCE K. ALTMAN

Federal officials suspended the troubled nationwide swine flu immunization program yesterday because of concern that the shots were possibly linked to recently reported cases of paralysis.

Since the end of last week, the Federal Centers for Disease Control in Atlanta, which runs the nationwide immunization program, has been investigating reports from at least 14 states of 94 cases, four of them fatal, of a form of paralysis called the Guillain-Barré syndrome.

Federal epidemiologists said that they could neither prove nor disprove the possible connection between the paralysis and the swine flu shots.

But to be on the safe side, Federal officials ordered the program halted late yesterday afternoon.

Of the 94 reported cases of paralysis, 51, including the four deaths, involved persons who had received swine flu shots between one and three weeks before the onset of paralytic symptoms. Thirty-one victims of the paralysis had not been vaccinated, and the status of the remaining 12 victims could not be established, Federal officials said.

In the metropolitan area, 18 cases were reported in New Jersey, 11 in Connecticut and none in New York.

The decision to suspend the swine flu program was announced in Washington by Dr. Theodore Cooper, Assistant Secretary of Health, Education and Welfare.

## "In the Interests of Safety"

Dr. Cooper said that he was acting "in the interests of safety of the public, in the interest of credibility, and in the interest of the practice of good medicine."

After meeting with President Ford, Dr. Cooper declined in a news conference to concede that the swine flu program was doomed as a result of this latest complication. But Dr. Cooper acknowledged that it would be "difficult to get the public to take flu shots again" unless there was a flu epidemic this season.

Dr. Cooper said it would be a minimum of a month before all epidemiologic studies could be completed and the flu vaccination program resumed.

The halt over the paralysis issue was the latest in a series of blows to the $135 million program. Last spring, the program was delayed six weeks when Parke Davis and Co., one of the four manufacturers, produced two million doses of the wrong kind of vaccine.

Then all drug companies threatened to stop production completely until Congress protected them from lawsuits by people who suffered side effects from the vaccinations. Children were excluded because the vaccine tests did not show it to be as effective as expected among young people.

And then less than two weeks after the delayed program got started, the program was suspended while epidemiologists investigated the deaths from heart attacks of three elderly people who had received shots within the same hour at the same clinic in Pittsburgh. No link was found between the vaccine and the deaths.

The possible connection between the swine flue vaccine and the Guillain-Barré paralytic syndrome apparently was first recognized in Minnesota last week.

Dr. David Sencer, the director of the Centers for Disease Control, said that Federal epidemiologists "have not proven any association with the vaccine and the Guillain-Barré syndrome, but we are not able with the available data to rule out the possibility of an association."

On Wednesday, center officials had announced that there was no apparent connection between swine flu vaccine and the paralytic syndrome, which usually starts in the legs and, over a period of several days to weeks, ascends to involve the nerves controlling the muscles in the upper part of the body.

Patients usually recover, but if the paralysis involves the breathing muscles, the patient may need treatment with a mechanical respiratory device. Deaths of three of the four victims in the current situation were attributed to respiratory paralysis. The fourth patient died from a blood clot in the lung, a condition that can complicate the Guillain-Barré syndrome.

The syndrome has been known to doctors since 1916 when Drs. Guillain, Barré and Strohl reported it. It is sometimes called the Landry-Guillain-Barré syndrome, and it can be difficult to diagnose.

Doctors usually test cerebral spinal fluid taken by a "needle inserted through the back to help make the diagnosis.

Guillain-Barré syndrome is not a disease that's ordinarily reported to health departments in this country. Officials of the National Institutes of Health said yesterday that upward of 5,000 cases occurred each year in this country.

The cause of the syndrome is unknown, but it has been reported to follow myriad situations, such as rabies immunization, viral infections and operations. There is no seasonal pattern, and the syndrome affects people of all ages.

The lack of precise statistics on the syndrome made the Federal epidemiologists' task more difficult. After learning of the cases, Atlanta officials asked epidemiologists in Alabama, Colorado, Minnesota and New Jersey, which have reputations for excellent reporting systems, to help clarify the questionable link between the syndrome and the vaccine. But the results of the quick four-state survey were inconclusive.

Yesterday morning, Atlanta officials held a conference telephone call with about 20 experts from the National Institutes of Health, the Bureau of Biologics, state epidemiologists and Dr. Edwin Kilbourne, an internationally respected influenza vaccine expert at Mount Sinai Medical School here.

"The absence of any [swine] influenza activity was really an important factor in making the decision today," one of the conference call participants said in an interview.

*December 17, 1976*

# Genetic Material of Virus From 1918 Flu Is Found

By GINA KOLATA

A group of Defense Department researchers has found genetic material from the notorious Spanish flu virus that killed at least 20 million people worldwide in the influenza pandemic of 1918.

Fragments of the virus were found lurking in a formaldehyde-soaked scrap of lung tissue from a 21-year-old soldier who died of the flu nearly 80 years ago. And now, medical experts say, investigators at last hope to answer a question that has troubled them for decades: what made this virus so deadly?

One part of the answer is that the Spanish flu virus passed from birds to pigs and then to humans, a mode of transmission that is thought to produce the most dangerous strains of influenza viruses. Indeed, fear of a swine flu epidemic in 1976 caused President Gerald R. Ford to mobilize the nation to immunize against a flu strain that infected soldiers at Fort Dix, N.J. That particular virus, however, turned out not to be a threat.

The search for the 1918 virus is of more than historical interest, said Dr. Jeffery K. Taubenberger at the Armed Forces Institute of Pathology in Washington, the leader of the team whose report is being published today in the journal *Science*. Dr. Taubenberger and other researchers hope that understanding the genetic code of the Spanish flu virus might help scientists prepare for the next influenza pandemic, which many scientists think is coming soon.

The Spanish flu epidemic seems to have begun in the United States in late spring and early summer of 1918, when doctors reported scattered outbreaks in military installations where recruits were reporting for training before going to France.

By September, when schools opened, the epidemic was roaring through the entire population and spreading rapidly to every corner of the world, attacking the young and healthy and killing them, often within days.

The flu virus itself is gone, vanished with the epidemic. But scientists have repeatedly tried to find traces of it, studying autopsy specimens and even exhuming bodies buried in Alaska where, they hoped, the virus would have remained preserved.

Even now, an expedition is being proposed to Spitsbergen, a Norwegian archipelago in the Arctic Ocean about 400 miles north of Norway, to exhume the bodies of miners who died of the flu.

An epidemic like that of 1918 "can come again, and it will," said Dr. Robert Webster, chairman of viral and molecular biology at St. Jude's Children's Research Hospital in Memphis.

Dr. Joshua Lederberg, a geneticist and Nobel laureate who is president emeritus of Rockefeller University in New York, called influenza "the most urgent, patently visible, acute threat in the world of emerging infections." And, Dr. Lederberg added, "the sooner we can learn what to anticipate, the more likely we will be able to blunt the next appearance" of a deadly flu virus.

Dr. Taubenberger studied specimens from Spanish flu victims that are among the millions of autopsy specimens that the pathology institute has been storing in warehouses since the Civil War. But he said he doubted that the study would succeed in light of the dismal history of failed efforts to find the virus.

For example, in the 1950s, a group of scientists that included Dr. Maurice R. Hilleman, director of the Merck Institute in West Point, Pa., who was then directing viral research at the Walter Reed Army Institute in Washington, traveled to Nome, Alaska, in a secret mission to examine the exhumed bodies of Eskimos who had died of the 1918 flu.

When Eskimo flu victims died, Dr. Hilleman said, they were buried in the middle of winter, in the frozen ground. The Army thought that these bodies, buried in the permafrost, might have remained frozen and preserved. But, Dr. Hilleman said, "the bodies were in such an advanced state of deterioration that no live virus was found."

More recently several scientists, including Dr. Webster, examined autopsy tissue from the Armed Forces Institute of Pathology but were unable to find viruses.

Dr. Taubenberger decided to go ahead anyway. Looking in the computerized records, he requested autopsy slides of the lungs of 198 soldiers who died of the Spanish flu.

In examining the slides, he looked for a particular type of pathology. Since the flu virus stops replicating within a couple of days after a person is infected, Dr. Taubenberger and his team wanted lung tissue from someone who died quickly, within a week after becoming ill, so that there might still be virus particles present.

That was possible, Dr. Taubenberger said, because the 1918 influenza strain was so deadly.

"The lungs of some who died in a few days were completely filled with fluids, as if they had drowned," he said. "No one has ever seen that before or since. It was a unique pathology."

Of the 198 cases that Dr. Taubenberger requested, 7 met his criteria. But only one had other features that led the researchers to believe that the flu virus was actively replicating when the man died.

The man was a private from New York State stationed at Fort Jackson, S.C., when he caught the flu.

"He was a healthy 21-year-old male with no medical history until he got this," Dr. Taubenberger said.

The soldier died within five days of infection, on Sept. 26, 1918, and in October his lung tissue was shipped to Washington, where it was stored, undisturbed, for nearly 80 years.

With the soldier's lung tissue in hand, the researchers began the tedious process of trying to extract the viral genetic material. The virus carries its genes in eight pieces of RNA that are packaged together in a protein coat. But over the years of storage, the 15,000 nucleotides that make up the viral RNA had broken apart into shards about 200 nucleotides long.

The researchers spent nearly two years amplifying the tiny segments of viral RNA so that they would have enough to analyze and assemble like a jigsaw puzzle. In their paper in *Science,* they report on the sequences of nine fragments of the virus that include pieces of its major genes.

The group has analyzed only about 7 percent of the virus, Dr. Taubenberger said, although he expects that he will eventually be able to complete the job. Others, like Dr. Webster, agree, but say it is still uncertain whether even that will reveal the secret of the virus's lethality.

But with his preliminary analysis, Dr. Taubenberger and his colleagues have already ruled out two hypotheses on why the virus was so deadly.

One was based on an analysis of a chicken influenza virus that swept through flocks of chickens in the early 1980s, killing them overnight.

The chicken virus was peculiar. One of its proteins had three basic amino acids at a spot where the host's enzymes had to break that protein in order for the virus to infect a cell. Ordinarily, there was only one such amino acid at that spot. So, investigators thought, maybe the three basic amino acids were a clue to lethality, and maybe they were a feature of the Spanish flu virus.

But, Dr. Taubenberger found, that was not the case. There was nothing unusual about the amino acids at that position in the Spanish flu virus.

Another hypothesis was that the flu had gone directly from birds to humans. Ordinarily, human flu viruses spread only in humans, but genetically distinct flu viruses also fester, independently, in birds, which do not become ill when they are infected. Occasionally, viruses from birds infect animals like pigs, and then jump to people. Even worse, some researchers proposed, might be a virus that jumped directly from birds to humans.

Antibodies of survivors of the 1918 epidemic indicated that the virus had lived in pigs before infecting humans. But the antibody evidence was indirect, and some thought it might be incorrect. The genetic analysis, however, indicated that the virus had, indeed, come to humans from pigs.

"I can't hold up one gene fragment and say, 'This is the reason,'" Dr. Taubenberger said. "This is the beginning of the story."

But it raises additional questions, the most immediate of which is whether the planned expedition to Norway should go forward.

The trip was proposed by Dr. Kirsty Duncan, who studies medicine and geography at the University of Windsor in Ontario. Dr. Duncan learned that seven miners who were digging coal in Spitsbergen died of the flu in 1918 and were buried there. She and her colleagues have been working with Dr. Nancy Cox, the chief of the influenza branch at the Centers for Disease Control and Prevention in Atlanta, to plan the trip to Norway.

Dr. Duncan said the team would meet in Atlanta. "We'll be debating how to proceed," she said.

Dr. Cox said the study of viral RNA from autopsy specimens might reveal all of the virus's secrets.

The question, of course, is whether it is worthwhile to risk unleashing live viruses that might still be in the frozen tissue of the miners.

*March 21, 1997*

CHAPTER 12

# Genome

# Clue to Chemistry of Heredity Found

A scientific partnership between an American and a British biochemist at the Cavendish Laboratory in Cambridge has led to the unraveling of the structural pattern of a substance as important to biologists as uranium is to nuclear physicists. The substance is nucleic acid, the vital constituent of cells, the carrier of inherited characters and the fluid that links organic life with inorganic matter.

The form of nucleic acid under investigation is called DNA (deoxyribonucleic acid) and has been known since 1869.

But what nobody understood before the Cavendish Laboratory men considered the problem was how the molecules were grooved into each other like the strands of a wire hawser so they were able to pull inherited characters over from one generation to another.

## Further Tests Slated

The two biochemists, James Dewey Watson, a former graduate student of the University of Chicago, and his British partner, Francis H. C. Crick, believe that in DNA they have at last found the clue to the chemistry of heredity. If further X-ray tests prove what has largely been demonstrated on paper, Drs. Watson and Crick will have made biochemical history.

Dr. Watson has now returned to the United States, where he intends to join Dr. Linus Pauling, of California, who has done most of the pioneer work on the problem.

[In Pasadena, Calif., Dr. Pauling said that the new Crick-Watson solution appeared to be somewhat better than the proposal for the structure of the nucleic acids worked out by Dr. Pauling and associates at the California Institute of Technology. The California solution was published in the February, 1953, issue of the *Proceedings of the National Academy of Sciences*.]

Dr. Crick may leave Britain, too, when he has done some more work on the problem. Right now, he said, it "simply smells right" and confirms research in many institutions, particularly the Rockefeller Foundation in the United States and at King's College in London.

The acid DNA, Dr. Crick explained is a "high polymer"—that is, its chemical components can be disentangled and rearranged in different ways.

DNA is the essential constituent of the microscopic life-threads called chromosomes that carry the genes of heredity like beads on a string.

In all life cells, including those of man, DNA is the substance that transmits inherited characters such as eye color, nose shape and certain types of blood and diseases. The transmission occurs at the vital moment of mitosis or cell division when a tangle of DNA containing chromosomes becomes thicker and the cell separates into two daughter cells.

## Forming of Molecular Chain

Although DNA has never been synthesized, Drs. Watson and Crick knew it was composed of horizontal hook-ups of bases (sugars and phosphates) piled one above the other in chain-like formations. The problem was to find out how these giant molecules could be fitted together so they could duplicate themselves exactly.

By a method of scientific doodling with hand-drawn models of the molecules, Drs. Watson and Crick worked out which molecules could be joined together with regard to the fact that some molecules were more rigid than others and had critical angles of attachment. Some months ago they decided that the only possible interrelation of the molecules was in the form of two chains arranged in a double helix—like a spiral staircase, with the upper chain resembling the staircase handrail and the lower resembling the outside edge of the stairs.

New evidence for double DNA chains in helical form now has been obtained from the King's College Biophysics Department in London, where a group of workers extracted crystalline DNA from the thymus gland of a calf and bombarded it with X-rays.

The resulting X-ray diffraction photographs showed a whirlpool of light and shade that could be analyzed as the components of a double helix.

Dr. Crick emphasized that years of work still must be applied to the helical carriers of life's characteristics. But a working model to aid in the genetical studies of the future now has been laid out in blueprint form by Drs. Watson and Crick—or so most biochemists here believe.

## Looks Good, Pauling Says

Reached by telephone in Pasadena, Dr. Pauling said last night that the Crick-Watson proposal for the structure of the nucleic acids "looks very good." Dr. Pauling has just returned from London where he talked with Dr. Crick and with Dr. Watson, who was formerly a student at California Institute of Technology.

Dr. Pauling said that he did not believe the problem of understanding "molecular genetics" had been finally solved, and that the shape of the molecules was a complicated matter. Both the California and the Crick-Watson explanations of the structure of the substances that control heredity are highly speculative, he remarked.

*June 13, 1953*

# After 10 Years' Effort, Genome Mapping Team Achieves Sequence of a Human Chromosome

By NICHOLAS WADE

After a decade of preparation, scientists have for the first time decoded the information in a human chromosome, the unit in which the genetic information is packaged.

The achievement, by a public consortium of university centers in Britain, the United States and Japan, is a milestone in the human genome project, an initiative started in 1990 with the goal of deciphering all of human DNA by 2005.

The success in decoding the first chromosome, even though it is the second-smallest of the 23 pairs in every human cell, validates the approach chosen by the public consortium and bolsters the chance that it can complete the full human genome as planned. In the last 18 months the consortium's strategy has been challenged by a private company, the Celera Corporation of Rockville, Md., which asserts it can sequence the genome faster by a different method.

"A new era has dawned—we have fulfilled the dreams of Mendel, Morgan, Watson and Crick, and Sanger, as we now have the essentially complete structure of the first human chromosome," said Dr. Bruce Roe of the University of Oklahoma, a member of the decoding team, referring to the principal architects of today's knowledge about genetics.

Understanding the human genome is expected to yield vast medical benefits, because almost every disease has a genetic component.

The central feature of each chromosome is an enormously long DNA molecule. The chromosome on which the latest work was done is called Chromosome 22, which, small as it is, contains 43 million units of DNA, of which researchers have now decoded 33.5 million. Though there is still much left to be done, the Chromosome 22 team believes that it has sequenced all regions of major interest to biomedical researchers—that is, the regions that contain the protein-making genes.

The fruit of the team's labors is an eye-glazing march of A's, C's, G's, and T's, as the four chemical units are abbreviated, which would take up 949 pages of this newspaper if printed in ordinary type.

Techniques for analyzing such vast molecules have only recently been developed. Two industrial-scale laboratories, at the Sanger Centre in England and Washington University in St. Louis, are the principal powerhouses in the public consortium's

252

campaign. The team working on Chromosome 22 also included scientists at Keio University in Japan and the University of Oklahoma. The team's leader is Dr. Ian Dunham of the Sanger Centre, where the bulk of the sequence was completed. The results are reported in today's issue of *Nature*, and the genome sequence will be posted on the Internet at www.genome.ou.edu/Chr22.html.

Dr. Roe estimated the total cost of sequencing the chromosome at $15 million to $20 million. The human genome project as a whole is budgeted at $3 billion.

So far, the Dunham team has identified 545 genes—each of which is composed of thousands of chemical units—and altogether there are probably 1,000 or so genes strung out along the chromosome. The total number of human genes is still unknown and estimates vary widely, from 60,000 to 120,000.

If there is a pattern in the types of genes nature has chosen to store on Chromosome 22, it has escaped the researchers. The genes appear to be a random assortment, including a large set of genes involved in the immune system and more than 20 genes that cause known human diseases when defective, such as DiGeorge and cat eye syndromes. In addition, one of the genes suspected of contributing to schizophrenia is believed to lie on Chromosome 22 but has not yet been identified.

Besides the interest in specific genes, biologists can also see for the first time the full architecture of a human chromosome. Their immediate reaction is in some cases pure awe at the daunting complexity of the structure and the distance yet to travel before its features are understood.

"I don't often pick up a scientific paper and find myself getting chills, as I did when I saw this whole chromosomal landscape," said Dr. Francis Collins, director of the human genome project at the National Institutes of Health. "This is a phenomenal historical moment, to see a full chapter of the human instruction book."

Although the goal of the human genome project is to sequence every one of the three billion letters in human DNA, the sequence of Chromosome 22 is not yet complete. There are 11 gaps, all of known length and fairly short. These are mostly regions that could not be cloned in bacteria, the standard way of amplifying long segments of human DNA for further analysis.

In addition, the team has not sequenced the DNA in two important features of the chromosome. One is the centromere, a region that helps the chromosome get copied correctly to each daughter cell when the cell divides. The other is the chromosome's short arm—a length of DNA on the other side of the centromere—which in Chromosome 22's case contains only multiple copies of genes involved in protein manufacture.

Dr. Collins said that completing every letter in the human genome was still the public consortium's goal but that at a recent meeting participants agreed that chromosomes could be declared essentially complete provided that the researchers had done everything possible with available techniques and had defined the size of any remaining gaps.

But the intent is to close every gap when better techniques are developed, he said, as "one should not declare victory just because one got tired of the problem."

*December 2, 1999*

# Genetic Code of Human Life Is Cracked by Scientists

## By NICHOLAS WADE

In an achievement that represents a pinnacle of human self-knowledge, two rival groups of scientists said today that they had deciphered the hereditary script, the set of instructions that defines the human organism.

"Today we are learning the language in which God created life," President Clinton said at a White House ceremony attended by members of the two teams, Dr. James D. Watson, co-discoverer of the structure of DNA, and, via satellite, Prime Minister Tony Blair of Britain.

The teams' leaders, Dr. J. Craig Venter, president of Celera Genomics, and Dr. Francis S. Collins, director of the National Human Genome Research Institute, praised each other's contributions and signaled a spirit of cooperation from now on, even though the two efforts will remain firmly independent.

The human genome, the ancient script that has now been deciphered, consists of two sets of 23 giant DNA molecules, or chromosomes, with each set—one inherited from each parent—containing more than three billion chemical units.

The successful deciphering of this vast genetic archive attests to the extraordinary pace of biology's advance since 1953, when the structure of DNA was first discovered and presages an era of even brisker progress.

Understanding the human genome is expected to revolutionize the practice of medicine. Biologists expect in time to develop an array of diagnostics and treatments based on it and tailored to individual patients, some of which will exploit the body's own mechanisms of self-repair.

The knowledge in the genome could also be used in harmful ways, particularly in revealing patients' disposition to disease if their privacy is not safeguarded, and in causing discrimination.

The joint announcement is something of a shotgun marriage because neither side's version of the human genome is complete, nor do they agree on the genome's size. Neither has sequenced—meaning to determine the order of the chemical subunits—the DNA of certain short structural regions of the genome, which cannot yet be analyzed.

With the rest of the genome, which contains the human genes and much else, both sides' versions have many small gaps, although these are thought to contain few or no genes. Today's versions are effectively complete representations of the genome but leave much more work to be done.

The two groups even differ on the size of the gene-coding part of the genome. Celera says it is 3.12 billion letters of DNA; the public consortium that it is 3.15 billion units, a letter difference of 30 million. Neither side can yet describe the genome's full size or determine the number of human genes.

The public consortium has also fallen somewhat behind in its goal of attaining a working draft in which 90 percent of the gene-containing part of the genome was sequenced. Its version today has reached only 85 percent, suggesting it was marching to Celera's timetable.

Today's announcement heralded an unexpected truce between the two groups of scientists who have been racing to finish the genome. Veering away from the prospect of asserting rival claims of victory, the two chose to report simultaneously their attainment of different milestones in their quest.

Celera, a unit of the PE Corporation, has obtained its 3.12 billion letters of the genome in the form of long continuous sequences, mostly about 2 million letters each, but with many small gaps.

A less complete version has been reported by the Human Genome Project, a consortium of academic centers supported largely by the National Institutes of Health and the Wellcome Trust, a medical philanthropy in London. Dr. Collins, the consortium's leader, said its scientists had sequenced 85 percent of the genome in a "working draft," meaning its accuracy will be upgraded later.

Both versions of the human genome meet the important goal of allowing scientists to search them for desired genes, the genetic instructions encoded in the DNA. The consortium's genome data is freely available now. Celera has said it will make a version of its genome sequence freely available at a later date.

In their remarks at the White House, Dr. Collins and Dr. Venter both sought to capture the wider meaning of their work in identifying the eye-glazing stream of A's, G's, C's and T's, the letters in the genome's four-letter code.

"We have caught the first glimpses of our instruction book, previously known only to God," Dr. Collins said. Dr. Venter spoke of his conviction from seeing people die in Vietnam, where he served as a medic, that the human spirit transcended the physiology that is controlled by the genome.

The two genome versions were obtained through prodigious efforts by each side, involving skilled management of teams of scientists working around the clock on a novel technological frontier.

Spurring their efforts was the glittering lure of the genome as a scientific prize, and a rivalry fueled by personal differences and conflicting agendas.

Dr. Venter, a genomics pioneer whose innovative methods have at times been scorned by experts in the consortium's camp, has often cast himself, not without reason, as an outsider battling a hostile establishment.

The consortium scientists were halfway through a successful 15-year program to complete the human genome by 2005, when Dr. Venter announced in May 1998 that as head of a new company, later called Celera, he would beat them to their goal by 5 years.

His bombshell entry turned an academic pursuit into a fierce race. Dr. Collins responded by moving his completion date forward to 2003 and setting this month as the target for a 90 percent draft.

"These folks have pulled out all the stops," he said of his staff in an interview last week. "They have achieved a ramp-up that is beyond anything one would have imagined possible."

The 15-year cost of the Human Genome Project, which began in 1990, has been estimated at $3 billion, but includes many incidental expenses. The consortium has spent only $300 million on sequencing the human genome since January 1999, when its all-out production phase began. Celera has not released its costs, but Dr. Venter said a year ago that he expected Celera's human genome to cost $200 million to $250 million.

The race opened with mutual predictions of defeat. The consortium's senior scientists predicted in December 1998 that Dr. Venter's method of reassembling the sequenced fragments of genomic DNA was bound to fail. In May 1999, Dr. Venter, confident of Celera's impending success, observed that the National Institutes of Health and the Wellcome Trust were "putting good money after bad."

The groups were divided by political as well as technical agendas. The consortium's two principal scientists, Dr. John E. Sulston of the Sanger Center in England and Dr. Robert Waterston of Washington University in St. Louis, insisted that the genome data should be published nightly, an unusually generous policy because scientists generally harvest new data for their own discoveries before sharing it.

Both of the consortium's administrative leaders, Dr. James D. Watson, and his successor, Dr. Collins, made a point of seeking out international partners so that the rest of the world would not feel excluded from the genome triumph. Thus even though centers in the United States and Britain have done most of the heavy lifting, important contributions to the consortium's genome draft have been made by centers in Germany, France, Japan and China.

Academic scientists have felt some chagrin that an altruistic, open and technically successful venture like the Human Genome Project should be upstaged by a commercial rival financed by the company that made the consortium's DNA sequencing machines.

But though Celera seeks to profit by operating a genomic database, Dr. Venter also believed that he could make the genome and its benefits available a lot sooner. He has succeeded in doing so, and in spurring the consortium to move faster.

Today's truce between the two teams offers several advantages. For Celera to claim victory over the consortium would risk alienating customers in the academic community. For the consortium, the surety of opting into a draw now may have seemed better than the risks of claiming victory with a complete genome much later.

Celera's version of the genome depends on the consortium's data. And the many small gaps in Celera's sequence will probably be filled by the consortium's scientists, adding further to their claim on credit for the final product.

The present truce between the sides is limited to today's announcement and an agreement to publish their reports in the same journal, although the details remain to be worked out. A joint workshop will be held to discuss the genome versions.

The versions of the human genome produced by the two teams are in different states of completion because of the different methods each used to determine the order of DNA units in the genome.

The consortium chose first to break the genome down into large chunks, called BAC's, which are about 150,000 DNA letters long, and to sequence each BAC separately. This BAC by BAC strategy also required "mapping" the genome, or defining short sequences of milestone DNA that would help show where each BAC belonged on its parent chromosome, the giant DNA molecules of which the genome is composed.

BAC's are assembled from thousands of snippets of DNA, each about 500 DNA letters in length. This is the longest run of DNA letters that the DNA sequencing machines can analyze. A computer pieces together the snippets by looking for matches in the DNA sequence where one snippet overlaps another.

But the BAC's do not assemble cleanly from their component snippets. One reason is that human DNA is full of repetitive sequences—the same run of letters repeated over and over again—and these repetitions baffle the computer algorithms set to assemble the pieces.

The stage the consortium has now reached is that all its BAC's are mapped, making the whole genome available in a nested set of smaller jigsaw puzzles. But the BAC's are in varying stages of completion. The BAC's covering the two smallest human chromosomes, numbers 21 and 22, are essentially complete. But many other BAC's are in less immaculate states of assembly. Many consist of assembled pieces no more than 10,000 units long, and the order of these pieces within each BAC is not known.

The sum of the assembled pieces in each BAC now covers 85 percent of the genome. This working draft, as the consortium calls it, is maybe not a thing of beauty but is of great value to researchers looking for genes and represents a major accomplishment.

Celera's genome has been assembled by a different method, called a whole genome shotgun strategy. Following a scheme proposed by Dr. Eugene Myers and Dr. J. L. Weber, Celera skips the time-consuming mapping stage and breaks the whole genome down into a set of fragments that are 2,000, 10,000 and 50,000 letters long. These fragments are analyzed separately and then assembled in a single mammoth computer run, with a handful of clever tricks to step across the repetitive sequence regions in the DNA.

The approach ideally required sequencing 30 billion units of DNA—10 times that in a single genome. Dr. Venter seems to have taken a considerable risk by starting his assembly at the end of March this year when he possessed only a threefold coverage of the genome. He has since raised his total to 4.6-fold coverage.

The decision may have been influenced by Celera's rate of capital expenditure— the company's electric bill alone is $100,000 a month—and by the need to sequence the mouse genome as well so as to offer database clients a two-genome package. The mouse genome is expected to be invaluable for interpreting the human genome, and Dr. Venter said today that Celera would finish sequencing it by the end of the year.

Because of having relatively little of its own data, Celera made use of the consortium's publicly available sequence data and, indirectly, of the positional information contained in the consortium's mapped set of BAC's. The consortium can justifiably share in the credit for Celera's version of the genome, another cogent factor in the logic of today's truce.

## Biotech Shares Rise and Fall

Stocks of biotechnology companies rose early yesterday after a White House announcement that the first survey of the human genome had been completed, but investors cashed in some of their profits before trading ended, causing several issues to fall.

Biotechnology shares peaked in March in a speculative frenzy, before backsliding sharply. In recent weeks, they again posted significant increases in anticipation of the genome announcement.

The Celera Genomics unit of the PE Corporation, which participated in the mapping project and has been one of the highest fliers, dropped $12.25, to $113 yesterday. The stock of the company, based in Rockville, Md., hit a record high of $252 a share on Feb. 25. Although well off its high, Celera shares are still up 1,400 percent from this time last year.

*June 27, 2000*

# The Quest for the $1,000 Human Genome

By NICHOLAS WADE

As part of an intensive effort to develop a new generation of machines that will sequence DNA at a vastly reduced cost, scientists are decoding a new human genome—that of James D. Watson, the co-discoverer of the structure of DNA and the first director of the National Institutes of Health's human genome project.

Decoding a person's genome is at present far too costly to be a feasible medical procedure. But the goal now being pursued by the N.I.H. and by several manufacturers, including the company decoding Dr. Watson's DNA, is to drive the costs of decoding a human genome down to as little as $1,000. At that price, it could be worth decoding people's genomes in certain medical situations and, one day, even routinely at birth.

Low-cost decoding may bring the genomic age to the doctor's office, but it will also raise quandaries about how to safeguard and interpret such a wealth of delicate and far-reaching personal information.

The first human genome decoding, completed by a public consortium of universities in 2003, cost more than $500 million. With the same technology, dependent on DNA sequencing machines made by Applied Biosystems, a human genome could probably now be decoded for $10 million to $15 million, experts say.

Much greater efficiency is expected from the new generation of DNA sequencing machines, based on different, highly miniaturized technologies. One machine, made by 454 Life Sciences, has been on the market since March 2005. Another, made by Solexa, will start shipping this summer. Applied Biosystems will start marketing its own next-generation machine next year.

Last month, at a training course organized by the Cold Spring Harbor Laboratory on Long Island, researchers were learning how to use the DNA decoding machines made by 454 Life Sciences. Looking like a hybrid between a washing machine and a giant iPod, the machines cost $500,000 each, not counting the computer software needed to analyze the results.

At their heart lies a plate of light-sensitive chips, the same as those used in telescopes for detecting faint light from distant stars. On top of the plate sits a glass slide pitted with thousands of tiny wells, each containing a fragment of the DNA to be decoded.

261

As each unit of DNA is analyzed in a well, a flash of light is generated by luciferase, the enzyme that fireflies use to make themselves glow. The telescope plate records the twinkling lights from each well and, at the end of the run, which lasts four or five hours, the sequence of units in each well's DNA fragment has been recorded. The fragments are about 100 units in length, and from their overlaps a computer can then be set to piece together the entire genome they come from.

In the training course, the project was to analyze DNA from a Tasmanian devil, a marsupial afflicted with a mysterious malady called devil facial tumor disease. The researchers found that the genome was laden with a virus that had integrated its sequence into the devil's DNA.

The 454 machine can assemble small genomes like those of bacteria, which perhaps accounted for the presence at the course of three scientists from the Department of Homeland Security. But the human genome is about 600 times larger than a bacterium's and includes many repetitive sequences that, like identical pieces in a jigsaw puzzle, make the solution much harder.

At the Cold Spring Harbor course, researchers heard Dr. Watson, the laboratory's chancellor, say that 454 Life Sciences had asked to sequence his genome with their new machine. Only two human genomes have been sequenced to date. The genome sequenced by the public consortium was a mosaic of DNA from several anonymous people. The consortium's rival, Celera Genomics, prepared a draft sequence, most of it from the genome of its former president, Dr. J. Craig Venter.

Dr. Watson told the students that he had given the company permission to publish the sequence of his genome, "provided they didn't release to the world that I have some disease I don't want to know about."

Genomic information can already reveal a lot and will reveal much more as the roles of new genes are discovered.

"I think that personal genetic information should ordinarily be kept secret," Dr. Watson said. "But I have said that 454 can put mine out there, even though it's saying something about my sons."

So far, however, 454 Life Sciences has not published Dr. Watson's genome, and it is not clear how much progress the company has made. Christopher K. McLeod, its chief executive, said, "Technically, we've done a lot of good work on it." But, he added, "I don't think we want to discuss where we are."

Mr. McLeod expressed reservations about releasing personal genetic information, despite having Dr. Watson's permission to do so. "Jim feels there are certain things he'd be comfortable releasing," he said. "I'm not sure we would agree."

Another factor may be that the company is developing a more powerful model of its machine that will be able to read DNA fragments that are 200 or even 400 units in length. These longer-read lengths should make it more feasible to decode large genomes, like those of people.

The 454 machine is at present being bought chiefly by researchers and by the large genome sequencing centers established by the public consortium. But it has begun to show promise for the clinic. One new use is in screening tumors for genes known to be mutated in cancer, a task that existing machines do not do well. Spotting which mutation has occurred in a patient's tumor can help in the choice of chemotherapy.

Although the 454 model is the only next-generation DNA sequencing machine on the market, it will be joined this summer by the machine from Solexa. The Solexa instrument, which will cost $400,000, works on somewhat similar principles but uses fluorescent dyes to visualize the structure of DNA. And next year Applied Biosystems will introduce its next-generation machine, based on a technology developed by George Church of Harvard, said Dennis A. Gilbert, the company's chief scientific officer.

Each of the manufacturers claims special advantages for its technology, ensuring that researchers will have a rich choice.

David Bentley, Solexa's chief scientist, said that the company's DNA sequencing machine had already decoded several bacterial genomes and that he was planning to sequence a human genome—that of an anonymous man from the Yoruba people of Nigeria. An African genome was chosen because there is greater genetic diversity in African populations, Dr. Bentley said.

The demand for whole genome sequencing is a long way off, in Dr. Bentley's view, but not so distant that it is too early to think about the consequences of generating such information. He advocates that two people should control access to a person's genome sequence—the patient and the physician.

Why not the patient alone? Dr. Bentley said genomes would be so difficult to analyze correctly that interpretation should stay within the medical profession. Otherwise, freelance services will spring up, offering to predict whether a person will get heart disease or their age of death. This potential for misinformation "would have a huge adverse impact on the medical use of genetic information," Dr. Bentley said.

A recent example of genetic misinformation occurred last month when a DNA testing genealogy company, Oxford Ancestors, told Thomas R. Robinson, an accountant at the University of Miami, that he was a descendant of Genghis

Khan. Only because Mr. Robinson sought a second opinion did he find that the information was incorrect.

Technology, not medicine, is the immediate force behind the quest for the $1,000 human genome. The new decoding machines are being developed because they are possible, not because hospitals are demanding them. But the makers expect that demand will grow as researchers develop new uses.

"As we drop the price and increase the capability, there are applications that couldn't be done before," like a researcher being able to screen a thousand patients for cancer mutations, Dr. Gilbert said.

At present, only a handful of genes are monitored by doctors in clinical practice, and specific tests for these genes make it unnecessary to decode a person's entire genome. But at some point, the new machines or their successors may make genome decoding a routine medical test.

Already, every newborn baby endures its heel being pricked to draw a few drops of blood, which are tested for a handful of enzymic deficiencies. But when genomes can be decoded for $1,000, a baby may arrive home like a new computer, with its complete genetic operating instructions on a DVD.

*July 18, 2006*

# In Good Health? Thank Your 100 Trillion Bacteria

By GINA KOLATA

For years, bacteria have had a bad name. They are the cause of infections, of diseases. They are something to be scrubbed away, things to be avoided.

But now researchers have taken a detailed look at another set of bacteria that may play even bigger roles in health and disease: the 100 trillion good bacteria that live in or on the human body.

No one really knew much about them. They are essential for human life, needed to digest food, to synthesize certain vitamins, to form a barricade against disease-causing bacteria. But what do they look like in healthy people, and how much do they vary from person to person?

In a new five-year federal endeavor, the Human Microbiome Project, which has been compared to the Human Genome Project, 200 scientists at 80 institutions sequenced the genetic material of bacteria taken from nearly 250 healthy people.

They discovered more strains than they had ever imagined—as many as a thousand bacterial strains on each person. And each person's collection of microbes, the microbiome, was different from the next person's. To the scientists' surprise, they also found genetic signatures of disease-causing bacteria lurking in everyone's microbiome. But instead of making people ill, or even infectious, these disease-causing microbes simply live peacefully among their neighbors.

The results, published on Wednesday in *Nature* and three PLoS journals, are expected to change the research landscape.

The work is "fantastic," said Bonnie Bassler, a Princeton University microbiologist who was not involved with the project. "These papers represent significant steps in our understanding of bacteria in human health."

Until recently, Dr. Bassler added, the bacteria in the microbiome were thought to be just "passive riders." They were barely studied, microbiologists explained, because it was hard to know much about them. They are so adapted to living on body surfaces and in body cavities, surrounded by other bacteria, that many could not be cultured and grown in the lab. Even if they did survive in the lab, they often behaved differently in this alien environment. It was only with the advent of relatively cheap and fast gene sequencing methods that investigators were able to ask what bacteria were present.

Examinations of DNA sequences served as the equivalent of an old-time microscope, said Curtis Huttenhower of the Harvard School of Public Health, an investigator for the microbiome project. They allowed investigators to see—through their unique DNA sequences—footprints of otherwise elusive bacteria.

The work also helps establish criteria for a healthy microbiome, which can help in studies of how antibiotics perturb a person's microbiome and how long it takes the microbiome to recover.

In recent years, as investigators began to probe the microbiome in small studies, they began to appreciate its importance. Not only do the bacteria help keep people healthy, but they also are thought to help explain why individuals react differently to various drugs and why some are susceptible to certain infectious diseases while others are impervious. When they go awry they are thought to contribute to chronic diseases and conditions like irritable bowel syndrome, asthma, even, possibly, obesity.

Humans, said Dr. David Relman, a Stanford microbiologist, are like coral, "an assemblage of life-forms living together."

Dr. Barnett Kramer, director of the division of cancer prevention at the National Cancer Institute, who was not involved with the research project, had another image. Humans, he said, in some sense are made mostly of microbes. From the standpoint of our microbiome, he added, "we may just serve as packaging."

The microbiome starts to grow at birth, said Lita Proctor, program director for the Human Microbiome Project. As babies pass through the birth canal, they pick up bacteria from the mother's vaginal microbiome.

"Babies are microbe magnets," Dr. Proctor said. Over the next two to three years, the babies' microbiomes mature and grow while their immune systems develop in concert, learning not to attack the bacteria, recognizing them as friendly.

Babies born by Caesarean section, Dr. Proctor added, start out with different microbiomes, but it is not yet known whether their microbiomes remain different after they mature. In adults, the body carries two to five pounds of bacteria, even though these cells are minuscule—one-tenth to one-hundredth the size of a human cell. The gut, in particular, is stuffed with them.

"The gut is not jam-packed with food; it is jam-packed with microbes," Dr. Proctor said. "Half of your stool is not leftover food. It is microbial biomass." But bacteria multiply so quickly that they replenish their numbers as fast as they are excreted.

The bacteria also help the immune system, Dr. Huttenhower said. The best example is in the vagina, where they secrete chemicals that can kill other bacteria and make the environment slightly acidic, which is unappealing to other microbes.

Including the microbiome as part of an individual is, some researchers said, a new way to look at human beings.

It was a daunting task, though, to investigate the normal human microbiome. Previous studies of human microbiomes had been small and had looked mostly at fecal bacteria or bacteria in saliva in healthy people, or had examined things like fecal bacteria in individuals with certain diseases, like inflammatory bowel disease, in which bacteria are thought to play a role.

But, said Barbara B. Methé, an investigator for the microbiome study and a microbiologist at the J. Craig Venter Institute, it was hard to know what to make of those studies.

"We were stepping back and saying, 'We don't really have a population study. What does a normal microbiome look like?'" she said.

The first problem was finding completely healthy people for the study. The investigators recruited 600 subjects, ages 18 to 40, poking and prodding them. They brought in dentists to probe their gums, looking for gum disease, and pick at their teeth, looking for cavities. They brought in gynecologists to examine the women to see if they had yeast infections. They examined skin and tonsils and nasal cavities. They made sure the subjects were not too fat and not too thin. Even though those who volunteered thought they filled the bill, half were rejected because they were not completely healthy. And 80 percent of those who were eventually accepted first had to have gum disease or cavities treated by a dentist.

When they had their subjects—242 men and women deemed free of disease in the nose, skin, mouth, gastrointestinal tract and, for the women, vagina—the investigators collected stool samples and saliva, and scraped the subjects' gums and teeth and nostrils and their palates and tonsils and throats. They took samples from the crook of the elbow and the folds of the ear. In all, women were sampled in 18 places, including three sites in the vagina, and men in 15. The investigators resampled subjects three times during the course of the study to see if the bacterial composition of their bodies was stable, generating 11,174 samples.

To catalog the body's bacteria, researchers searched for DNA with a specific gene, 16S rRNA, that is a marker for bacteria and whose slight sequence variations can reveal different bacterial species. They sequenced the bacterial DNA to find the unique genes in the microbiome. They ended up with a deluge of data, much too much to study with any one computer, Dr. Huttenhower said, creating "a huge computational challenge."

The next step, he said, is to better understand how the microbiome affects health and disease and to try to improve health by deliberately altering the microbiome.

But, Dr. Relman said, "we are scratching at the surface now."

It is, he said, "humbling."

*June 13, 2012*

# In Treatment for Leukemia, Glimpses of the Future

### By GINA KOLATA

Genetics researchers at Washington University, one of the world's leading centers for work on the human genome, were devastated. Dr. Lukas Wartman, a young, talented and beloved colleague, had the very cancer he had devoted his career to studying. He was deteriorating fast. No known treatment could save him. And no one, to their knowledge, had ever investigated the complete genetic makeup of a cancer like his.

So one day last July, Dr. Timothy Ley, associate director of the university's genome institute, summoned his team. Why not throw everything we have at seeing if we can find a rogue gene spurring Dr. Wartman's cancer, adult acute lymphoblastic leukemia, he asked. "It's now or never," he recalled telling them. "We will only get one shot."

Dr. Ley's team tried a type of analysis that they had never done before. They fully sequenced the genes of both his cancer cells and healthy cells for comparison, and at the same time analyzed his RNA, a close chemical cousin to DNA, for clues to what his genes were doing.

The researchers on the project put other work aside for weeks, running one of the university's 26 sequencing machines and supercomputer around the clock. And they found a culprit—a normal gene that was in overdrive, churning out huge amounts of a protein that appeared to be spurring the cancer's growth.

Even better, there was a promising new drug that might shut down the malfunctioning gene—a drug that had been tested and approved only for advanced kidney cancer. Dr. Wartman became the first person ever to take it for leukemia.

And now, against all odds, his cancer is in remission and has been since last fall.

While no one can say that Dr. Wartman is cured, after facing certain death last fall, he is alive and doing well. Dr. Wartman is a pioneer in a new approach to stopping cancer. What is important, medical researchers say, is the genes that drive a cancer, not the tissue or organ—liver or brain, bone marrow, blood or colon—where the cancer originates.

One woman's breast cancer may have different genetic drivers from another woman's and, in fact, may have more in common with prostate cancer in a man or another patient's lung cancer.

Under this new approach, researchers expect that treatment will be tailored to an individual tumor's mutations, with drugs, eventually, that hit several key aberrant genes at once. The cocktails of medicines would be analogous to H.I.V. treatment, which uses several different drugs at once to strike the virus in a number of critical areas.

Researchers differ about how soon the method, known as whole genome sequencing, will be generally available and paid for by insurance—estimates range from a few years to a decade or so. But they believe that it has enormous promise, though it has not yet cured anyone.

With a steep drop in the costs of sequencing and an explosion of research on genes, medical experts expect that genetic analyses of cancers will become routine. Just as pathologists do blood cultures to decide which antibiotics will stop a patient's bacterial infection, so will genome sequencing determine which drugs might stop a cancer.

"Until you know what is driving a patient's cancer, you really don't have any chance of getting it right," Dr. Ley said. "For the past 40 years, we have been sending generals into battle without a map of the battlefield. What we are doing now is building the map."

Large drug companies and small biotechs are jumping in, starting to test drugs that attack a gene rather than a tumor type.

Leading cancer researchers are starting companies to find genes that might be causing an individual's cancer to grow, to analyze genetic data and to find and test new drugs directed against these genetic targets. Leading venture capital firms are involved.

For now, whole genome sequencing is in its infancy and dauntingly complex. The gene sequences are only the start—they come in billions of small pieces, like a huge jigsaw puzzle. The arduous job is to figure out which mutations are important, a task that requires skill, experience and instincts.

So far, most who have chosen this path are wealthy and well connected. When Steve Jobs had exhausted other options to combat pancreatic cancer, he consulted doctors who coordinated his genetic sequencing and analysis. It cost him $100,000, according to his biographer. The writer Christopher Hitchens went to the head of the National Institutes of Health, Dr. Francis Collins, who advised him on where to get a genetic analysis of his esophageal cancer.

Harvard Medical School expects eventually to offer whole genome sequencing to help cancer patients identify treatments, said Heidi L. Rehm, who heads the molecular medicine laboratory at Harvard's Partners Healthcare Center for

Personalized Genetic Medicine. But later this year, Partners will take a more modest step, offering whole genome sequencing to patients with a suspected hereditary disorder in hopes of identifying mutations that might be causing the disease.

Whole genome sequencing of the type that Dr. Wartman had, Dr. Rehm added, "is a whole other level of complexity."

Dr. Wartman was included by his colleagues in a research study, and his genetic analysis was paid for by the university and research grants. Such opportunities are not available to most patients, but Dr. Ley noted that the group had done such an analysis for another patient the year before and that no patients were being neglected because of the urgent work to figure out Dr. Wartman's cancer.

"The precedent for moving quickly on a sample to make a key decision was already established," Dr. Ley said.

Ethicists ask whether those with money and connections should have options far out of reach for most patients before such treatments become a normal part of medicine. And will people of more limited means be tempted to bankrupt their families in pursuit of a cure at the far edges?

"If we say we need research because this is a new idea, then why is it that rich people can even access it?" asked Wylie Burke, professor and chairwoman of the department of bioethics at the University of Washington. The saving grace, she said, is that the method will become available to all if it works.

## A Life in Medicine

It was pure happenstance that landed Dr. Wartman in a university at the forefront of cancer research. He grew up in small-town Indiana, aspiring to be a veterinarian like his grandfather. But in college, he worked summers in hospitals and became fascinated by cancer. He enrolled in medical school at Washington University in St. Louis, where he was drawn to research on genetic changes that occur in cancers of the blood. Dr. Wartman knew then what he wanted to do—become a physician researcher.

Those plans fell apart in the winter of 2002, his last year of medical school, when he went to California to be interviewed for a residency program at Stanford. On the morning of his visit, he was nearly paralyzed by an overwhelming fatigue.

"I could not get out of bed for an interview that was the most important of my life," Dr. Wartman recalled. Somehow, he forced himself to drive to Palo Alto in a drenching rain. He rallied enough to get through the day.

When he returned to St. Louis, he gave up running, too exhausted for the sport he loved. He started having night sweats.

"I thought it might be mono," he said. "And I thought I would ride it out."

But then the long bones in his legs began to hurt. He was having fevers.

He was so young then—only 25—and had always been so healthy that his only doctor was a pediatrician. So he went to an urgent care center in February 2003. The doctor there thought his symptoms might come from depression, but noticed that his red and white blood cell counts were low. And Lukas Wartman, who had been fascinated by the biology of leukemia, began to suspect he had it.

"I was definitely scared," he said. "It was so unreal."

The next day, Mr. Wartman, who was about to graduate from Washington University's medical school, went back there for more tests. A doctor slid a long needle into his hip bone and drew out marrow for analysis.

"We looked at the slide together," Dr. Wartman said, recalling that terrible time. "It was packed with leukemia cells. I was in a state of shock."

Dr. Wartman remained at the university for his residency and treatment: nine months of intensive chemotherapy, followed by 15 months of maintenance chemotherapy. Five years passed when the cancer seemed to be gone. But then it came back. Next came the most risky remedy—intensive chemotherapy to put the cancer into remission followed by a bone-marrow transplant from his younger brother.

Seven months after the transplant, feeling much stronger, he went to a major cancer meeting and sat in on a session on his type of leukemia. The speaker, a renowned researcher, reported that only 4 or 5 percent of those who relapsed survived.

"My stomach turned," Dr. Wartman said. "I will never forget the shock of hearing that number."

But his personal gauge of recovery—how far he could run—was encouraging.

By last spring, three years after his transplant, Dr. Wartman was running six to seven miles every other day and feeling good. "I thought maybe I would run a half marathon in the fall."

Then the cancer came back. He remembered that number, 4 or 5 percent, for patients with one relapse. He had relapsed a second time.

This time, he said, "There is no number."

His doctors put him on a clinical trial to try to beat the cancer with chemotherapy and hormones. It did not work.

They infused him with his brother's healthy marrow cells, to no avail.

## A Clue in RNA

Dr. Wartman's doctors realized then that their last best hope for saving him was to use all the genetic know-how and technology at their disposal.

After their month of frantic work to beat cancer's relentless clock, the group, led by Richard Wilson and Elaine Mardis, directors of the university's genome institute, had the data. It was Aug. 31.

The cancer's DNA had, as expected, many mutations, but there was nothing to be done about them. There were no drugs to attack them.

But the other analysis, of the cancer's RNA, was different. There was something there, something unexpected.

The RNA sequencing showed that a normal gene, FLT3, was wildly active in the leukemia cells. Its normal role is to make cells grow and proliferate. An overactive FLT3 gene might be making Dr. Wartman's cancer cells multiply so quickly.

Even better, there was a drug, sunitinib or Sutent, approved for treating advanced kidney cancer, that inhibits FLT3.

But it costs $330 a day, and Dr. Wartman's insurance company would not pay for it. He appealed twice to his insurer and lost both times.

He also pleaded with the drug's maker, Pfizer, to give him the drug under its compassionate use program, explaining that his entire salary was only enough to pay for 7½ months of Sutent. But Pfizer turned him down, too.

As September went by, Dr. Wartman was getting panicky.

"Every day is a roller coaster," he said at the time, "and everything is up in the air."

Desperate to try the drug, he scraped up the money to buy a week's worth and began taking it on Sept. 16. Within days, his blood counts were looking more normal.

But over dinner at a trendy St. Louis restaurant, he picked at his chicken and said he was afraid to hope.

"Obviously it's exciting," he said. "But Sutent could have unanticipated effects on my bone marrow." Maybe his rising red blood cell counts were just a side effect of the drug. Or maybe they were just a coincidence.

"It's hard to say if I feel any different," Dr. Wartman said.

And the cost of the drug nagged at him. If it worked, how long could he afford to keep taking it?

The next day, a nurse at the hospital pharmacy called with what seemed miraculous news: a month's supply of Sutent was waiting for Dr. Wartman. He did not know at the time, but the doctors in his division had pitched in to buy the drug.

Two weeks later, his bone marrow, which had been full of leukemia cells, was clean, a biopsy showed.

Still, he was nervous. The test involved taking out just a small amount of marrow. Cancer cells could be lurking unseen.

The next test was flow cytometry, which used antibodies to label cancer cells. Again, there were no cancer cells.

But even flow cytometry could be misleading, Dr. Wartman told himself.

Finally, a yet more sensitive test, called FISH, was done. It labels cancer cells with fluorescent pieces of DNA to identify leukemia cells. Once again, there were none.

"I can't believe it," his awe-struck physician, Dr. John DiPersio, told him.

Dr. Wartman, alone in his apartment, waited for his partner, Damon Berardi, to come home from work. That evening, Mr. Berardi, a 31-year-old store manager, opened the door with no idea of Dr. Wartman's momentous news. To his surprise, Dr. Wartman was home early, waiting in the kitchen with champagne and two flutes he had given Mr. Berardi for Christmas. He told Mr. Berardi he should sit down.

"My leukemia is in remission," he said. The men embraced exultantly, and Dr. Wartman popped open the champagne.

"I felt an overwhelming sense of relief and a renewed vision of our future together," Mr. Berardi said. "There were no tears at that moment. We had both had cried plenty. This was a moment of hope."

## Hunches and Decisions

Dr. Wartman and his doctors had fateful decisions to make, with nothing but hunches to guide them. Should he keep taking Sutent or have another bone-marrow transplant now that he was in remission again?

In the end, Dr. DiPersio decided Dr. Wartman should have the transplant because without it the cancer might mutate and escape the Sutent.

Meanwhile, Pfizer had decided to give him the drug. Dr. Wartman has no idea why. Perhaps the company was swayed by an impassioned plea from his nurse practitioner, Stephanie Bauer.

Dr. Wartman's cancer is still gone, for now, but he has struggled with a common complication of bone-marrow transplants, in which the white blood cells of the transplanted marrow attack his cells as though they were foreign. He has had rashes and felt ill. But these complications are gradually lessening, and he is back at work in Dr. Ley's lab.

His colleagues want to look for the same mutation in the cancer cells of other patients with his cancer. And they would like to start a clinical trial testing Sutent to discover whether the drug can help others with leukemia, or whether the solution they found was unique to Lukas Wartman.

Dr. Wartman himself is left with nagging uncertainties. He knows how lucky he is, but what does the future hold? Can he plan a life? Is he cured?

"It's a hard feeling to describe," he said. "I am in uncharted waters."

*July 7, 2012*

CHAPTER 13

# Germ Theory

# Dr. Koch's Discovery

The public may justly complain of the slowness of the secular and scientific press to recognize the news value of the highly important results of Prof. Koch's discovery of the parasitical source of tubercular disease.

Prof. Tyndall's letter to the London *Times*, which we published on Wednesday morning, first made known to the English-speaking world the facts stated in Dr. Koch's address, delivered nearly a month earlier before the Physiological Society of Berlin. Yet it is safe to say that the little pamphlet which was left to find its way through the slow mails to the English scientist outweighed in importance and interest for the human race all the press dispatches which have been flashed under the Channel since the date of the delivery of the address—March 24. The rapid growth of the Continental capitals, the movements of princely noodles and fat, vulgar Duchesses, the debates in the Servian Skupschina, and the progress or receding of sundry royal gouts are given to the wings of the lightning; a lumbering mail-coach is swift enough for the news of one of the great scientific discoveries of the age. Similarly, the gifted gentlemen who daily sift out for the American public the pith and kernel of the Old World's news leave Dr. Koch and his bacilli to chance it in the ocean mails, while they challenge the admiration of every gambler and jockey in this Republic by the fullness and accuracy of their cable reports of horse-races.

In its purely scientific aspects, Dr. Koch's discovery that pulmonary consumption and all tubercular diseases are produced by a "minute rod-shaped parasite" is one of the most impressive and striking achievements of the human mind. This young German physiologist, as Prof. Tyndall sketches him, carrying on a series of masterly investigations in the intervals of attendance upon such cases of croup and measles as his "modest country practice" brought him; afterward, favored by Government patronage, extending his researches and perfecting his methods of observation and experiment until with his microscope, his rabbits, dogs, and guinea pigs, and his wonderful breeding establishments for the bacilli, he had built up for his discovery a scientific basis such as Darwin was accustomed to construct for his own before he gave them to the world—the man and his work furnish a new and shining illustration of what can be done for humanity by that modern science which elderly orthodox gentlemen are fond of declaring is made up half of empiricism and half of the bravado of reckless self-assertion. In pushing one step further our knowledge of the pathology of the human body, Dr. Koch has given science a new title to its honors, and imbued with new force and meaning the command, "Know thyself."

But science has yet much to do to seize the results of this discovery and apply them to the alleviation and cure of disease. We cannot doubt that every intelligent reader of Prof. Tyndall's abstract of Dr. Koch's lecture instantly recognized the importance of the proof it affords that consumption is contagious. It cannot be said, therefore, that for the present the new knowledge we have gained is void of practical interest. But to draw from it its great possible benefits is the work of the future, and, fortunately, a work which the physiologist and physician may hopefully undertake. The popular interest in the little parasite Dr. Koch has introduced to the world will deepen in proportion as medical science demonstrates its power to annihilate him or rob him of his fatal power. Tubercular diseases, it is said, are the cause of one-seventh of the deaths of the human race. In this country pulmonary consumption is a scourge of such distressing prevalence and mortality that it may be reckoned first among the maladies which our changeable climate is supposed to foster. And it is a disease against which medical skill contends with but slight hope of success. Whether this will be true for all time, in spite of Dr. Koch's observations of habits of bacilli, cannot be foretold. But the analogy of that other dreaded scourge—small-pox—affords ground for hope that its melancholy ravages may be stayed by some form of artificial inoculation.

Two hundred years ago almost everybody had the small-pox. Court chronicles mention its disfiguring effects upon the faces of Kings and nobles, and half the advertisements for runaway slaves contained the statement that the fugitive was "deeply pitted with small-pox." But the small-pox bacillus has been tamed and made a comparatively harmless little creature by a modifying transplantation to the bodies of cattle, whence he is voluntarily received into the human system, as a safeguard against the invasion of his kinsman of the original type. Dr. Koch's experiments have thus far failed to produce any modification in the character of the tubercular bacillus sufficient to warrant the experiment of inoculation upon a human subject. We may be very sure, however, that the attempt will not be given up by physiologists until it is proved to be hopeless or the supply of rabbits and guinea pigs gives out. But inoculation for consumptive diseases is not the only end science will strive for. What can be done to stay the ravages of the bacilli when they have already fastened upon the system? Do they sometimes lie dormant for years in the lungs? Is it the bacillus itself, the germ of consumption that is, or only a tendency to the disease that a consumptive parent transmits to the child? Why do atmospheric conditions so visibly stay or favor the work of the parasite in many cases? These and a hundred other kindred questions are yet to be answered.

*May 7, 1882*

CHAPTER 14

# Heart Disease

# Can Dreaded Hardening of Arteries
# Now Be Cured?

The study of diseases of the heart and blood vessels has received a great impetus in the last year or two. The result has been a noteworthy improvement in the methods of diagnosis, a better understanding of the circulatory system, the invention of many mechanical aids to cardiac therapeutics, and the discovery of a successful remedy for some of the lesions which heretofore have baffled the skill of the medical profession.

In addition, the daring operations on heart, arteries, and veins should not be forgotten; operations which were unheard of a few short years ago, but which have become matters of routine practice. Surgery of the thorax, which includes the heart and the adjacent blood vessels, has assumed such importance that in one hospital at least in this city, the German Hospital, a special operating room has been constructed for this kind of work, so that the air pressure can be regulated to the exigencies of the case.

Prominent among the items of news of a scientific nature recently cabled from Europe was the announcement that Prof. Arthur Keith, the eminent English physician, has been demonstrating at the Royal College of Surgeons, London, some remarkable advances which have been made lately in the knowledge of the structure, functions, and diseases of the heart. One of the most remarkable of these, it is said, is the detection of a small mass of peculiar tissue, which has been named the heart's "pacemaker," because apparently within it the beat of the heart has its origin. The announcement probably refers to the localization of a nerve centre.

The structure, it appears, was first recognized five years ago by Prof. Keith and Dr. Martin. Then Prof. Thomas Lewis of University College found that the site of the new structure was also the point at which the heart-beat first appears. Prof. Lewis fixed the localization by means of an electrical device.

Although this point is the chief centre for the activity and regulation of the heart, there are apparently many secondary centres which can take over the initiating of the heart-beat. It is said that the suggestion which led to the discovery of Prof. Keith was made by a Japanese pupil named Towara in Prof. Aschoff's laboratory.

The most dreaded of all the ills of the cardiac and vascular systems nowadays seems to be arteriosclerosis, or hardening of the arteries. It is an old axiom that a man is as old as his arteries." This simply means that it is possible for a man of forty to have arteries in a condition which should not be encountered normally in persons under seventy years of age. The hard or hardening artery means increased blood pressure, with a consequent increased strain on the heart.

This may lead to a long train of distressing symptoms, and, of course, ultimate death.

The public is beginning to know a good deal about "hardening of the arteries." The term figures often—too often—in obituary notices. Heart disease, according to statistics, is carrying off a greater percentage of persons than formerly. This fact cannot be denied, and it is attributed largely to worry, the abnormal rush of the life of to-day, and sometimes to faulty methods of eating and bad nutrition.

Dr. M. Herz of Vienna, an authority on diseases of the heart and blood vessels, commented as follows last Summer on arterio-sclerosis:

"In the United States there is not, so far as we know, any widespread fear of arteriosclerosis. The public recognizes that people are ill from 'hardening of the arteries,' and that they often die with, if not from, this condition.

"In Austria, however, there is an exaggerated fear of this condition, which in medical men is amounting to a phobia, and the great frequency or suddenly fatal angina pectoris and cardio-renal (heart and kidney) disease seems largely responsible for this fear. The author [Dr. Herz] thinks arteriosclerosis may have undergone a change of type; and in response to a circular of inquiry addressed to several thousand physicians in reference to possible new causal elements, it appears that psychic trauma (mental injury) and excessive bodily labor are leading factors, and that a combination of the two is especially in evidence.

"All individuals now labor under forced pressure, due, as the author terms it, to conditions having become Americanized. There is a continued succession of psychic traumatism with physical overstrain, and as a matter of fact the cause is practically that of neurasthenia, and the treatment should be mainly psychic in so-called premature cases, the production of a cheerful frame of mind."

The anxiety and fear concerning arteriosclerosis in Austria may have some bearing on the fact that out of Austria has come a man, Dr. Bruno Fellner Jr., of Franzenbad, near Carlsbad, to tell of what seems to be a fairly successful remedy he discovered for the disease while working in the laboratory with Prof. Franz Müller at Berlin, head of the Physiological Institute there. Dr. Fellner arrived in New York a few days ago, and will demonstrate his treatment in a number of hospitals in this city and throughout the country, and explain it to various medical societies.

Dr. Fellner appeared before the Medical Society of the Greater City of New

York last Monday evening and delivered an address on the subject. Here is a part of his paper:

"A number of years have been devoted by the author to the study of blood pressure, in the human body, especially to its abnormal increase (hypertension) as it is found in its most universal and specific representative, arteriosclerosis. These studies were pursued in Vienna at the clinics of Prof. Nothnagel and Prof. von Noorden, and in Munich with Prof. Friedrich Müller.

"For years it has been my aim to find a remedy which would counteract or neutralize or remove the contraction of the peripheral arteries, which is the main factor in the production of increased resistance to the heart's action and obstruction of free circulation of the blood, both symptoms of increased blood pressure. Such a remedy would be expected to regulate the circulation in two ways: Gradual persistent reduction of pressure and by distinct enlargement of the peripheral vessels.

"All drugs known to be vaso-dilators (dilators of blood vessels) or which exert favorable action on any of the symptoms of arteriosclerosis were subjected to trial without satisfactory results, until Prof. Franz Müller of Berlin and myself decided to utilize the former's brilliant researches on the vaso-dilatory and pressure-reducing action, of yohimbin, which, derived from the bark of a tree indigenous to Kamerun, in Africa, had hitherto only been known as a drug of doubtful value in another class of ailments.

"Intravenous injections of yohimbin in cats was found to produce a pronounced reduction of blood pressure, dilatation of the peripheral vessels, and increased volume of blood in the extremities and in the brain. This action also occurred in remote arteries, i.e., when heart and brain were excluded, and was, therefore, undoubtedly due to direct irritation of the peripheral vaso-motor nerves and the muscular coats of the vessels.

"The question then occurred to me whether and in what manner the results of these experiments could be applied to cases of hypertension, that is, arteriosclerosis. The hypodermic administration of the drug was found the only method which insured good results. Yohimbin alone, however, was found impractical on account of its injurious action upon the respiratory centres and its irritating action upon the sacral plexus (of nerves).

"Numerous combinations with other drugs were tried with the view of excluding this latter peculiarity without success. Finally, however, it was discovered that the only combination in which it would retain its vaso-dilatory property and lose its irritating action was that of nitrate of yohimbin with uretan. In this new medicament, called vasotonin, the disagreeable properties of yohimbin have been completely neutralized.

"Vasotonin is dispensed in sterile vials of two cubic centimetres, each containing a single dose, and the injection into the arms is painless and can be done without interfering with the patient's daily work, although it will be wise to administer the first dose at the patient's home, followed by a rest of one hour. As a rule injections are made every other day, except in cases with very grave symptoms, when they are practiced daily. About twenty injections are necessary. It is very desirable to observe the patient closely, not alone for the improvement of his symptoms, but also of the blood pressure with the aid of proper apparatus.

"Prof. Müller and myself made the first public report of the results of our experiments with this drug at the Congress for Internal Medicine held at Wiesbaden in 1909; later, in the Medical Society of Berlin. Since that time the remedy has been used in numerous hospitals, in clinics, and in private practice, so that up to date the number of cases treated amounts to about 5,000.

"I will now submit to you an impartial, unbiased report of these cases, limiting it to my personal experience and to those published in recent literature by well-known reliable authors. My own cases number 120; 100 of arteriosclerosis, 20 of hypertension from other causes. The increased blood pressure fell considerably in 90 per cent, which result was obtained in from two to six weeks, and lasted from four to fifteen months.

"Increase of circulation in the peripheral blood vessels could be easily demonstrated. Furthermore, it was observed that there was a considerable reduction in the size of the dilated heart, especially of the left ventricle, and also a more or less complete disappearance of various cerebral and nervous symptoms due to the sclerotic process.

"Fifteen cases of angina pectoris remained absolutely free of symptoms for weeks and months. Upon return of that painful condition, a second course of treatment had a favorable influence, lasting from six to twelve months. The precordial pressure, air hunger, vertigo, spasms of vessels, and other sclerotic symptoms disappeared. The patient would regain his courage and take a renewed interest in life.

"Of course, I do not propose to claim a permanent cure of this formidable organic disease, but I do maintain that in 80 per cent of my cases there was a distinct and lasting improvement, 10 per cent were benefited but slightly, and in 10 per cent, while the remedy made no impression upon the disease, there was absolutely no bad effect in any manner.

"The following reports are taken front current literature, especially the German.

During a discussion following the reading of a paper by Prof. Müller and myself, Prof. Herz recommended the use of vasotonin, especially in cases of presclerosis and in cases of angina pectoris, but deprecated the reduction of blood pressure à tout prix, although he did not agree with Krehl, who saw absolutely no benefit in arteriosclerosis from pressure-reducing therapy. He extolled the practical results obtained with vasotonin, in which he was joined by Prof. Senator.

"Stachelin of the first medical division of the Charity Hospital of Berlin makes the first extensive and painstaking report. His especial object was to determine whether, when blood pressure was reduced by vasotonin, other symptoms usually accompanying this condition were also favorably influenced, which is denied by Krehl. He declares that with the aid of the sphygmomanometer he was able to demonstrate distinct dilatation of the peripheral vessels, accompanied by considerable diminution of the pressure.

"This reduction varies considerably. The dilatation may be observed in the arm after eight hours. There was also considerable improvement in all subjective symptoms, which would last some time. After fifteen to thirty injections given in the course of four to six weeks, Stachelin saw great relief in cases of angina pectoris, which is afforded by no other known remedy. It is this success in this most grave and painful form of arteriosclerosis which induces Stachelin to consider the immediate use of vasotonin as the foremost indication in the treatment of that affliction.

"Other subjective symptoms, such as vertigo, headache, dyspnoea (shortness of breath), precordial pressure (pressure in front of the heart), and pain were greatly relieved, so that Stachelin advocates the use of vasotonin also in these cases, whether accompanied by hypertension or not. Nephritis (Bright's disease) furnishes no counter indication.

"These results obtained in hospitals are supported by experience gathered in private practice. Grabi, after observations made upon himself and others who had suffered from this disorder for years, declares that none of the hitherto employed means to reduce pressure showed such a continued action as vasotonin. The most various angio-sclerotic disorders are removed.

"Similar favorable results have been obtained by Schlattenstein in the policlinics at Rosin. Rosendorff of the Jewish Hospital writes of absolute failure to obtain positive results. This is not easily explained, although it is an interesting fact that different observers employing the self-same material occasionally arrive at opposite results. Then we have Bennecke and Lommel of Jena using the same material at that hospital, the former deriving no better results from the use of vasotonin than from the customary hospital treatment, while the latter writes of similar favorable results as obtained by Stachelin and myself.

"Another observation made in my first cases was the favorable influence this remedy had upon sclerotic disturbances in the brain. Experiments upon the animal showed this to be due to a distinct dilatation of the cerebral vessels, and this fact was further beautifully illustrated by Hirschfelder in Liehen's clinic in a patient who had a considerable loss of substance of the bony vault of the skull. The brain was examined by the plethymograph during the administration of vasotonin. Hirschfelder found after a double dose of vasotonin there was considerable elevation of the plethymogram, showing a great increase in the quantity of blood circulating in the brain.

"This improvement in the cerebral circulation after reduction of hypertension has caused Hirschfelder, Stachelin, and myself to consider it indicated in such cases of cerebral arteriosclerosis, in direct opposition to Tobias.

"Liehen bases his use of vasotonin in cases of depressive melancholia on this very action of vasotonin. His results are to be published in greater detail in the near future. Again, it has been asserted that in cases of apoplectic injury to the brain vasotonin has caused a rapid subsidence of the alarming symptoms and an early disappearance of the accompanying paralysis.

"The blood supply of the sensory organs is also powerfully influenced by this drug. A perceptible dilatation of the retinal vessels has been observed, and researches as to its use in various affections of the eye are now being made.

"Stein and myself at the policlinic of Prof. Alexander in Vienna have tried it in those aural disturbances due to arteriosclerosis of the labyrinth. Such patients often exhibit no other symptoms of arteriosclerosis except those referred to the ear, such as vertigo, ringing of the ears, deafness, and headache. The sphygmomanometer, however, will always show an increased arterial tension.

"A dozen of these cases, in which every other therapeutic measure had failed to give relief, were treated with full doses of vasotonin, which invariably caused a subsidence of these troublesome symptoms as soon as the pressure-reducing action of the blood became evident. Vertigo was always the first to disappear, as shown by the aid of the revolving chair. The deafness was affected in a lesser degree, while the ringing was much improved.

"In bronchial asthma it affords much relief, cutting short the attacks, but the improvement does not endure as in cases due to arteriosclerosis. However, Jacobs of Krause's clinic, has had very gratifying results in these cases.

"When the tension and pressure in the boiler of a machine are dangerously high, one must open the safety valve as well as other communications to allow the surplus steam to escape. We will, therefore, consider the best remedy, one which will reduce the blood pressure by appealing to vasomotor nerves which govern and regulate the smallest vessels, causing them to open wide, thus increasing their calibre, which will admit of more abundant circulation of blood through them with greater rapidity; the pressure will fall, and the heart and other organs will receive a greater amount of the nourishing fluid.

"At best the treatment of arteriosclerosis is of doubtful success, certainly almost hopeless until this remedy was discovered, which has been shown experimentally and practically to reduce blood pressure, to dilate the blood vessels (accelerating the coursing through them of the blood), to dissolve spasm of the walls of the vessels. It meets the requirements of the theories hitherto accepted of the causation of arteriosclerosis.

"May we not, therefore, hope that this increased flow through the contracted vessels will assist materially by furnishing new nourishment in the recovery of the rigid, degenerated coats of the arteries?"

Dr. Fellner will appear before other medical societies in this city to discuss this new remedy.

The use of the sphygmomanometer has contributed in a large measure to the improvement in methods of diagnosis and in observing the progress of diseases affecting the circulatory system. It is an instrument for measuring the pressure of the blood. It is fastened about the wrist, rather tightly, and the impetus of the pulse is transmitted to mercury in a tube, and the mercury rises proportionately to the blood pressure, which is measured by the marks on the glass, in a manner similar to the registration of temperature by the thermometer.

Another remarkable instrument which is employed now in the diagnosis of cardiac ailments is the electrocardiograph. The impulse of the heart causes tracings to be made, and from these tracings the physician is able to tell whether or not the heart is in a normal condition and position. The accompanying illustrations of electrocardiograms, and X-ray pictures with electrocardiograms, show the difference in tracings resulting from normal positions, malpositions, and pathological conditions of the heart.

These two aids to diagnosis have become well-nigh indispensable to physicians, whether general practitioners, specialists, or insurance examiners.

Dr. J. W. Fisher of Milwaukee says in the insurance department of the *Medical Record*:

"No practitioner of medicine should be without a sphygmomanometer. He has in this instrument a most valuable aid in diagnosis. The sphygmomanometer is indispensable in life insurance examinations, and the time is not far distant when all progressive life insurance companies will require its use in all examinations of applicants for life insurance."

A notable feature of surgical work with the blood vessels to-day is the great improvement in the methods of the transfusion of blood. Formerly it was transferred from the donor to the recipient through a glass or metal tube. The operator could never be certain of the value of the procedure, inasmuch as some change was likely to, and often did, occur in the blood while it was passing through the tube, so that it was ineffectual for the purpose for which it was required when it reached the recipient.

This obstacle is now overcome. Direct transfusion is the method of to-day. The artery of the donor is severed and the free end is applied directly to the opened vein of the recipient. The blood flows directly into the vein, and its value is unimpaired in the transmission.

A new method of combating gangrene resulting from arteriosclerosis has been devised. It is a surgical procedure, and consists in a change of circulation by cutting into the affected limb and uniting the main artery with the main vein. It has proved successful in arresting the destructive process in several cases.

A stimulus to thoracic surgery, including necessary operations on the heart and on blood vessels in its vicinity, has been given in this city by the erection at the German Hospital of a new operating pavilion to be devoted solely to operations of this character. It was established as the result of the energy and enthusiasm of Dr. Willy Meyer.

This pavilion has a wonderful air pressure system. In operations where it is necessary to open the chest cavity an air pressure different from the normal is often required, and in the new pavilion any desired pressure can be obtained.

"The German Hospital of New York," says Dr. Meyer, in a descriptive article written for the *Medical Record*, "appears thus thoroughly equipped for the performance of thoracic surgery by the transpleural route. It is not limited to the use of the apparatuses which I have provided, but affords facilities for the use of any other thoracic apparatus and the employment of all methods appearing at all promising.

"For, looking broadly at the prospective evolution of thoracic surgery, I expect practice to prove that surgical work in the thorax will have to be done along the general lines of surgical work in other parts of the body.

"There is no one apparatus and no one method covering every contingency. They should all be employed wherever indicated and should be ready for immediate use when required. It is on these comprehensive lines that the new thoracic department of the German Hospital has been conceived and constructed."

*November 26, 1911*

# Dr. Meltzer Perfects Devices to
# "Raise the Dead"

Something more than a year ago a group of famous scientists organized to study the effects of electric shock in the hope of lessening the number of casualties resulting from accidents in the industrial world. The immediate object sought was an improved method of resuscitation.

The commission named for this purpose was composed of members of the American Medical Association, the National Electric Light Association, and the American Institute of Electrical Engineers. Prominent among the members of the commission nominated by the American Medical Association was Dr. Samuel J. Meltzer of the Rockefeller Institute for Medical Research. Among this scientist's well-known achievements was the perfection of the intra-tracheal insufflation method of artificial respiration (in conjunction with Dr. Auer), which is of great value in the administration of general anaesthetics where operations extending over a long period have to be performed. It has also saved the lives of many who were practically dead. There is an instance described by Dr. Meltzer in the article to be quoted from later in which a man took 15 grains of morphine by hypodermic injection (enough to kill fifteen men) and then turned on the gas. To all intents and purposes he was dead when discovered, but he "came to life" again after intra-tracheal insufflation had been practiced for twelve hours. This story was denied when printed exclusively in *The Times* last Fall, but now it receives official confirmation.

## First Experiments

As soon as Dr. Meltzer assumed his responsibilities as a member of the commission he set to work to discover a simple means of artificial respiration by pharyngeal insufflation (the forcing of air into the lungs through the channels of mouth and pharynx) which would be readily available in emergency cases in all kinds of industrial plants. The results of a series of brilliant experiments were announced two months later in the *Journal of the American Medical Association* on May 11, 1912. In the course of his report Dr. Meltzer made this statement:

"I have made also a few experiments on animals which were killed purposely either by etherization or by illuminating gas. In these cases the pharyngeal insufflation was not instituted until all traces of respiration and heart beats disappeared. So far, only two recoveries can be recorded. No serious attempt, however, has yet been made to study those problems in a proper manner."

A brief paragraph will be sufficient to outline the method proposed by Dr. Meltzer at that time. It consisted of the introduction of a catheter into the pharynx, pulling out the tongue, forcing the back part of the tongue against the roof of the mouth by pressure applied far back under the chin, putting a weight on the abdomen to keep air from being forced into the stomach, connecting the catheter with a bellows, and pumping air into the lungs.

Now, a year later, Dr. Meltzer says (*Journal of the American Medical Association,* May 10, 1913) that while this method was successful in animals it did not stand the crucial test when applied to human beings. This did not discourage the scientist, however, for he declares in the same paragraph that he has overcome the difficulties met with and obtained the desired end, not by one method alone but by two! The methods are extremely simple and can be used by laymen in factories after a few instructions. Dr. Meltzer's latest report on this subject is issued from the Department of Physiology and Pharmacology of the Rockefeller Institute for Medical Research, and is entitled "Simple Devices for Effective Artificial Respiration in Emergencies."

"The method thus described," says the author, referring to his earlier report of a year ago, "which worked well in four species of animals (dogs, cats, rabbits, and monkeys), has since been tried on living as well as on dead human beings. Here, however, the method failed to work. In human beings, pressure on the suprahyoid region (above the hyoid bone) does not restrict effectively the free escape of air through the mouth; neither is the entrance into the nasopharynx sufficiently blocked by the pressure of the flexible pharyngeal tube. The air insufflated into the pharynx escapes freely through the mouth and nose and enters therefore into the lungs with too little force to overcome the resisting elasticity of the lungs and the thoracic walls and thus to cause an inspiration.

"In other words, the simple arrangement which is so efficient a method of artificial respiration for animals proved to be unsatisfactory when applied to man because of the difference in the anatomic construction.

"I then set out to develop the method further, so as to make it applicable to human beings. I believe that I now have attained that end. In the following I shall describe two methods which have caused effective respiration (that is, effective rhythmic entrance of air into the lungs) even in human cadavers stiff in rigor mortis or frozen stiff. I shall designate the respective methods of artificial respiration as the pharyngeal and the mask device. I shall describe the pharyngeal device first and in greater detail.

"The pharyngeal tube to be used in human beings is made of metal. It measures transversely 38 millimeters and vertically 27, and is about 18 centimeters long. The lower (tongue) side is flat, the upper (palate) side is round. At the pharyngeal end the upper side is longer by about four centimeters than the tongue side; when the tube is inserted through the mouth into the pharynx, the end of the upper side has to reach the posterior wall of the pharynx, while the lower side may end somewhere between the radix (root) of the tongue and the posterior wall of the pharynx.

"For an adult of medium size the dimensions of the tube are sufficient to fill out the entrance into the pharynx so as to prevent the escape of air through the mouth; it also blocks reliably the entrance into the nasopharynx. Of course, tubes of various dimensions may be had at hand, so as to fit the individual sizes. The outer end of the tube carries, in the first place, a hollow neck-like projection to connect the tube with the insufflation apparatus. It has, besides, a round hole, through which a large stomach tube may be introduced into the esophagus and the stomach, when necessary; this hole is usually kept closed by a movable plate."

## The Respiratory Valve

"The outer end of the pharyngeal tube is connected by a short heavy piece of rubber tubing with a little device which I designate as respiratory valve. It is a small tube about 10 centimeters long and 3 centimeters in diameter, which carries a valve inside and a ring outside. By means of that ring the valve may be moved from side to side. When it is moved to the right side, it connects the insufflating apparatus with the pharyngeal tube and air or oxygen is driven into the pharynx and the lungs. When the ring is moved to the left side, the current of air or oxygen is shut off; at the same time an opening is established through which the expired air may now readily escape. The respiratory valve may be conveniently held in the hand and the ring moved from side to side by the thumb. The ring moving the valve is not in the middle, but near one end of that little device, the end which should be connected with the pharyngeal tube.

"The other end of the respiratory valve should be connected by means of strong rubber tubing with glass-blower foot bellows which should be worked so as to give an approximately continuous current of air; or it may be connected with an oxygen tank. Between the respiratory valve and the bellows (or oxygen cylinder) a 'safety valve' should be interpolated in order that the air or oxygen should not be driven into the pharynx with too high pressure.

"The safety valve may be of such a simple kind as I described in the recently appeared sixth volume of Keen's work on surgery for the intratracheal insufflation apparatus. It consists simply of a calibrated tube dipping in mercury. The pressure should be arranged for not less than 20 millimeters mercury, and may be even 25 millimeters; the pharyngeal system of insufflation will always permit an escape of some air through any of the exits."

## How It Works

"Heavy weights to be placed on the abdomen, a broad belt to reinforce the pressure on the abdomen, and a large stomach tube, about 33 French, complete the outfit.

"The pharyngeal insufflation apparatus for artificial respiration consists, then, of a metal pharyngeal tube, the respiratory valve, foot bellows, or an oxygen tank and a safety valve. In addition, there should be on hand a tongue forceps, a stomach tube, heavy weights and a belt. The procedure is as follows:

"After a heavy weight is placed on the abdomen, the tongue should be pulled out by means of an appropriate forceps and the pharyngeal tube inserted into mouth and pharynx as far as it may go. For the sake of being in readiness, the respiratory valve should be kept attached to the pharyngeal tube. The free end of the respiratory valve should now be connected with the foot bellows or the oxygen tank, to either or which a safety valve is attached.

"Now the oxygen tank should be opened, or the foot bellows started working, while the respiratory valve is taken in the right hand and the ring moved by the thumb from side to side, keeping it for two or three seconds at each place. The same man who works the bellows with his foot may work at the same time the respiratory valve with his hand.

"When the ring rests at the right side, the air from the bellows or the oxygen from the tank is insufflated into the pharynx with a force of 20 millimeters of mercury and unavoidably enters the lungs, causing an inspiration. On account of the pressure on the abdomen the inspiration causes essentially distension of the thorax; when the ring is turned to the left the insufflation is cut off and the elastic recoil of the ribs and of the abdominal viscera causes an efficient expiration.

"The rubber tubing connecting the pharyngeal tube with the respiratory valve should be short, in order to cut off the dead space and during expiration eliminate carbon dioxide as much as possible. Rebreathing is surely undesirable. All tubing employed for connections should have thick walls to prevent kinking. The tongue should be kept pulled out in order to keep the epiglottis raised. After the pharyngeal tube is inserted the tongue may be kept in proper position by tying it (not too tight) to the tube; the forceps may be then taken off. The tying of the stretched tongue to the tube may even assist the latter in remaining in position.

"The weight on the abdomen prevents the entrance of air in any considerable quantity into the stomach and the little which gets there escapes again when the insufflation is cut off; it never gets into the intestines. The pressure on the abdomen has still another significance. In patients with completely abolished respiration usually the blood pressure is also very low and most of the blood may be accumulated in the abdominal viscera. The heart is then scantily filled, and not enough arterial blood is sent to peripheral organs. Under such circumstances a good pressure on the abdomen may raise the blood pressure by even as much as 30 millimeters of mercury; the heart is filled more efficiently and sends more blood to the medulla oblongata, arousing there the activities of the respiratory and vasomotor centres. Figure 1 shows the effect of abdominal pressure on the blood pressure."

## In Special Cases

"For this reason I recommend to have a belt on hand to reinforce the pressure. With a belt alone not much success can be obtained. In cases of accidents, when it might happen that no suitable weight is at hand, the individual who handles the respiratory valve may sit down on the abdomen of the victim.

"There might be conditions which do not permit the placing of weights on the abdomen; for instance, when a collapse occurs during a laparotomy. Under this circumstance a stomach tube of a large diameter should be introduced through the esophagus into the stomach. The tube restricts to a sufficient degree the entrance of air into the stomach, and the air which enters there escapes readily through the tube as staged before. In the anterior end of the pharyngeal tube is an opening for that purpose which is usually kept closed by a movable plate.

"A stomach tube of a 33 French diameter fits exactly into this opening. I am of the opinion that it is preferable to have in every instance, even when pressure on the abdomen is exerted, also a tube in the stomach. Since the apparatus may have to be used in some emergency cases by laymen, however, the latter might be loath to handle a stomach tube. And since the experiments have shown that very good results may be had with the pressure alone, I do not feel like insisting on the simultaneous use of the stomach tube in all simple cases.

"Besides the metal pharyngeal tube, I studied also the availability of the use of insufflation with the aid of a well-fitting mask. In this arrangement every other part is the same as in that for the pharyngeal tube, except that instead of introducing a tube into the pharynx, a mask is laid over mouth and nose and by bands tightly applied to the face. The mask has a hollow projection for the connection with the respiratory valve. I tested the mask method on various animals; as was previously found for the pharyngeal tube, it was established that also by means of the mask efficient artificial respiration can be carried on.

"With the aid of the mask method of artificial respiration, completely curarized (and anesthetized) animals were kept in an excellent condition for many hours. By this method, of course, some infectious matter may be driven into the trachea and perhaps cause infection; by this method, further pressure is exerted on the middle ear; neither does the mask method allow the introduction of a stomach tube. However, in dealing with emergency cases, with immediate danger to life, such considerations as the above methods are, comparatively speaking, mere trifles and can be hardly taken into account.

"I have tested also the effectiveness of insufflation through metal pharyngeal tubes on animals; it is even more satisfactory than with elastic rubber tubes. It works promptly; the introduction gives less trouble and the tube remains in position for hours.

"Both the pharyngeal and mask methods were tested also on human cadavers. Air entered into the lungs when insufflated by either of these methods, even if the dead bodies were in rigor or frozen stiff. In some cases unmistakable efficient respiratory movements of chest and abdomen were manifestly present. But even when the stiffness interfered with the free movements, auscultation proved conclusively the entrance of air into the lungs. Especially was this the case in a man who died under signs of pulmonary oedema; rales (rattling sounds) could be heard all over the chest.

"The accompanying sketches illustrate these methods better than they can he described. In Figure 2, the pharyngeal tube (P.T.) is shown connected with the respiratory valve (R.V.), the foot bellows (B.) and the safety-valve (S.V.). A stomach tube (S.T.) is pushed through the pharyngeal tube. In Figure 3, the mask (M.) is shown applied to the face. By means of an inflatable ring (Infl.), the mask is made air-tight. There is a weight on the abdomen and a belt around it. The respiratory and safety valves are the same as in Figure 2. The bellows are here replaced by an oxygen cylinder.

"In an emergency case no time should be lost on matters of less importance before starting the main act, and that is: the artificial respiration. When using the mask, for instance, no time should be lost in tying and fixing it properly; it should be pressed over mouth and face by the hand. After the insufflation is well on the way, some one may attend to the tying of the mask, the fixing of the tongue properly and the putting of the belt around the weight over the stomach. Regarding the fixing of the tongue, it may be, as stated before, tied to the pharyngeal tube, when using the same."

## Further Description

"When using the mask, the handle of the tongue forceps may be fixed to the victim's neck so as to keep the tongue stretched; or the tongue may be tied by means of tape or gauze bandage, pulled out well and the end of the tape or bandage tied around the victim's neck. It should be kept in mind that the pulling out of the tongue is an essential factor in any procedure for artificial respiration. In completely paralyzed individuals there is a tendency for the tongue to be kept somewhat firmly over the entrance into the larynx, caused, perhaps, by some final attempt at inspiration.

"I may say in passing that the demonstrations made with some machines for artificial respiration, for commercial and advertising purposes, on living and unanesthetized individuals, is entirely misleading and should not be taken as evidence of the efficiency of such machines in cases when individuals are unconscious and the respiratory mechanism paralyzed.

"It will be safer to have on hand a mask as well as a pharyngeal tube. When the latter should prove too small, the escape of the insufflated air alongside the tube may be remedied by tamponading the entrance into the pharynx around the tube with gauze. Besides, as I have indicated above, tubes of various sizes should be on hand.

"The foot bellows need not be large; smaller foot bellows worked a little more rapidly give a sufficiently strong, continuous current of air. The continuous air current is in the arrangement here described preferable to the interrupted current produced by hand bellows; it is difficult to have the rhythm of the bellows coincide properly with the rhythm in the respiration produced by the respiratory valve; it may occur that the bellows are compressed just when the valve is closed, &c., and the result might be an irregular and inefficient artificial respiration.

"It is evident that the methods of artificial respiration by devices here described can be readily combined with the Shäfer method of manual artificial respiration. The individual is then placed on his abdomen and the turning of the ring of the respiratory valve to the left has to coincide in time with the pressure on the lumbar muscles. Inspiration as well as expiration will thus be efficiently reinforced."

## The Emergency Bag

"While on the basis of my extensive experience I have reason to believe that the devices which are here described will answer the purpose satisfactorily in all cases in need of artificial respiration, it is safer to think of methods which are capable of improving the efficiency of the devices. Emergencies may arise of which we are unable to think of now; factors of safety are designated by some students of mechanics as factors of ignorance.

"The emergency bag should contain small foot bellows, the safety-valve, the respiratory valve and the pharyngeal tube all readily connected by rubber tubing. Further, a mask, a tongue forceps, a strong belt or cords, a stomach tube, a roll of tape or one-inch gauze bandages and scissors. Weights might increase too much the weight of the bag. Bricks, stones or pieces of heavy metal, &c., may be had at any place.

"Wherever oxygen can be had it should be used in preference to the air from the bellows. It should be remembered that according to Hill and Macleod, however, prolonged inhalation of oxygen may do harm to the lungs. When, therefore, prolonged artificial respiration is required, the use of air should be alternated with oxygen.

"The devices for artificial respiration here described are certainly simple and inexpensive. Their efficiency has been tested to a much greater extent than any other device I know of. The possibility of keeping up the circulation in a normal condition for hours while the voluntary respiration is completely abolished (by curare) is certainly a rigid test, which has not been applied to any other method of artificial respiration except to that used in experimental laboratories with tracheotomy as a prerequisite, and, as I may add, to the method of intra-tracheal insufflation.

"The last mentioned device, which has now been tested in nearly two thousand cases on human beings, would be, in my opinion, indeed the most ideal method for artificial respiration. It has been used, to my knowledge, in two human cases of severe poisoning (morphine fifteen grains subcutaneously combined with inhalation of gas, and smoking opium for two days with complete absence of respiration) for twelve hours continuously with complete recoveries. But this method requires some training and could never be left to the hands of laymen.

"The handling of the artificial respiration by means of the pharyngeal and mask devices which I describe here is so simple that laymen could well be trusted with its execution. And that was the main object of my endeavor to develop these devices."

The writer quotes this from a former article:

"There is the possibility that the actual cause of death might be, in one case or another, especially in acute cases, only of a temporary nature, so that efficient artificial respiration might assist in temporizing and thus prove occasionally life-saving indeed. Such possibilities, though they may be realized only once in a thousand times, justify the making of an attempt in each and every instance."

*May 18, 1913*

# Heart Surgery Made Safer by Invention of Cardioscope

At least one spectacular invention was announced at the recent meeting in Chicago of the American Association of Thoracic Surgeons. Dr. Durff S. Allen of George Washington University, a young surgeon, has the distinction of being the inventor of an instrument which he has named the cardioscope, the purpose of which is to illuminate and magnify the field in operations on the heart.

This implies, of course, the possibility of such operations; it implies, moreover, that the heart is by no means the tender organ that it was formerly considered to be, but is, in fact, a tough muscle so constructed as to be able to withstand the normal strain of a long life. The average rate of the human heartbeat is seventy-two times a minute. Thus in a lifetime of 100 years the heart beats 3,784,320,000 times. An organ that can stand the strain of these myriad pulsations, these alternate expansions and contractions, must be strong indeed; no man-made device can compare with it except the clock or watch, and they have to be wound, whereas the heart is a self-winder.

The cardioscope will facilitate those wonderful heart operations devised ten years ago by Dr. Theodore Tuffier and Dr. Alexis Carrel of the Rockefeller Institute for Medical Research. Inspiration, conviction and resolute daring enabled these two scientists to operate successfully on the valves of the hearts of animals. They widened them by cutting and narrowed them with surgical stitches.

One is led to inquire how a surgeon can cut or sew with safety a beating heart. The answer to that is: The surgeons stilled the heartbeats by applying clamps to the blood vessels leading to and away from the organ, thus relieving it temporarily of its chief functions of propelling blood through the body and drawing it back again. "While the operations were in progress mechanical respiration was maintained by intratracheal insufflation, a method devised by the late Dr. Samuel J. Meltzer, who was also connected with the Rockefeller Institute.

## Epochal Operations

The specific operation which the two physicians reported was for enlargement of the pulmonary orifice of the heart to permit the free flow of blood and thus relieve or prevent congestion. Here is what they said about it:

"The operation will be much less dangerous in the future because the details of the technique have now been thoroughly established. These experiments show that it is possible to perform an operation which will increase the circumference of the pulmonary orifice without involving much danger to the life of the animal. It is probable that operations of this type may be employed in the treatment of stenosis (stoppage) of the pulmonary artery in man."

Bight dogs were subjected to the experiments, which involved patching of the pulmonary arteries. Two of the animals died; the others recovered without shock and six months later were reported to be well.

Dr. Carrel reported other experimental operations on the sigmoid valves of the heart, the organ being rendered quiescent for several minutes by clamps, as in the other cases.

It is in the diagnosis of such conditions as these and in subsequent operations for their relief that Dr. Allen's cardioscope will prove invaluable. As its name implies, it is an instrument with which to look at the heart. It is described as a small apparatus, in bulk about the size of a pocket flash lamp. It has a strong magnifying lens and is equipped with an electric light. An incision having been made through the tissues over the section of the organ to be observed, the small instrument is introduced so that a magnified view of the diagnostic and possible operative field is obtained. In other words, the surgeon is enabled to obtain visual proof of existing pathological conditions. He can verify or reject a diagnosis which had depended upon symptoms alone, and thus fortify his opinion as to whether surgical interference is warranted.

The possibility of these radical surgical procedures settles the question as to whether or not the heart is a tender or a tough organ; it is unquestionably tough, yet is subject to grievous injury from diseases, from the emotions, from poisons, fatigue and the constant strain of our modern strenuous life.

## The First Stethoscope

The art and science of diagnostics, especially in diseases of the heart, have taken a mighty stride between the first primitive stethoscope and the cardioscope. One day in 1813, Laennec, the great French clinician, was on his way on foot to call upon a patient. He saw two boys playing a game at opposite ends of a wooden beam. One tapped on the wood; the other, his ear against the beam, listened. It gave Laennec an idea. Reaching the bedside of his patient, he rolled a sheet of stiff paper into a cylinder, placed one end over the patient's heart and listened at the other. The heart sounds were heard with much greater distinctness than when the physician applied his ear to the patient's chest. From this primitive stethoscope the modern instrument of that name was developed.

Laennec was not the first to conceive the possibilities of auscultation, for Hook wrote in 1703 in his book *Method of Improving Natural Philosophy* "Who knows but that, as in a watch, we may hear the beating of the balance, and the running of the wheels, and the striking of the hammers, and the grating of the teeth, and multitudes of other noises; who knows, I say, but that it may be possible to discover the motions of the internal parts of bodies, whether animal, vegetable or mineral, by the sound they make; that one may discover the works performed in the several offices and shops of a man's body, and thereby discover what engine is out of order? I have been able to hear very plainly the beating of a man's heart."

## Heart Strain in Modern Life

Just before the World War, eminent physicians in Europe and America turned their attention to combating heart disease. Activity in this direction was so marked as to attract worldwide attention. Scientists seemed to be working in concert, as if forewarned of the immediate necessity for action to offset the great strain that was about to be put on the hearts of mankind. Many new diagnostic appliances were brought into use at that time, and many new surgical procedures were developed. The operations on the heart valves mentioned above are examples. And promptly the heart strain came; few escaped it.

What of today? That strain is with us yet, accentuated, moreover, by our present mode of life, by our business methods, by our feverish habits of eating and drinking, and even by the manner in which we take our recreation; in a word, we are living in an age of speed; in an age in which a tremendous strain is daily being put upon our hearts. The result is inevitable; speed will have its toll of death and disability from weakened hearts.

A physician, with this thought in mind, made an automobile tour of Manhattan Island between the hours of 11 p.m. and 1 a.m. a week ago. He touched the limits of the Island in its four cardinal aspects. In avenues and side streets; to the north and south; on the east side and west side; in parks and out of them, the same conditions were found: congestion everywhere of vehicles and persons; evidences of strain on all sides; tense and unavoidable emotionalism that must prevail where the people will not rest. All of this artificiality of life tends to produce functional derangements of the vascular system—weakness of the heart.

Science coldly proves that alcohol, tobacco, coffee and tea are capable of producing heart weakness. Persons who turn midnight into noon for pleasure, after the work of the day is done, habitually consume greater quantities of these four agents than those who do not. There can be no doubt, physicians say, that the night life of the New York of the present is highly conducive to heart strain. What can be done about it? Nothing, unless the doctors can point to a moral and drive it home convincingly enough to actuate the population of the city to go to bed when bedtime comes.

Heart disease and heart strain are two different things. Statistics are variously interpreted. One set of figures has it that 2 per cent of the population, or more than 2,000,000 persons in the United States, suffer from serious heart disease. Others interpret the figures in another light. For instance, a keeper of vital statistics will explain that the term "heart disease" on a death certificate may cover different ailments, such as those of the blood vessels, and that the term is used merely for convenience. It was reported that in 1920 there died from organic heart disease in this country 151,000 persons. On the other hand, Sir James Mackenzie of London, long distinguished as an authority on this subject, says that heart disease is not common.

## Preventing Heart Trouble

"Whether common or not, physicians, school clinics and health boards happily have the means of checking it, so that the probabilities are that the future will see less of actual organic heart disease rather than more. For it is a fact that the seeds of heart disease are sown in the young, and science has learned how and where. In many cases the seeds of heart disease are germs that locate in spongy tonsils and adenoids, in bad teeth and in gums. School medical inspection is doing much to clean up these sources of infection. Then we have inflammation of the interior of the heart from rheumatic and other infections, and heart disease may follow diphtheria or scarlet fever.

The germs are swept from tonsil or infected tooth or joint into the blood stream. They reach the heart and may form fungus-like colonies on the heart's valves. There they cause scars which are in evidence in the form of warped distortions of the edges of the valves so that they no longer fit the orifices they were designed to close tightly. The heart muscle is likewise equipped with blood vessels for its own nourishment, and the wandering germs carried through these find lodgment in the muscle itself, where they produce damaging scars. One of the varieties of germs which frequently reach the heart by the medium of the defective tonsils is the streptococcus viridans, which is the active agent in the so-called septic sore throat, often epidemic and often attributed to a faulty milk supply.

Robert Louis Stevenson strolled in the village of Saranac on a Winter night for purposes of meditation. Later he wrote of his contemplations: "'Come,' said I to my engine, 'let us make a tale.'" The result was *The Master of Ballantrae*. By his "engine," he, of course, referred to his brain. Had he mentioned his heart, doubtless, he would have called it his "pump." It is often spoken of as a pump and sometimes as a power chamber.

The analogy of the pump is a striking one. Many of us have manipulated the handle of a suction-pump. When it was in full working order water gushed from its spout in a smooth, unbroken stream; when it was old, with leaky and patched valves, the water oozed from around the edges of the valves; the stream from the spout was broken and irregular, and the whole action of the apparatus was labored. So it is in the case of valvular heart disease. And it is this condition that advanced surgery, reinforced by the cardioscope, aims to remedy.

## What Makes the Heart Beat

We have spoken of the heart as a power chamber; in the light of modern knowledge we can more exactly term it an electrical power chamber. In the course of a long life the heart potentially dies 3,000,000,000 or more times. There is a brief pause after each heartbeat; that infinitesimal hesitation is the potential death of the organ. How is it revived again? Science has learned that it is by self-generated electricity—the never-failing mystery of life. Today physicians speak confidently of the electrical centres of the heart. They are fairly numerous, but their exact distribution is uncertain. "With the expiring movement of the heart one or other of these tiny living batteries springs into action and explodes. For the moment this particular one is the pacemaker; the others follow in rapid succession. This is what we mean when we say that the heart is the self-winder; it is also a self-starter after the initiation of the primary impulse.

If one wishes to get an idea of this mysterious, irregular action of the electric centres of the heart, he has only to visualize a glass jar containing a dozen fireflies. Placed in the dark, the points of light are seen intermittently in different parts of the container as one would see, if they were visible, the discharges of the electric impulses in the heart.

Already science has utilized the conductivity of this heart-generated electricity in the diagnostic field. The electrocardiograph, an instrument attached to the body, receives the different heart impulses and records them by tracings on paper. Dr. Robert H. Halsey used it in the Post-Graduate Hospital in this city more than ten years ago. With these tracings before him the properly trained physician is able to translate them into terms of the cardiac conditions which give rise to them, with the same facility with which he can interpret blood conditions from a report on the analysis of the patient's blood.

Other diagnostic devices are the polygraph, which records impulses from various blood vessels, and a remarkable instrument which, by the utilization of Einthoven's string galvanometer, is able to photograph the sounds of the heart. The latter apparatus was used in the laboratory of the College of Physicians and Surgeons of Columbia University a decade ago, and was attached for diagnostic purposes to patients in Roosevelt Hospital on the opposite side of the street.

It should be explained that it is the belief of scientists that the heart's revivifying electric impulses are generated by the contraction of the organ; and that the five links in the chain of cardiac integrity by which it is able to carry on its work are its functions of rhythmicity, excitability, conductivity, contractility and tonicity.

Other diagnostic inventions are the sphygmomanometer, by which the blood pressure in the arteries is determined, and radiography, by which the size and shape of the heart can be seen by means of the X-ray.

All of these aids to differential diagnosis are of comparatively recent origin. Their use and the concerted campaign against heart disease during the last decade, carried on in this city by the Association for the Prevention and Relief of Heart Disease and several cooperating organizations, have served to bring heart ailments sharply to public attention. It may be that there is no greater amount of organic heart disease than formerly; there seems to be more because of its more general recognition. The amount can unquestionably be reduced by education of the young and beneficent propaganda; also by the concerted efforts of the association for its prevention and relief and the great convalescent work being done in the splendid hospital of the Burke Foundation at White Plains, where so many heart patients are sent from the hospitals in this city. Dr. Frederic Brush presides over this institution, which is the largest and most modern for convalescents in the world. Dr. Brush advocates dancing among other exercises for the cardiac convalescent.

The remedy for modern heart strain lies with the people. There is only one remedy—a return to sane methods of living.

*June 10, 1923*

# Heart-Lung Machine Is Used Successfully for the First Time in a Medical Case

## By WALDEMAR KAEMPFFERT

What is said to be the first successful use in this country of a heart-lung machine on a human patient was reported at last week's meeting of the American Association for Thoracic Surgery. The machine ("dispersion oxygenator" is its technical name) was developed at the Fels Research Institute for the Study of Human Development, Antioch College. It is one of about twenty that have been constructed here and abroad, all alike in principle though widely different in design. The all-glass Fels machine is probably the least expensive of the lot. It cost just $60.

The patient in the case was a former fireman who suffered from fibrosis (scarring) of both lungs. He could breathe only with difficulty, so that he became "blue." Besides, his heart was unable to meet the demands made upon it. His blood was sent from a leg vein through the Fels machine, enriched with oxygen (normally the function of the lungs), was rid of carbon dioxide, and returned to the body through a vein in the arm. The machine was primed with three pints of blood. A little heparin prevented it from clotting.

In this case the blood was oxygenated for seventy-five minutes. The patient's color changed from blue to a near-normal pink. Since the machine served as a lung he did not have to strain himself by breathing in short gasps. No anesthetic was necessary. After the machine had done its work the man slept soundly for the first time in weeks.

## Experiments

All this was the successful outcome of a project in which the Fels Institute was joined by the University of Cincinnati's Medical School. Not until a year's experience had been gained with dogs was the machine tried in a human case.

There was no surgical operation. The ex-fireman did not have his chest opened to expose the heart, which is what happens to experimental dogs that survive the operation and that run about days later as if nothing had happened to them. The fireman's lungs and his heart were still functioning. The machine did most of their work.

So far a heart-lung machine has not been used when it was necessary to open the chest and to by-pass heart and lungs completely. Dr. A. M. Dogliotti, Professor of Surgery of the University of Turin, Italy, came the nearest to this last year. He reported at the fourteenth congress of the International Society of Surgeons that in August, 1951, he had used a heart-lung machine on a 50-year-old man who was dying because a tumor was interfering with the heart's action. Dr. Dogliotti opened the man's chest, connected the heart-lung machine and cut out the tumor. When last heard from the patient was alive and well. Dr. Dogliotti made it plain that he used the machine only as a partial substitute for the heart. A 6-year-old child was operated on in this country last year with the aid of a heart-lung machine, but died because the case was hopeless.

## Bubble Danger

In all heart-lung machines the formation of bubbles must be avoided as oxygen is introduced into the blood. Bubbles mean death. To prevent them from forming, a turbulence is created in the blood reservoirs of some machines, just as some of us stir up a Scotch and soda to make it "fizz" more. In the Fels machine oxygenated blood is broken up and with it larger bubbles by passing it upward through beads coated with silicone. In addition there is a bubble trap.

The all-glass oxygenator of the machine was invented by Dr. C. Clark Jr. He and Dr. James Helmsworth of the University of Cincinnati worked together on the fireman.

*May 11, 1952*

# A Balloon Device Averts Surgery for Coronary Disorders

By LAWRENCE K. ALTMAN

To spare many patients painful and costly surgery, doctors are turning to a technique that involves inflating a balloon in arteries clogged by fatty deposits from arteriosclerosis.

The balloon, inflated after being introduced into the damaged area of a blood vessel, compresses obstructions and allows more oxygen-rich blood to flow to an organ. In some instances, the technique is relieving cramps and saving legs by removing obstructions to the blood supply to the lower limbs. In others, it relieves the obstructions that produce the chest discomfort called angina and might also lead to heart attacks.

In addition, this method (known technically as percutaneous transluminal angioplasty) is treating, and even curing, some cases of a type of high blood pressure that results from blockage of an artery feeding the kidneys. Although such blockages cause only a small percentage of all cases of high blood pressure, the therapy can be dramatically successful, freeing the patient entirely from drug therapy.

Until four years ago, radiologists who were experienced in using angioplasty for several ailments were unable to flatten obstructions in the coronary arteries, which are the ones that nourish the heart. Heart attacks can result when coronary arteries are blocked by fatty substances.

Now this technique, in addition to all its other applications, is becoming more commonly used to compress obstructions in coronary arteries. Although coronary angioplasty generally is still considered experimental, it is becoming a standard practice at a few hospitals.

Three doctors who have compressed obstructions in the coronary arteries of more than 1,100 patients have the longest experience with the technique. They are Dr. Andreas Gruntzig, who devised the technique at the University of Zurich and now works at Emory University in Atlanta; Dr. Simon H. Stertzer at Lenox Hill Hospital in New York; and Dr. Richard K. Myler at St. Mary's Hospital in San Francisco.

A few doctors at other hospitals have done about 100 cases, and many more are learning the technique by attending tutorial courses and by observing their more experienced colleagues. Beyond learning the actual procedure, the doctor must also learn how to deal with the variety of life-threatening complications that can develop at any step, particularly in the coronary arteries.

Because of those potential complications, wherever coronary angioplasty is used, there must be a back-up team ready on an instant's notice to do open-heart surgery.

Angioplasty removes the blockage caused by atherosclerotic plaques, or the accumulation of fatty substances on the inside wall of an artery. Precisely what happens to the compressed plaque and extruded material remains a mystery, but early fears that extruded plaque material might produce some new problem somewhere else have not been realized.

The chief practical problem now with this procedure is that the blood supply in an artery can stop suddenly for any of several reasons—an arterial spasm, a blood clot—threatening a heart attack or sudden death unless the problem is relieved by emergency open-heart surgery.

Until recently, use of the balloon in coronary arteries was limited to removing single obstructions, and for that reason, only about 10 percent of the estimated 100,000 patients eligible for coronary by-pass operations each year in this country were expected to benefit from the balloon technique.

However, the sausage-shaped balloon devices are being made longer and stronger. A few doctors are testing them to compress more than one obstruction in a single coronary artery or single obstructions in more than one artery. Future modifications in the equipment may allow doctors to compress, as they cannot yet, obstructions that have become hardened from natural calcification.

Further, some doctors are doing angioplasty in patients who have had coronary by-pass operations and then developed further obstructions in the veins that were grafted in the by-pass operation.

As the technology and experience improve, the number of patients who may benefit from the technique could become much larger. And whether there is a potential limit to the number of obstructions that can be removed is not known.

In about four of five patients, the balloon technique removes the obstruction and immediately relieves the symptoms. And about 84 percent of such patients will maintain their success after three years, according to data collected in a registry at the National Institutes of Health and reported at a meeting of the American Heart Association in Dallas two weeks ago.

However, the blockage may recur and close down the artery in about 16 percent of patients. Such recurrences usually happen within the first six months following angioplasty. A second angioplasty, or a by-pass operation, or both, may be needed in these cases.

According to the most recent report, emergency surgery is performed on 6.9 percent of coronary angioplasty patients. The death rate among all coronary angioplasty patients as a result of the procedure is 0.8 percent, about the same as for coronary by-pass operations done by experienced surgeons.

The angioplasty technique was devised in 1964 by Dr. Charles T. Dotter and Dr. Melvin P. Judkins at the University of Oregon, where they used it to relieve leg cramps and other problems that had resulted from arteriosclerotic plaques that blocked the arteries that nourish the pelvis and legs in nine patients. Last year, Dr. Dotter reported that the artery in one of those patients was still open without further surgery 14 years later.

The Oregon technique gained wider acceptance in European than American hospitals for compressing plaques in the arteries that supply blood to the legs. But it was not until 1977 that Dr. Gruntzig, working with engineers in Switzerland, succeeded in developing miniaturized tubes, small enough to compress an obstruction in a coronary artery. About 15,000 angioplasties have been done to date in all arteries throughout the world.

The technique, simple as it may sound, involves plenty of medical technology, including the use of a fluoroscope, at least two sets of coronary angiogram X-rays (before and after the balloon does its work), injection of several drugs during the procedure, and Teflon-coated tubes.

At Lenox Hill Hospital last Wednesday, Dr. Stertzer successfully compressed a plaque in a coronary artery of a 57-year-old-man. A few days earlier, coronary angiograms showed that his angina pain was due to an obstruction measuring less than one inch in length in a major coronary artery.

As Dr. Stertzer scrubbed his arms before beginning the procedure, he told a visiting physician: "In anyone's first 75 cases, the complication rate is on the high side and the success rate on the low side. Now my complication rate is decreasing and my success rate increasing."

Dr. Stertzer, a cardiologist, was aided by four attendants, including a heart surgeon, Dr. Eugene Wallsh, who stood by in case a complication might arise during the procedure, which lasted a little more than one hour.

Dr. Stertzer began by injecting a local anesthetic into the patient's right elbow crease and used a scalpel to cut to the artery. He injected heparin, a blood-thinning drug, into the artery to help prevent the formation of potentially dangerous clots.

Then he pierced the artery with a long thin tube. At the tip was a guide wire. Two passages ran the length of the tube. One was to collect blood to record data such as the pressure within the artery as well as to allow injection of radio-opaque substances to outline the anatomy of the heart's blood vessels. Through the second passage, an assistant would later use a hand device to inflate the balloon with fluid to crush the plaque.

Before Dr. Stertzer could align the balloon with the plaque in the left anterior descending coronary artery, he had to push the tube through the arteries in the upper arm, shoulder and into the aorta, the main artery leading from the heart.

Among the limiting factors of the technique are the tortuosity and angulation of the blood vessels as well as the nooks and crannies of the anatomy, which vary according to the individual and the degree of damage produced by arteriosclerosis.

Dr. Stertzer injected a dose of nitroglycerine to help prevent a potentially dangerous spasm of the coronary arteries. When he wanted to outline the arteries, he squirted a small amount of radio-opaque dye through the tube and observed the pattern on a fluoroscopic screen directly in front of him.

Dr. Stertzer worked patiently, but in a moment of frustration, he commented that the balloon tube "almost always goes where you don't want it to go."

From time to time, Dr. Stertzer removed the tube from the patient's heart to reshape the tip of the guide wire so that he could more easily follow the anatomy of the coronary arteries. At one point, he left the room to check the location of the blockage on an angiogram.

Shortly thereafter, he passed the balloon through the obstructed portion of the artery. A technician rapidly inflated the balloon for a few seconds, then deflated it. They repeated the step three times. Each time, they increased the pressure in the balloon, thereby decreasing the amount of pressure gradient.

Then, the doctors took another series of X-rays and removed the tubes. As Dr. Stertzer sutured the incision in the elbow crease, he told the patient that he would rest in his hospital room overnight, go home to have Thanksgiving dinner with his family, and return to have exercise testing as an outpatient.

Meanwhile, the patient's angina pain is gone, and so is his need for medication— at least for now—all without a coronary by-pass operation and at about one-fifth of the $15,000 a by-pass operation costs.

*December 1, 1981*

309

# Dentist, Close to Death, Receives First Permanent Artificial Heart

By LAWRENCE K. ALTMAN

S ALT LAKE CITY—For the first time in history, surgeons early today implanted a permanent artificial heart to replace a dying human heart.

The operation, which lasted seven and a half hours, was performed at the University of Utah Medical Center here by a team headed by Dr. William C. DeVries.

The patient was Dr. Barney B. Clark, a 61-year-old retired dentist from the Seattle area. Dr. Clark, who was described as bedridden and on the verge of death from heart failure just before the operation, was reported in critical but stable condition tonight. If he recovers, he is destined to spend the rest of his life tethered to 6-foot-long hoses connected to an air compressor that powers the artificial heart. The compressor sits in what his doctors call "a grocery cart."

## Indicates He Is Not in Pain

Doctors at a news conference late today said Dr. Clark was able to recognize his wife, signal yes or no in response to questions and move his arms and legs. His doctors said he had indicated to them that he was not in pain.

He was also said to have given a note to a nurse asking for a drink of water, which he cannot have yet. He cannot speak because his breathing is being maintained for now by an artificial respirator that is connected to a tube in his windpipe.

Dr. DeVries declared the operation "a success" and expressed cautious optimism about Dr. Clark's prognosis. "He looks like any other patient coming out of open-heart surgery," Dr. DeVries said. His recovery, he added, "is not over yet; it's just beginning."

The surgeon said that "last night, all the doctors on the team believed he would be dead" without the operation, "and he isn't." The operation was described as a dazzling technical achievement. But its value in the treatment of the estimated 50,000 Americans each year who might need it will depend partly on how long and how well Dr. Clark and other recipients live. Moreover, if the procedure proves successful, it will raise difficult questions about who should receive the hearts and the nation's willingness to pay the price. The device itself cost $16,450.

The doctors frequently adjusted the rate of Dr. Clark's artificial heartbeat after the operation ended shortly after 7 a.m. today. It was beating at 116 times each minute at latest report. The heartbeat for healthy people varies considerably but is usually within the range of 65 to 80 beats a minute. The doctors do not know what the appropriate rate for Dr. Clark will ultimately be.

In the complex recovery process, Dr. Clark faces many potential complications, including pneumonia, other infections, collapsed lungs and blood clots. But the possibility of rejection, which has been the bane of human heart transplantation, does not exist in this case because there is no foreign tissue to set off the body's attack mechanism.

Dr. Clark was described as an ideal candidate to be the first recipient of the experimental heart because he was psychologically well-adjusted and had excellent support from his family. Moreover, as a medical professional, he understood that doctors could do nothing else for him and that he had no other option but death.

The artificial heart, made largely of molded polyurethane, is called the Jarvik-7 after its developer, Dr. Robert K. Jarvik, who is a member of the surgical team. The device is somewhat larger than a human heart but weighs about the same. Powered by the compressor, it makes a soft clicking sound that is audible through Dr. Clark's chest wall.

Dr. Chase N. Peterson, vice president of health affairs for the University of Utah, described Dr. Clark and the surgical team as "on the threshold of something that is as exciting and thrilling as has ever been accomplished in medicine."

## "Striking Out for New Territory"

"This man is no different than Columbus," he said. "He is striking out for new territory." For the last three years, Dr. Clark has suffered from a condition of unknown cause called idiopathic cardiomyopathy, which is a primary disease of the heart muscle. It resulted in congestive heart failure, in which an insufficient supply of blood is circulated through the body.

There were anxious moments in the operation, although they were not considered life-threatening. One part of the mechanical heart was defective and had to be replaced by a spare part. Another difficulty was that Dr. DeVries had to work with heart tissue that was paper-thin because of earlier steroid therapy.

Dr. DeVries expressed hope that Dr. Clark could leave the hospital in a few weeks. He would then live with his family in a specially equipped house in Salt Lake City.

Dr. DeVries made it clear that he would not proceed with another similar operation until the results of this one were clear.

## Was No Definitive Treatment

Until the recent licensing of a drug called captopril, there has been no definitive treatment for the condition Dr. Clark suffered from. In addition, many other drugs are part of the standard medical regimen for heart failure. Coronary bypass and other operations are of no value in remedying Dr. Clark's condition.

Dr. Clark's physicians in Seattle and here had treated him with steroids because they suspected he might have a condition called myocarditis that resulted from a viral infection.

At the time of the operation, his diseased heart was no longer responding to the standard drugs. Dr. Clark was selected as the first recipient of an artificial heart largely because he was born in Utah and commuted here from Seattle to visit members of his family. His cardiologists, Dr. Terence A. Block in Seattle and Dr. Jeffrey L. Anderson here, worked as a team and eventually referred him to the Utah medical center as a possible candidate for the operation.

As Dr. Clark's condition deteriorated, his physical activity was increasingly curtailed. In recent weeks he was confined to bed as the heart failure approached its terminal stages.

## Operation Was Put Off

He was reported to have put off the operation until now partly because he wanted to put his affairs in order. He was not eligible as a candidate for a heart transplant at Stanford Medical Center because doctors there have decided not to do the operation on people older than 50.

Dr. Clark's condition worsened last weekend. More fluid accumulated in his legs and abdomen because his dying heart could not pump enough blood. His breathing became more difficult because fluid accumulated in the lungs.

Had Dr. Clark not been a candidate for the artificial heart, Dr. DeVries said, he probably would have died at home. Instead, he was admitted to the hospital Monday afternoon. Shortly thereafter, he signed a so-called informed consent form permitting the experimental operation. He signed it again 24 hours later in accordance with regulations of the Federal Food and Drug Administration, which regulates devices such as the artificial heart.

In the intervening 50 or so hours, the doctors prescribed even larger doses of the drugs he was taking to prepare him for the operation. The doctors also worked to correct abnormalities in his blood clotting system and other bodily functions resulting from the heart failure. Tests of his critically important kidney function were reported within normal limits. The other worrisome conditions responded well enough for the doctors to proceed.

The operation had been scheduled to begin at 8 a.m. today, but it was advanced to late last night because the doctors felt they could wait no longer.

His cardiac output, a critical test of heart function, was one liter instead of the customary five liters, Dr. Peterson said.

There were several urgent concerns. One was that Dr. Clark would suffer a stroke or serious brain damage overnight, thereby making the operation worthless. Another was that with further deterioration the hazards of surgery would have been even greater than they generally are for an experimental operation.

In the operation, about two-thirds of the heart was removed. The surgeons removed the bottom two chambers, the left and right ventricles. But they left the top two chambers, the left and right atria, as an anchor for the artificial heart.

*December 3, 1982*

# Race Is On to Develop Nonsurgical Ways to Unclog Arteries

## By SANDRA BLAKESLEE

As millions of Americans cope with the pain and danger of clogged arteries, physicians are striving to develop improved nonsurgical techniques for cleaning out the arteries safely and permanently.

In experiments at hospitals all over the country, patients are having their arteries reamed out with hot lasers that boil away the clogs, or blasted out with "cold" lasers. Others are having their arteries cleaned with mechanical devices that shave or gouge away the clogging material, called plaque. Some patients are having mesh-like wires implanted into their freshly cleaned arteries to prevent new obstructions from forming.

Doctors say many patients, lured by the notion that lasers perform miracles and by hospital advertising, are specifically requesting such procedures instead of today's conventional nonsurgical treatment, balloon angioplasty.

### Some Experts Are Worried

This worries some experts. While some new methods may prove helpful in saving lives, some proponents are making unsubstantiated claims about their experimental systems and especially about lasers, said Dr. George Abela, a cardiologist at the University of Florida School of Medicine in Gainesville who is a pioneer in the field. "Unfortunately, if these claims are not borne out, both the public and the scientific community will be put off the technology."

Dr. Tom Robertson, chief of the cardiac disease branch of the National Heart, Lung and Blood Institute in Bethesda, Md., said: "The public should consider these techniques to be experimental. We do not yet have enough information to know if the benefits outweigh the risks."

Experts said the lure of huge profits was driving the boom in improved methods for cleaning arteries, especially clogged coronary arteries that can lead to heart attack.

Until a decade ago, the only treatment for blocked arteries was bypass surgery. In a long operation, blood is detoured around the blocked section of an artery with a section of vein taken from the leg or with a nonessential artery from the chest.

In the late 1970s a nonsurgical technique, balloon angioplasty, was introduced in which an ultra-thin guidewire is inserted into a major leg artery and threaded through the circulatory system to an obstruction. Only a minor incision is required.

Doctors track the wire on a special screen with an image similar to an X-ray. Dye is injected into the patient's arteries so they are highlighted on the screen. Next, a long thin tube called a catheter, with a deflated balloon on one end, is passed along the guidewire to the obstruction. When the tip of the catheter reaches the blockage, the balloon is inflated, pressing plaque against the arterial walls and opening a channel through which blood can flow more freely.

The major drawback is that 30 percent of all coronary arteries and 40 to 50 percent of leg arteries develop new obstructions within six months of the balloon treatment, doctors say.

Surgeons are not surprised by the high recurrence rate, said Dr. Nicholas Kouchoukos, a cardiologist at Washington University in St. Louis. "When you take plaque and mash it up against the wall of an artery, you split layers of the vessel itself," he said. "That trauma invites problems."

Doctors say the balloon often leaves a jagged edge, with flaps of tissue hanging loose from the artery's inner lining. Most balloon angioplasties are done with a surgical team standing by so that if an artery clogs soon after the balloon is removed, an emergency bypass operation can be performed. Another drawback is that totally blocked arteries and arteries with many obstructions are not amenable to the technique.

Given these problems and the vast market, dozens of companies are developing techniques to improve conventional balloon angioplasty.

The sexiest systems from a marketing standpoint use lasers to vaporize or destroy plaque. Lasers are devices in which atoms or subatomic particles are jostled to generate highly concentrated energy beams. The three being developed for use in arteries are based on different ways of exciting the atoms of a variety of gases or matter. These include argon, a synthetic garnet crystal and a mixture of reactive gases. Each operates at different energy levels.

The main risk of using lasers is perforation. Coronary arteries are notoriously difficult to work with. Small and fragile, they move with each heart beat and take tortuous turns. The sac around the heart will fill up with blood a minute after a vessel is broken, stopping the heart. Lasers can also burn arterial walls, causing them to shrink and lose water.

Most laser angioplasty systems today are being tested in long, straight leg arteries. Only a few are being tested in the coronary arteries.

One leading system, the hot tip, makes use of a laser to heat a bullet-shaped metal or sapphire cap at the end of a catheter. The tip, 750 degrees Fahrenheit, is moved back and forth through the blockage. After the tissue swells up from the heat injury, a balloon widens the vessel.

Another system employs a hot laser to destroy tissue, then relies on conventional balloon angioplasty to further open the artery. In June, a team at the St. Francis Hospital in Evanston, Ill., was first to open a totally blocked coronary artery using laser-assisted balloon angioplasty.

Researchers are also working on a "cold," or excimer, laser, which operates at ultraviolet wavelengths with extremely high energy levels. Molecules are driven apart by light rather than heat. The excimer cuts precisely, leaving a smooth unburned surface. Balloon angioplasty may not be needed as a follow-up.

Another experimental procedure uses two types of laser. After a catheter reaches a blockage, a low-power laser is used to identify the type of tissue in the target. Then a high-powered laser blasts away the tissue.

## Laser-Balloon Techniques

Perhaps the newest technique is balloon-laser welding. An artery is first widened by conventional balloon angioplasty. On the last balloon inflation a laser is turned on, heating the surrounding tissue. The temperature is not hot enough to destroy tissue, but the artery walls are stretched and welded into a smooth surface. Because the procedure is painful, patients are briefly anesthetized.

Some doctors are testing new mechanical devices. An artherectomy catheter shaves plaque out of an artery. Other devices suction the plaque or gouge it out. In addition, mesh-like metallic devices called stents are being placed in arteries to hold them open after balloon angioplasty.

Dr. Abela and others say that each new system for cleaning arteries may eventually find its own niche.

"We need to learn which device works best under which circumstances," he said.

*July 28, 1988*

# New Heart Studies Question the Value of Opening Arteries

By GINA KOLATA

A new and emerging understanding of how heart attacks occur indicates that increasingly popular aggressive treatments may be doing little or nothing to prevent them.

The artery-opening methods, like bypass surgery and stents, the widely used wire cages that hold plaque against an artery wall, can alleviate crushing chest pain. Stents can also rescue someone in the midst of a heart attack by destroying an obstruction and holding the closed artery open.

But the new model of heart disease shows that the vast majority of heart attacks do not originate with obstructions that narrow arteries.

Instead, recent and continuing studies show that a more powerful way to prevent heart attacks in patients at high risk is to adhere rigorously to what can seem like boring old advice—giving up smoking, for example, and taking drugs to get blood pressure under control, drive cholesterol levels down and prevent blood clotting.

Researchers estimate that just one of those tactics, lowering cholesterol to what guidelines suggest, can reduce the risk of heart attack by a third but is followed by only 20 percent of heart patients.

"It's amazing and it's completely backwards in terms of prioritization," said Dr. David Brown, an interventional cardiologist at Beth Israel Medical Center in New York.

Heart experts say they understand why the disconnect occurred: they, too, at first found it hard to believe what research was telling them. For years, they were wedded to the wrong model of heart disease.

"There has been a culture in cardiology that the narrowings were the problem and that if you fix them the patient does better," said Dr. David Waters, a cardiologist at the University of California at San Francisco.

The old idea was this: Coronary disease is akin to sludge building up in a pipe. Plaque accumulates slowly, over decades, and once it is there it is pretty much there for good. Every year, the narrowing grows more severe until one day no blood can get through and the patient has a heart attack. Bypass surgery or angioplasty— opening arteries by pushing plaque back with a tiny balloon and then, often, holding

317

it there with a stent—can open up a narrowed artery before it closes completely. And so, it was assumed, heart attacks could be averted.

But, researchers say, most heart attacks do not occur because an artery is narrowed by plaque. Instead, they say, heart attacks occur when an area of plaque bursts, a clot forms over the area and blood flow is abruptly blocked. In 75 to 80 percent of cases, the plaque that erupts was not obstructing an artery and would not be stented or bypassed. The dangerous plaque is soft and fragile, produces no symptoms and would not be seen as an obstruction to blood flow.

That is why, heart experts say, so many heart attacks are unexpected—a person will be out jogging one day, feeling fine, and struck with a heart attack the next. If a narrowed artery were the culprit, exercise would have caused severe chest pain.

Heart patients may have hundreds of vulnerable plaques, so preventing heart attacks means going after all their arteries, not one narrowed section, by attacking the disease itself. That is what happens when patients take drugs to aggressively lower their cholesterol levels, to get their blood pressure under control and to prevent blood clots.

Yet, researchers say, old notions persist.

"There is just this embedded belief that fixing an artery is a good thing," said Dr. Eric Topol, an interventional cardiologist at the Cleveland Clinic in Ohio.

In particular, Dr. Topol said, more and more people with no symptoms are now getting stents. According to an analysis by Merrill Lynch, based on sales figures, there will be more than a million stent operations this year, nearly double the number performed five years ago.

Some doctors still adhere to the old model. Others say that they know it no longer holds but that they sometimes end up opening blocked arteries anyway, even when patients have no symptoms.

Dr. David Hillis, an interventional cardiologist at the University of Texas Southwestern Medical Center in Dallas, explained: "If you're an invasive cardiologist and Joe Smith, the local internist, is sending you patients, and if you tell them they don't need the procedure, pretty soon Joe Smith doesn't send patients anymore. Sometimes you can talk yourself into doing it even though in your heart of hearts you don't think it's right."

Dr. Topol said a patient typically goes to a cardiologist with a vague complaint like indigestion or shortness of breath, or because a scan of the heart indicated calcium deposits—a sign of atherosclerosis, or buildup of plaque. The cardiologist puts the patient in the cardiac catheterization room, examining the arteries with an angiogram. Since most people who are middle-aged and older have atherosclerosis, the angiogram will more often than not show a narrowing. Inevitably, the patient gets a stent.

"It's this train where you can't get off at any station along the way," Dr. Topol said. "Once you get on the train, you're getting the stents. Once you get in the cath lab, it's pretty likely that something will get done."

One reason for the enthusiastic opening of blocked arteries is that it feels like the right thing to do, Dr. Hillis said. "I think it is ingrained in the American psyche that the worth of medical care is directly related to how aggressive it is," he said. "Americans want a full-court press."

Dr. Hillis said he tried to explain the evidence to patients, to little avail. "You end up reaching a level of frustration," he said. "I think they have talked to someone along the line who convinced them that this procedure will save their life. They are told if you don't have it done you are, quote, a walking time bomb."

Researchers are also finding that plaque, and heart attack risk, can change very quickly—within a month, according to a recent study—by something as simple as intense cholesterol lowering.

"The results are now snowballing," said Dr. Peter Libby of Harvard Medical School. "The disease is more mutable than we had thought."

The changing picture of what works to prevent heart attacks, and why, emerged only after years of research that was initially met with disbelief.

Early attempts to show that opening a narrowed artery saves lives or prevents heart attacks were unsuccessful. The only exception was bypass surgery, which was found to extend the lives of some patients with severe illness but not to prevent heart attacks. It is unclear why those patients lived longer; some think the treatment prevented their heart rhythms from going awry, while others say that the detour created by a bypass might be giving blood an alternate route when a clot formed somewhere else in the artery.

Some early studies indicated what was really happening, but were widely dismissed. As long ago as 1986, Dr. Greg Brown of the University of Washington at Seattle published a paper showing that heart attacks occurred in areas of coronary arteries where there was too little plaque to be stented or bypassed. Many cardiologists derided him.

Around the same time, Dr. Steven Nissen of the Cleveland Clinic started looking directly at patients' coronary arteries with a miniature ultrasound camera that he threaded into blood vessels. He found that the arteries were riddled with plaque, but almost none of it was obstructing blood vessels. Soon he began proposing that the problem was not the plaque that produced narrowings but the hundreds of other areas that were ready to burst. Cardiologists were skeptical.

In 1999, Dr. Waters of the University of California got a similar reaction to his study of patients who had been referred for angioplasty, although they did not have severe symptoms like chest pain. The patients were randomly assigned to angioplasty followed by a doctor's usual care, or to aggressive cholesterol-lowering drugs but no angioplasty. The patients whose cholesterol was aggressively lowered had fewer heart attacks and fewer hospitalizations for sudden onset of chest pain.

The study "caused an uproar," Dr. Waters said. "We were saying that atherosclerosis is a systemic disease. It occurs throughout all the coronary arteries. If you fix one segment, a year later it will be another segment that pops and gives you a heart attack, so systemic therapy, with statins or antiplatelet drugs, has the potential to do a lot more." But, he added, "there is a tradition in cardiology that doesn't want to hear that."

Even more disquieting, Dr. Topol said, is that stenting can actually cause minor heart attacks in about 4 percent of patients. That can add up to a lot of people suffering heart damage from a procedure meant to prevent it.

"It has not been a welcome thought," Dr. Topol said.

Stent makers say they do not mislead doctors or patients. Their new stents, coated with drugs to prevent scar tissue from growing back in the immediate area, are increasingly popular among cardiologists, and sales are exploding. But there is not yet any evidence that they change the course of heart disease.

"It's really not about preventing heart attacks per se," said Paul LaViolette, a senior vice president at Boston Scientific, a stent manufacturer. "The obvious purpose of the procedure is palliation and symptom relief. It's a quality-of-life gain."

*March 21, 2004*

CHAPTER 15

# Kidney Disease

# Machine Purifies Blood and Restores It to the Body

By VAN BUREN THORNE, M.D.

Three physicians, Dr. John J. Abel, Dr. Leonard G. Rowntree, and Dr. B. B. Turner, working in the pharmacological laboratory of Johns Hopkins University, in Baltimore, have elaborated an ingenious theory by which they have succeeded in taking all the blood out of the body of a living animal, "cleansing" it, and restoring it to the body without danger to the animal's life.

The word "cleansing" in this connection means that they are able to remove the diffusible constituents of the blood while it is outside the body. The wonderful apparatus which they have devised is so similar in its action to the kidney that they usually refer to it as the "artificial kidney."

The process of the elimination of undesirable constituents in the blood is called by the investigators "vivi-diffusion." The first demonstration before a body of physicians was made in Baltimore about fourteen months ago. The method was described in May last, before the Association of American Physicians in Washington, and last Summer demonstrations were given in London and in Groningen. More recently, it was brought to the attention of physicians in Philadelphia, while the current issue of the *Journal of Pharmacology and Experimental Therapeutics* contains a complete account of the laboratory experiments and a detailed description of the apparatus.

The title of this article, as well as that appearing in the *Transactions of the Association of American Physicians*, reads: "On the Removal of Diffusible Substances from the Circulating Blood of Living Animals by Dialysis."

## Astounding Possibilities

The physicians so far do not record attempts to apply their principle as a therapeutic measure for the relief of human ailments, but from what they have already made known the possibilities in this direction are astonishing. It is certain that poisons in the blood detrimental to human life, and which are impossible of elimination by inactive or badly diseased kidneys, can be removed from the body by means of this apparatus. Dogs weighing up to forty or fifty pounds have been used in the work, chiefly for the reason that all of the apparatus so far employed was only intended to take care of the quantity of blood contained in a body weighing fifty pounds or less.

The physicians are now constructing a machine capable of doing the work necessitated by a volume of blood circulating in a body weighing up to 200 pounds, and, inasmuch as they have determined to their own satisfaction that the procedure is not inimical to life, there is no reason why it should not be applied to human beings when the occasion arises.

Of course, the impression is not intended to be conveyed that the blood is all out of the body at one time, or that something is not supplied to the body to take the place of that which is temporarily absent. In order to make this point clear it is necessary to give a description of the apparatus and the manner in which it is employed. This will be done in the simplest possible way; and it will be seen that, despite the complicated apparatus used, the theory upon which its employment is based is as plain a physiological proposition as could well be thought of.

## Tapping the Arteries

Although prior to the time of Harvey—not so very long ago, as time is measured—no one was aware that the blood circulated throughout the body, every schoolboy knows nowadays that the heart pumps out blood through the arterial system to the most distant parts of the body; that it next passes through minute vessels called capillaries, and finally returns to the heart again through the venous system. In other words, it leaves the heart through the arteries and returns through the veins. These Johns Hopkins physicians conceived the idea of tapping one of the large arteries, allowing the blood to flow out, and returning it to a large vein when they had finished with it.

There were many difficulties to be overcome, but they finally made a system of tubes of a material porous enough to allow the substances they wished eliminated to escape through the sides as it passed through them. One end of the system of tubes was connected with an artery, which had been opened, by means of a single tube called a cannula. The other end of the system was joined to the receiving vein by another cannula. Now then we have blood coming out of an artery into a cannula, through the cannula into the system of tubes (whose various branchings and their significance will be explained later), through the system of tubes to the second cannula, and thence into the vein, and so back to the heart.

So far, we have merely described the method by which blood can be taken out of the body and restored to it without any great difficulty. This in itself is a simple procedure. We have not, however, shown what takes the place in the body of that volume of blood which is temporarily outside of it. The nearest approach to the blood serum of an animal is a mixture of salt and water in certain proportions, referred to in laboratory experimentation as a "normal saline solution." Before circulation in the apparatus is established, the system of tubes is filled with saline solution. "When blood flows out of the artery, through the cannula, and into the tubes, it forces the saline solution in front of it, through the tubes, the second cannula, the vein, and into the circulation in the body."

It will be readily seen, therefore, that as soon as the tubes are filled with blood an equal amount of saline solution is taking the place of the blood absent from the body. For instance, if the system of tubes will hold a volume of liquid equal to one-third of that circulating in an animal body, it will be seen that when circulation in the apparatus is properly established the animal is living minus a third of its blood, which has been replaced by saline solution. This is exactly the proportion of blood that was removed by the investigators in the course of some of their experiments.

It is now in order to explain how the diffusible constituents get out of the tubes while the blood is passing through them. As stated earlier, these tubes are made of a substance which permits certain solids to pass through it. The solids pass into a solution which surrounds the system of tubes, and may be collected therefrom and subjected to analyses which will reveal their nature and quantity. Blood passed through tubes as described, and from which certain constituents have been removed by passage through the walls of these tubes before it again enters the body, has been subjected to dialysis. The walls of the tubes are composed of a "dialyzing membrane," and the substances removed, to use the language of the laboratory, have been "dialyzed out."

Dialysis really means separation. A definition of the more formidable word:

"The separation of crystalloid from colloid substances in a solution by interposing an animal membrane between the solution and pure water; the crystalloid substances pass through the membrane into the water on the other side, the colloids do not." (Stedman)

As the investigators themselves say, the outer fluid may, of course, be water, but this leads very quickly to haemolysis (destruction) of the red corpuscles. If the experimenters desire to prevent any substance in the blood from "dialyzing out" they simply add the same proportion of that substance to the outer fluid as is contained in the blood itself. There is then a complete balance both within and without the system of tubes, so far as that substance is concerned, and, therefore, it will not pass through the walls of the tubes in either direction. The writers say:

"Where the object of the experiment is merely to remove from the blood abnormal constituents, as, for example, poisons, or constituents specifically secreted into the blood by a certain organ, normal serum from a similar animal may be used, thus insuring complete balance of all normal constituents, inside and out."

## Coagulation Overcome

One of the problems hitherto arising in connection with the removal of blood with the intention of using it to benefit a second person, as in transfusion, has been overcome by these investigators. It used to be said that blood was never the same once it left its natural environment, the blood vessels, if only for the briefest period. The change most to be feared, especially in blood transfusion, was coagulation. The Johns Hopkins experimenters have effectually overcome any tendency to coagulation by the injection of a substance derived from the medicinal leech and which is called hirulin.

These are some of the remarks of the investigators contained in their summary:

"A method has been devised by which diffusible constituents may be removed from the blood of a living animal, which does not involve any procedure prejudicial to life.

"Two animals have made rapid and complete recovery after being subjected to the procedure for two or three hours respectively.

"The method has been shown to be available for collecting from the blood under the ordinary conditions of physiological experimentation substances present only in small amount at one time.

"As an organ of elimination of abnormal substances (for example, poisons), quantitative results obtained with salicylic acid show that the apparatus in its present form compares not unfavorably with the kidney. The direction of improvement is indicated and experiments in this direction are in progress.

"Material has been collected in large quantity for the study of the non-proteid amino-bodies present in the blood. The chemical separation of these bodies is in progress and only preliminary results are here given.

"Directions in which the method may be utilized both for the study of problems in physiological chemistry, and as a promising therapeutic agent, have been indicated."

Elsewhere, in indicating the possible use of the apparatus as a therapeutic agent, the authors say:

"Again, there are numerous toxic states in which the eliminating organs, more especially the kidneys, are incapable of removing from the body at an adequate rate, either the autochthonous (aboriginal) or the foreign substances whose presence in excessive amount is detrimental to life processes.

"In the hope of providing a substitute in such emergencies, which might tide over a dangerous crisis, as well as for the important information which it might be expected to provide concerning the substances already referred to as normally present in the blood, and also for the light that might thus be thrown on intermediary stages of metabolism, we have devised a method by which the blood of a living animal may be submitted to dialysis outside the body, and again returned to the natural circulation without exposure to air, infection by micro-organisms, or any alteration which would necessarily be prejudicial to life. The process may be appropriately referred to as 'vivi-diffusion.'

"The apparatus constitutes what has been called an artificial kidney in the sense that it allows the escape of the diffusible constituents of the blood, but it differs from the natural organ in that it makes no distinction between these constituents, the rate of their elimination being presumably proportional to the coefficients of diffusion.

"It will be shown, however, that any given constituent of the blood, as urea, sugar, or sodium chloride (common salt), can be retained in the body by a simple expedient when so desired.

"The substitution in the animal's body of saline solution for an equal volume of blood leaves the physiological condition as nearly as possible unchanged and chemical results obtained by this method may be expected to represent normal conditions very closely, closer, for example, than when large quantities of blood are drawn off for analysis.

"When the circulation in the apparatus is established there is a fall in the blood pressure which is greater or less, according to the size of the apparatus in proportion to that of the animal, but there can be no other immediate symptoms. Rapid and complete recovery after an experiment lasting many hours may be obtained by due regard to asepsis and care in the use of the anaesthetic. Serious loss of blood is avoided by driving the greater part back into the animal's body at the end of the experiment. For purely chemical investigations the experiment is usually performed under complete chloretone anaesthesia."

## How Tubes Are Made

Lack of space does not permit a description of the details of manufacture of the tubes. They are made of a dialyzing substance called celloidin, and are molded inside glass tubes to which they conform. When dry they are pulled out. The dialyzing tubes are attached at the ends to glass tubes of like diameter, and the whole is contained in a glass jacket provided with an inlet and outlet for the outer fluid.

The reason so many tubes are used in the apparatus is to provide the maximum diffusing surface with as small a volume as possible. The apparatus for an animal of moderate size, like a dog, may have from about sixteen tubes up to "two or three times that number. Great care is taken in making the apparatus to avoid all sharp angles and sudden bends, and care must be taken that all branching channels are as nearly as possible of the same width, length and directness. These precautions are necessary in order to maintain a uniformity of flow, which is a very important consideration.

The first apparatus, which consisted of only four tubes, was used on a rabbit, and was connected with the carotid artery on the neck and the femoral vein (in the hind leg), and, consequently, about the length of the animal's body. The experimenters, however, have made a great improvement in practice by causing the blood in the apparatus to turn on itself after the manner of a U-tube, so that inflow and outflow tubes were at the same end and close together. This is the arrangement that is now carried out invariably, the result being that in present experiments the two cannulae are attached to the carotid artery and vein, or femoral artery and vein of the same, or usually of opposite sides.

Chloretone is used as the anaesthetic in these experiments because of its ability to produce prolonged and light anaesthesia with relatively little depression. The chemical name of this substance is tertiary, trichlor-butyl alcohol. It is administered by stomach tube about two hours before the operation. The powdered crystals are washed down with a little water. This usually produces the desired anaesthesia, but sometimes it is necessary to give a little ether at certain stages.

The investigators found that their experiments were costing a great deal of money on account of the high price of hirudin, the anti-coagulative principle of the medicinal leech. They had to pay $27.50 a gram for it, and sometimes it was necessary to use half a gram in a single experiment. They therefore resolved to extract their own hirudin, after buying leeches by the thousand, and they describe in detail their method of preparing the agent.

The experimenters declare in the most emphatic manner that the apparatus may be attached to an animal and the blood allowed to course through it for several hours without inducing any untoward effects or injuring the animal in any way. They give the details of two such experiments to prove their contentions. The hirudin is harmless and the substance of which the tubes is composed does not give up to the blood anything that affects the blood pressure.

## Quick Recovery

Both animals in the two experiments mentioned made a quick recovery, and in the weeks following, during which they were kept under observation, nothing abnormal was noted; on the contrary, as is usual in such cases, the animals improved in condition and took on weight because of the good care they received.

The experimenters selected salicylic acid with which to test the eliminating power of their apparatus, for the reason that quantitative estimations of this drug are easily made, that it is a substance of average diffusibility, and that, the time required for its complete elimination by the natural eliminating organ, the kidney, is known, During the first seven hours they recovered by means of the apparatus 19.1 per cent of the total amount given. As the manipulations involved in the separate hourly estimations unavoidably result in some loss, the authors assume that the actual output of salicylates in the apparatus is somewhat higher than that found.

Another interesting fact revealed in the experiments with salicylic acid is that the bladder is entirely free from the drug while the apparatus is dialyzing it out of the blood. A comparison of the rate of elimination of salicylic acid by the authors' apparatus with the rate of elimination by the kidneys of an animal that is not depressed by anaesthetic, or operative, procedures, showed that the animal actually eliminated in the natural way in six hours 1.6 per cent less than was removed by the dialyzer in seven hours. The writers say:

"These data show that the apparatus can already compete with the kidneys on favorable terms, at least, during the early hours of dialysis.

Here are the details of one experiment, as recorded by the physicians, indicating the amount of salicylic acid recorded hour by hour:

"Experiment B. May 2, 1913. Dog weighing 11.3 kgm. A small apparatus used (16 tubes), holding 260 cc. of blood. Apparatus attached to left carotid artery and right external jugular vein.

"12:45. Apparatus attached and hirudin solution (0.4 per cent) allowed to flow slowly into the apparatus the clip on the jugular vein being removed. About 40 cc. of hirudin solution used, more being injected later.

"1:02. Arterial clip removed.

"2:25. Dialysate removed and fresh solution introduced into the apparatus.

"2:30. 0.99 gram sodium salicylate in 20 cc. of water injected slowly into left femoral vein.

"3:40. Dialysate removed. Salicylic acid recovered (first hour) equals 24.12 mgm.

"4:55. Dialysate removed. Salicylic acid recovered (second hour) equals 15.22 mgm.

"5:55. Dialysate removed. Salicylic acid recovered (third hour) equals 13.23 mgm.

"6:55. Dialysate removed. Salicylic acid recovered (fourth hour) equals 11.40 mgm.

"8:20. Dialysate removed. Salicylic acid recovered (fifth hour) equals 10.50 mgm.

"9:05. Dialysate removed. Salicylic acid recovered (sixth period forty-five minutes) equals 9.63 mgm.

"It will be seen that the total amount of salicylic acid recovered by dialysis in the above experiment in five and three-quarters hours was 84.10 mgm., equaling 97.5 mgm. sodium salicylate. The average hourly output was, therefore, 17 mgm., which again does not compare so very unfavorably with rate of excretion by the kidney for a similar period when the drug is given by the mouth."

## Other Substances Eliminated

In conclusion, the experimenters mention some of the other substances that are known to be eliminated from the blood by the apparatus. Salicyluric acid is one of them. Many of the well-known constituents of the blood and urine also accumulate in the fluid surrounding the dialyzing tubes, among them sugar, urea, phosphates, and diastase. Ethyl sulphide is also freely eliminated. The writers add:

"Of more interest is the fact that we now have at our disposal a method for accumulating the non-proteid nitrogenous constituents of the blood other than urea in any desired amount, the quantity possible to be obtained depending on the size of the animal used, the dialyzing surface of the apparatus and the number of experiments performed.

"A wide field of investigation is opened up by the use of this apparatus in a comparative study of the blood flowing to and from various organs with reference both to the substances which they extract from, or add to, the general circulation and to the special active principles (hormones, &c.) which may be present in their internal secretions.

"A beginning in this direction has been made by attaching the apparatus to the portal vein (four experiments), the blood of which gave by diffusion considerably more amino-acids (determined by Van Slyke's method) than that of the carotid.

"Work in this direction, as well as in the improvement of the apparatus for the various purposes above outlined and accumulation of the experience necessary along these lines, is being pushed actively forward."

The statement of the investigators to the effect that the apparatus is still in a very imperfect state and is susceptible of great improvement, warrants the belief that ultimately it will aid in solving some of the most vexing problems of medical science.

*January 18, 1914*

# Panel Holds Life-or-Death Vote in Allotting of Artificial Kidney

By HAROLD M. SCHMECK JR.

One of the most dramatic stories of medical triumph and tragedy in recent history is being enacted daily in Seattle.

It means a longer life for a few but, because facilities for cure are limited, inevitable death of kidney disease for thousands of others.

A handful of men and women who should be dead, by normal medical criteria, are living and leading nearly normal lives. One of them, a young physics graduate student, was dying last summer. By fall he was well enough to go back to his studies and research. In December he was married.

Three weeks ago, at a scientific meeting, he gave a paper on the mathematics behind the device that keeps him alive. Few persons in the audience knew how intimately the research mattered to him.

The triumph—a new type of artificial kidney and mode of treatment—has been able to prolong life for some persons doomed because their kidneys would never function again.

The new kidney device is not a radical departure from earlier machines. But it has been modified to provide long-term use and to simplify its operation.

Like other such machines, its essential feature is a sandwich of cellophane sheets through which blood and a special chemical bath flow to purify the blood. The blood flows to the machines from tubes implanted in the patient's arm.

The chemical bath used by the new artificial kidney is considerably larger than for other such devices. It has a capacity of more than 100 gallons.

Other artificial kidneys have been designed for short-term emergency use, rather than for lasting performance.

The tragedy lies in the fact that while thousands of persons are dying of kidney diseases in the country only a few can be accepted for treatment at the Seattle center. Present facilities cannot care for more than the handful now being treated.

Consequently, as news of the Seattle group's dramatic results has spread through the Northwest, it has been found necessary to set up two committees to screen and choose among the applicants for treatment.

One of these is a medical committee. But because there are far more medically suitable candidates for the treatment than can be accepted, an anonymous committee of laymen has seen set up to narrow the selection further.

This group includes a bank president, a labor leader, a minster, two physicians, a housewife and a lawyer. It must choose who is to live and who is to die. Some of the criteria have to be arbitrary. Only persons who have lived in the state of Washington since last August are eligible. No one is accepted who is over 40 years old or who has no dependents.

But the full tragedy is not simply a need for additional centers, more space, more equipment, more manpower.

What has been accomplished to date has been research toward a goal, not the attainment of the goal itself.

The treatment devised by specialists at the University of Washington School of Medicine is experimental. It needs improvements, which are being developed. There may also be pitfalls that have not yet become evident. At present, too, the cost is great. It has been estimated that it takes roughly $10,000 a year to keep one patient on the treatment.

Because of all these factors there is a limit to the pace at which expansion can wisely be pursued. Currently about a dozen patients can potentially be handled by the facilities in Seattle.

By the end of another year, according to the leader of the research project, it should be sufficiently enlarged to handle about all of the most medically ideal candidates for the treatment who live in the State of Washington.

At the same time it must be borne in mind that an artificial kidney device will not do everything a real kidney does and the importance of this disparity over long-term treatment needs evaluation. Furthermore, some other medical centers have not been as successful with long-term treatment as has the Seattle group. Thus, the time for a full-scale program has not yet arrived, tragic though this fact is.

The leading figure in the research project in Seattle is Dr. Belding H. Scribner, Associate Professor of Medicine at the University of Washington School of Medicine. Last week in Atlantic City he gave a report on his experimental program to one of the nation's most respected medical research groups, the American Society for Clinical Investigation.

One specialist called it the meeting's most exciting report. The first four patients in Dr. Scribner's program began treatment during the winter of 1960. One died of a heart attack a year after the treatment began, but the three others are still alive, still being treated and leading comfortable lives. One is working full time.

## A Complete Substitute

The first patient, now entering his third year of treatment, has kidneys so damaged by disease that they do not function at all. His case proves that the treatment can substitute totally for the natural organ and do so for many months, Dr. Scribner said.

The two other patients have some residual kidney function, but not enough to keep them alive without artificial aid.

A main purpose of the human kidney is to filter from the blood chemical compounds and waste products that would be poisonous if they accumulated. These substances are carried from the body as urine.

No person can survive long if this cleansing action ceases. The patient dies after bouts of convulsions, vomiting and severe pain.

There are several disease conditions and types of poisoning in which the kidneys stop working temporarily. To carry patients through these crises of a few days artificial kidney devices were first developed during the mid-nineteen-forties.

Credit for being the first to build an artificial kidney machine suitable for treating human patients is given to Dr. W. J. Kolff of the Netherlands. He built his first device during the German occupation in World War II.

## Toxins Are Filtered

In the natural kidney, toxic products are filtered from the blood across thin membranes through which some substances will diffuse while others will not. In the artificial kidney, the process, called hemodialysis, is the same, though the equipment is bulky and huge compared with a human kidney.

In the artificial devices thin films of blood from the patient flow over thin cellophane sheets. Flowing on the other side of each membrane is a chemical bath. The toxic substances from the blood pass through the pores of the membrane and are carried away. The cleansed blood flows back into the patient's circulation.

The process is continuous. The blood flows steadily into the device, is cleansed of impurities and flows steadily back into the patient's blood stream.

The techniques and equipment for doing this job on a short-term basis for medical emergencies have been thoroughly developed since World War II. To do it often enough, regularly enough and in a routine manner so that a patient's blood may be cleansed periodically over many months is a far more taxing problem.

## Duration Limited

Furthermore, for technical reasons, a patient could not be subjected repeatedly, for months on end, to some phases of the normal hemodialysis procedure.

Because of these serious problems much of the medical profession has been apathetic toward the possibilities of the routine use of artificial kidneys, to maintain patients with chronic incurable disease.

Dr. Scribner's report last week gave hopeful evidence that the many obstacles could be overcome. For a few selected patients many months of added life have been given through the agency of medical science and several thin sheets of cellophane.

The Seattle equipment and techniques have been designed purposely for routine operation. They differ considerably from those of centers where the artificial kidney is used for a short emergency.

One crucial factor, Dr. Scribner said, has been the development of cannulae (small tubes) that can be implanted permanently in the patient. Through these, the patients are "plugged in" quickly and efficiently for each of their twice-weekly hemodialysis sessions. The tubes are made of special silicone rubber. Their development has been an engineering feat in itself, in Dr. Scribner's view.

Ordinarily they are implanted in one of the patient's arms—one tube connected with an artery, the other with a vein. When not in use on the artificial kidney the two ends are joined in a shunt so that blood continues to flow rapidly, and without clotting, through the cannulae.

This shunt, of horseshoe shape, projects an inch or two outside the patient's arm and is kept closed by medical tape. It can readily be opened at treatment time.

Experience has shown that these shunts can be kept in place without interfering with the patient's activities and that ordinary precautions keep them free from infection.

The ordinary precautions failed with one patient who dug clams with his cannulae in place. It was found, in his case, that the tubes could also be placed in a leg, with equally good results.

The other special features of the Seattle procedure include these points:

• The blood is fed from one of the patient's arteries rather than from a vein. Therefore the artificial kidney needs no pump and no priming with donated blood.

- The chemical bath into which the body "poisons" filter during dialysis is large enough so that it need not be changed during a full twelve- to sixteen-hour blood-cleansing session.

- The bath and dializer are kept cold to minimize the danger that bacteria will grow and invade the blood during the long session. The blood is rewarmed before returning to the body.

## Treatment Simplified

The sum effect of the modifications is that a procedure, normally highly technical and requiring the continual presence of a physician, has now been simplified to the point at which one nurse can supervise the treatment of three patients at once. Dr. Scribner considers this accomplishment the key to making the treatment practical for long-term chronic use.

When the program began, each patient was given one twenty-four hour dialysis one day each week. It was found that two shorter periods were more effective.

The work is done at two centers set up for the purpose; one at the university and the other at a community center where the program is financed by the John A. Hartford Foundation. Dr. Scribner's research is supported by a grant from the National Institute of Health.

One line of research now in progress may make it possible eventually to do without the cellophane sandwich device altogether. In the alternative technique, the patient's own peritoneum, the inner lining of the abdominal cavity, would do the filtering now accomplished by the cellophane sheets.

This method is used at some centers for short-term dialysis. The chemical bath is pumped into the peritoneal cavity and then pumped out again after it has drawn the impurities from the blood across the natural membrane.

If this technique could be perfected for routine night-time use, by the patient in his own home, for example, the day would be at hand when thousands of persons with serious kidney disease might lead normal lives despite their otherwise fatal illnesses.

It is difficult to say how far in the future such a possibility may be, Dr. Scribner said.

Even the success so far achieved, however, has brought medical science a step closer to one of the strangest and gravest choices that has ever confronted the medical profession.

The traditional concept of all medicine is to preserve the patient's life. Through the artificial kidney and other devices (the artificial heart pacemaker, for example) it is becoming possible to keep a person alive despite fatal and irreparable defects in one or more of his major organs.

In some cases, this extra life granted by the accomplishments of science can be almost normal. In others, it is, at best, invalidism for which there is no cure.

The question that many physicians are beginning to ask is this:

How may a physician make the choice and where must he draw the line between artificially prolonged life and natural death?

*May 6, 1962*

# Aid to Kidney Patients

By HOWARD A. RUSK, M.D.

As reported in this column last Sunday, each year 6,000 Americans with kidney disease die whose lives could be saved if sufficient resources were available to provide kidney dialysis.

Last November the White House received a report from a special committee on chronic kidney disease that recommended the Federal Government spend about $1 billion during the next six years to save their lives.

Currently there are about 7,000 terminal uremic patients each year who could benefit from dialysis, the process in which a "mechanical kidney" is used to remove the poisonous waste that accumulates in the blood. There are only, however, facilities for accommodating about 1,000.

In New York City and Westchester County, for example, there were only 66 beds in November, 1967, although it is expected this number will double by January, 1969.

The committee therefore pointed out that about 25,000 lives could be saved during the next six years under the program it recommends.

Currently the Federal Government supports dialysis through Public Health Service Demonstration Grants to a number of states and through vocational rehabilitation in some states.

The Veterans Administration also has a program for patients eligible for its services.

## Johnson Recommendation

Last year, President Johnson recommended amending Title 18, the Medicare section of the Social Security Act, to cover persons who, regardless of age, were permanently disabled.

Congress, however, rejected the proposed amendment.

Had it been adopted, terminal uremic patients who could benefit would have been eligible for dialysis care.

Unfortunately, the Public Health Service Demonstration Grants for dialysis are running out.

New York State, however, last year voted to establish a kidney disease center with satellites throughout the state and a special committee has been established to advise the State Department of Health on the implementation of this legislation.

Dialysis costs are constantly being lowered and will continue downward with technological improvements and increased use.

Currently, dialysis in a hospital costs about $14,000 per year, but following initial hospitalization, patients can be transferred to a home dialysis program at a cost of about $3,000 to $4,000 per year.

As Dr. Norman Deane, director of the dialysis program at New York City's Lenox Hill Hospital, has pointed out in a booklet, "Hemodialysis at Home," there are many other advantages to home dialysis.

Dr. Deane also warns against general public feeling that the problem is merely "shortage of hardware." He also points out that there are many patients with kidney disease who are not suitable for dialysis because of other complications.

He urges that all patients in the early stages of kidney disease should be sent to qualified specialists for evaluation and treatment that may prevent or delay the patient's reaching the stage of irreversible uremia that may be terminal.

Copies of the booklet may be obtained on request from Dr. Norman Deane, Lenox Hill Hospital, 77th Street and Park Avenue, New York, N.Y., 10021.

In its report the committee on chronic kidney disease pointed out its belief that kidney transplantation is the preferred therapeutic route. Today, about 2,000 kidney transplants have taken place with approximately 75 per cent chance of function for more than a year if a related donor is used. The chances are significantly lower if the kidney is obtained from a nonrelative or a cadaver.

## Advanced Typing Methods

With advanced typing techniques there has been a steady increase in the chances of success. The chances of finding a compatible donor through typing techniques is good as the recipient can be sustained indefinitely on dialysis while a search is conducted for a compatible donor.

The transplant patient, if the graft takes, is essentially a well person with few restrictions on his activities. In contrast the dialysis patient must be hooked up to his machine for several hours twice weekly.

The experts report also that a person who receives a transplant can expect to live twice as long as a patient on dialysis. As facilities for kidney transplantations are extended the need for dialysis will increase as each transplant patient requires an average of three months of preoperative dialysis plus further treatment on the dialyzer if his graft fails.

A small but growing voluntary agency, the National Kidney Foundation, 315 Park Avenue South, New York, N.Y., 10010, is seeking to improve the current treatment of kidney disease patients, control and reduce its occurrence by means of detection programs and increase support for research.

The Administration is now being pressed by Congress to cut nonmilitary spending by $4 billion to $6 billion before it will consider the President's request for an increase in income taxes.

The fate of the 6,000 Americans with kidney disease who now die each year is squarely in the hands of those responsible for these budget cuts.

Unfortunately, unless this program receives financial support new knowledge developed in the laboratory cannot be used at the bedside and individual physicians must continue to make the decision as to who will live and who, unfortunately, will die, with the ability to pay being a primary consideration.

*June 2, 1968*

# Concern Rising Over Costs of Kidney Dialysis Program

By RICHARD D. LYONS

Congressmen and Government officials have become increasingly concerned over the rocketing costs of a Federal program that is sustaining the lives of an increasing number of Americans, now about 40,000 people, who are suffering from acute kidney disease.

In Britain meanwhile, several thousand people suffering from the same class of diseases have died each year recently because the Government refused to give the socialized health system the funds necessary to pay for the medical technology needed to prevent them from dying.

Some of the legislators and administrators here who supported the kidney dialysis program for humanitarian reasons when it was first enacted six years ago now are having second thoughts about it because the costs are becoming enormous.

It is now likely that the Federal Government will be paying $1 billion in the next fiscal year to keep sufferers of incurable kidney disease alive, an amount that is from three to six times the cost that was anticipated when Congress enacted the bill in 1972.

## Threat of Poison Averted

Kidney dialysis is a process in which the circulatory system of a person whose kidneys have been destroyed by disease is connected to a machine that cleanses the blood of impurities in a manner similar to the functioning of normal kidneys. People without functioning kidneys usually must be dialyzed two or three times a week or they would be fatally poisoned by their own wastes.

The kidney dialysis legislative provision, which directed that the Medicare program pay most of the costs of treatment even for persons under the age of 65, was tucked inside an enormous Social Security reform bill. It was months after passage by overwhelming votes of both houses of Congress that its true implications became known.

No one has seriously suggested that Congress vote to take away Medicare coverage for kidney dialysis, but last year an attempt—apparently unsuccessful—was made to brake the cost increases through a bill introduced by two members of the House Ways and Means Committee, Representative Dan Rostenkowski, Democrat of Illinois, and Representative Charles A. Vanik, Democrat of Ohio.

The key point at issue in the dispute over the costs of kidney dialysis is where the procedure should be performed—at home, at an average yearly cost of from $8,000 to $12,000, or at an institution, where costs range from $15,000 to $30,000 a year.

## Comparison of Nations

About 90 percent of Americans undergo dialysis at an institution, whereas in Canada the ratio is 40 percent, and in Britain it is 35 percent.

"The reason is that the United States is an island of socialism in a sea of free enterprise," said Dr. Arthur Shimizu, the director of the Canadian Renal Failure Registry in Hamilton, Ontario.

Dr. Shimizu said that cost increases had also plagued the Canadian dialysis program but that they were being brought under control there "because we have better Government regulation of health care." As a result, he said, the number of persons in Canada being treated institutionally is falling.

"We are using such incentives for home dialysis as paying the spouse of a person suffering from kidney disease to run the machine, and having such supplies as new needles and chemicals delivered to the home," he added.

## Curb on Institutional Care

The Rostenkowski-Vanik bill contained a host of such incentives to avoid institutional dialysis, plus a provision that would have forced half of all dialysis to be done either in the home or in a relatively low-cost self-care dialysis center by 1980.

"The lobbyists gutted the hell out of it," was the way one official of the Social Security System described the House action. Rather than setting a ceiling of 50 percent on those persons who could be dialyzed in an institution, the version adopted by the House last September merely set 50 percent as "a national goal."

Further, the Senate version that passed earlier this month, also without a formal vote, even deleted the language calling for a national goal. In effect, the attempt at cost containment had been killed.

Perhaps the one organization that has the most to gain by the deletion of home dialysis directives is National Medical Care Inc., a Boston-based company that has 86 profit-making dialysis centers and clinics that took in $91 million last year, most of it from the Federal Government.

## Role of Ex-Reagan Aide

John Sears, the former campaign manager for Ronald Reagan, is the Washington lobbyist for the company. According to Congressmen whom he has lobbied in favor of institutionalized dialysis, Mr. Sears's sales pitch was, "What's wrong with making a profit?"

Dr. Eugene Schupak of Rockleigh, N.J., the company's president, insisted that his centers performed more cheaply than most, about $102 per dialysis. This is partly borne out by Canadian costs of about $125 per dialysis.

Further, Dr. Schupak argued that it is much more convenient and esthetically preferable for a kidney disease sufferer to undergo treatment away from his home. The machine itself is cumbersome and the procedure may be disruptive within a home since it may take from four to six hours.

*April 28, 1978*

CHAPTER 16

# Mental Health

# Dreams of the Insane Help Greatly in Their Cure

There has been a revolution in the last few years in the method of treating the insane and those persons suffering from nervous affections bordering on insanity. The new mode of procedure is based on the remarkable studies of Prof. Dr. Sigmund Freud of Zurich, who has devoted his energies to a field of investigation practically untouched by other research workers engaged in elucidating the mysteries of the disordered mind.

Freud's method is known as psychanalysis, which bears the same relation to mental and nervous diseases that the microscope does to pathology. Abnormal mental conditions had been judged hitherto practically by mere superficial inquiry and observation. Freud and his pupils literally turn the minds of their patients inside out.

Those patients hovering on the borderline of insanity are made to see the absurdity of their fears, delusions, and obsessions, and by the force of logic are restored to mental health. Even in cases of real insanity the persistent application of the Freud methods results in a great deal of benefit to large numbers of patients.

Freud's reasoning has made such a profound impression on those engaged in the treatment of the nervous and insane that his principles are being applied in State institutions throughout the civilized world, as well as in private practice. Psychanalysis is now a part of the routine practice in the Institution for the Insane on Ward's Island, as well as in other State institutions.

Prof. Freud has written several books dealing with various phases of his theories and their practical application. One of his pupils, Dr. A. A. Brill of this city, who is well known as a neurologist, and who has translated many of Freud's articles into English, has written a book on the subject which is a lucid and comprehensive review of the whole matter. This work is entitled *Psychanalysis, Its Theory and Practical Application*. It has just been issued by the W. B. Saunders Company of Philadelphia and London.

In his preface, Dr. Brill gives some interesting and welcome information relative to the advance that has been made in the last few years in the treatment of the insane in New York and elsewhere. He says:

"Like many others in the field of mental and nervous work, I received my training in the State Hospital for the Insane (Ward's Island). It was my fortune to enter the hospital service at a very important period of its development. Dr. Frederick

Peterson was then President of the Commission in Lunacy, and it was mainly through his untiring energy that the New York State hospitals were thoroughly modernized and put on a firm scientific basis. It was mostly through his efforts that Dr. Adolf Meyer became Director of the Pathological Institute at Ward's Island, N.Y.

"The advent of Dr. Meyer marks a new epoch in the New York State Hospital service. An accomplished neurologist and psychiatrist of long experience, he soon instilled new life and interest into the work by giving regular courses of lectures and demonstrations on the theories and methods then in vogue. The old way of writing a one-line note about the patient's mental and physical condition every three or six months had to stop, despite the grumbling of the 'old-timers,' and we were required to make frequent and comprehensive examinations of our patients and to note carefully what we found.

"These examinations were made in accordance with a scheme thoroughly worked out by Dr. Adolf Meyer, the underlying principles of which were the teachings of Kraepelin, Wernicke, and Ziehen. This good work has continued up to the present with excellent results.

"Since I left the State service I have visited and worked in some of the best psychiatric clinics in Europe, and I am glad to say that all things considered the work of the New York State Hospital compares very favorably with the work done in most of the hospitals of its kind.

"What I say in reference to the New York State Hospital can be readily applied with some modifications to most of the hospitals for the insane in this country. It is well known that within the last ten to twelve years the management and treatment of the insane in this country have undergone a marked transformation, which is of great benefit to the patient, the doctor and the public.

"The State Hospitals are now treating the patients as patients in the true sense of the word; they are rapidly filling up an enormous gap in the medical profession by training doctors how to treat the insane, and they are gradually abolishing the popular prejudices against hospitals for the insane. The medical schools, too, are now paying more though not enough attention to mental diseases; and last, but not least, excellent and commendable work is being done by the Social Service Departments and the National Society for Mental Hygiene.

"The progressive evolution in the study of mental diseases has called attention to another neglected field in which the most important work is still to be done. I refer to the so-called 'border-line' cases, the neuroses and mild psychoses who never reach the State hospitals, but form the greatest proportion of clinic and dispensary practice. In the ten years from 1900 to 1909, 21,290 patients were examined by the assistants in the neurological department of the Vanderbilt Clinic, New York, and about 20 per cent of this number were diagnosed as neurasthenia, psychasthenia, hysteria and as mild forms of the functional psychoses.

"Although I am not ready to give statistics, I do not hesitate to assert that the same conditions prevail in almost every clinic and dispensary. A striking feature in these border-line cases is the fact that the great majority run a chronic course. Up to recent years no real effort has been made to understand these unfortunates. It is gratifying to note, however, that a complete change has taken place in this direction. Physicians now realize that the old adage *mens sana in corpore sano* is not to be taken in the strict sense, and hence do not rely on physical treatment alone. All enlightened and progressive physicians recognize psychotherapy as an important therapeutic agent in the treatment of these border-line cases of mental diseases.

"Now, as there is a demand for psychotherapy, the question naturally arises as to which is the method of preference. Without entering into the merits and demerits of the different systems of psychotherapy, admitting that in competent hands they are all good and useful, and that I myself employ them in certain cases, I do not hesitate to assert that psychanalysis is the most rational and effective method of psychic therapy. I say this after I have practiced for years the existing psychotherapeutic methods.

"Psychanalysis is the only system of psychotherapy that deals with the neuroses as entities instead of treating symptoms as do hypnotism, suggestion, and persuasion. To hypnotize a patient because he suffers from obsessions or phobias is equivalent to treating the cough or fever regardless of the disease of which it is but one of the manifestations. Hypnotism takes no cognizance of personality; it simply imposes blind obedience which at best lasts until worn off. Psychanalysis always concerns itself with the individual as a personality and enters into the deepest recesses of the mind. It is for that reason that the results of psychanalysis are most effective; and it is only through psychanalysis that we can hope to gain a real insight into the neuroses and psychoses, a thing of prime importance in the study of mental prophylaxis.

"These assertions are not based merely on the reading of a few scattered papers, but on about six years of hard work and most constant occupation with the subject. For it is only through hard work and long experience that one can acquire a thorough knowledge of Freud's psychology. Recently I had the pleasure of talking to some who claimed to have used psychanalysis in the treatment of patients and who spoke rather discouragingly, saying that it produced no result.

"Such statements readily show the gross misunderstanding of the work. For it is not the treatment of a few hours, weeks or even months that cures; it is the psychic elaboration accomplished during a long period by one thoroughly conversant with the work. I do not think that it is too much to ask of one who wishes to make use of a certain technical method that he should first learn its basic principles. One cannot expect to become proficient in psychanalysis unless he has mastered at least Freud's theories of the neuroses, the interpretation of dreams, the sexual theories, the psychopathology of everyday life, and his book on wit, and last but not least, who has not had a training in nervous and mental work.

"Besides these qualifications one must know how to select his cases. It has been wrongly supposed that we claim to be able to cure everything. Neither Freud nor any of his pupils has ever advanced such claims. On the contrary, Freud has repeatedly emphasized that psychanalysis has a limited field, and that it should be used only in limited cases. Let us hear what he says:

"'The former value of the person should not be overlooked in the disease, and you should refuse a patient who does not possess a certain degree of education, and whose character is not in a measure reliable. We must not forget that there are also healthy persons who are good for nothing, and that if they only show a mere touch of the neurosis, one is only too much inclined to blame the disease for incapacitating such inferior persons.

"'I maintain that the neurosis does not in any way stamp its bearer as a dégénéré, but that, infrequently enough, it is found in the same individual associated with the manifestations of degeneration. The analytic psychotherapy is, therefore, no procedure for the treatment of neuropathic degeneration, on the contrary it is limited by it. It is also not to be applied in persons who are not prompted by their own suffering to seek treatment, but subject themselves to it by order of their relatives.

"'If one wishes to take a safe course he should limit his selection to persons of a normal state. Psychoses, confusional states, and marked (I might say toxic) depressions are unsuitable for analysis, at least, as it is practiced to-day. I do not think it at all impossible that with the proper changes in the procedure it will be possible to disregard this contraindication, and thus claim a psychotherapy for the psychoses.

"'The age of the patient also plays a part in the selection for the psychoanalytic treatment. Persons near or over the age of fifty lack, on the one hand, the plasticity of the psychic processes upon which the therapy depends—old people are no longer educable—and on the other hand, the material which has to be elaborated, and the duration of the treatment is immensely increased. The earliest age limit is to be individually determined; youthful persons are excellent subjects for analysis.'

"As the actual working method will be described later, I shall confine myself here to a few facts, which, although strictly speaking, belong to the epilogue, may nevertheless be worth mentioning in this connection. With the beginning of the analysis I investigate the patient's dream life. I instruct him to write down his dreams on awakening. This is very important, because dreams give us the most reliable information concerning the individual, and they invariably show some relation to the symptoms. I never attempt, however, to analyze a dream before knowing the patient for at least two weeks. Dreams cannot be analyzed unless one has the full co-operation of the dreamer, and this is only possible after certain rapport has been established between the doctor and the patient."

"It is this rapport, or the transference, as we will call it, with which one must start. Nothing can be done without it, and unless this is properly managed little can be done for the patient. One may get excellent results in surgery or in any other specialty without seeing the patient's face, but psychanalysis presupposes an intimate acquaintanceship. There must be a mutual understanding and liking between doctor and patient. One must, however, be on his guard lest the transference be carried too far."

As an instance of the importance of Freud's studies, it may be stated that societies have been formed in the majority of the medical centres solely for the purpose of studying his theories and reporting the results of the practical application of his ideas. Such a society exists here. It is called the New York Psychoanalytic Society.

It is not the purpose of this article to enter into a discussion of the psycho-neuroses, the actual neuroses, the psychological mechanisms of paranoia, or any of the morbid mental states. The public is more interested in the practical application of actual Sherlock Holmes methods to the mental operations, both conscious and unconscious, of the patients of Freud and his disciples. Like Kipling's wonderful harper who performed for the King and then said to him, "I hae harpit your secret soul in three," Freud and his followers literally tear hidden secrets from the bewildered minds of their patients, and the latter do not know that they are revealing them. This is done largely through the interpretation of dreams.

"So far as I know," says Dr. Brill, "no author has solved the problem of the dream so ingeniously and successfully as Prof. Freud. As mentioned previously in developing his psychology of the psychoneuroses, Freud found that the dream plays a very important part in the psyche of the individual. The dream is not a senseless jumble, but a perfect mechanism, and when analyzed it is found to contain the fulfillment of a wish; it always treats of the innermost thoughts of a personality, and for that reason gives us the best access to the unconscious.

"No psychanalysis is complete, nay possible, without the analysis of dreams. The dream not only helps us to interpret symptoms, but is often an invaluable instrument in diagnosis and treatment. The causative factors of many neuroses are extremely vague and usually unconscious to the patient, and it is by means of the dream that the underlying etiological factors are disclosed."

Here is a typical instance to illustrate the relation of the dream to the neurosis. It occurred in Dr. Brill's practice:

"Case: Miss G., 28 years old, American, came to me in January, 1908, because she had been 'very nervous' for about three months. Her family history showed that her father died of nephritis and had a 'stroke' (left hemiplegia) a few months before he died. She had been well until three months before. Since then she had suffered from insomnia, irritability, loss of appetite, constipation, headache, uncalled for worry, crying spells and anxious expectation. Her mother stated that she had entirely changed, that she expressed pessimistic ideas, often repeating that she would like to die. Examination showed all the symptoms enumerated. The patient was pretty, she showed no stigmata and was above the average in intelligence. While inciting her story she showed the typical indifference often found in hysteria. She smiled when I asked her why she felt so depressed and could give no reason for it. She knew that she really had nothing to worry about and that she had everything to live for, yet she could not 'shake off the blue feeling.'"

One of the most distressing thoughts was that something might happen to her mother.

"To those acquainted with the language of hysteria this means just the opposite. It was merely a reaction of the wish that she might lose her mother, and, as we shall see later, there was a reason for that wish. Physically there was nothing worth mentioning. I diagnosticated the case as a mild anxiety hysteria with imperfect conversion.

"I saw her a number of times, but made no progress in the treatment. To my question she always answered: 'I feel about the same.' I then thought of psychanalysis and with that in view I asked her to write out her dreams and bring them to me. She was sure that she never dreamed except when her stomach was out of order, but promised to comply with my request if ever she should and one day brought me the following dream:

"'I dreamed that I was in a lonely country place and was anxious to reach my home in Liconow or Liconor Bay, but could not get there. Every time I made a move there was a wall in the way. It looked like a street full of walls. My legs were as heavy as lead. I could only walk very slowly as if I were very weak or very old. Then there was a flock of chickens, but that seemed to be in a crowded city street, and they—the chickens—ran after me and the biggest of all said something like "Come with me into the dark."'

"This dream seems absurd enough and as the dreamer remarked: 'It is so ridiculous that I am ashamed to tell it. Whoever heard of such a thing as chickens talking?' She was assured that it must mean something and the analysis proceeded.

"It would be too long and immaterial for the purposes of this work to give here the whole analysis which, when recorded, covered over eight pages of foolscap. Only the principal associations and symbolic expressions necessary to explain the dream will be enumerated.

"On asking the dreamer what the most vivid part of the dream was she answered that it was the second part relating to the chickens. When asked to repeat the thoughts evoked by concentrating her mind on the word 'chickens,' she gave the following: 'I could only see the biggest chicken, all the others seemed blurred; it was unusually big and had a very long neck and it spoke to me—the street recalls where I used to go to school—I graduated from public, school when I was thirteen—the block was always crowded with children from school'—she then began to blush and laugh and when asked to explain her actions, said:

"'It recalls the happy school days when I was young and had no worries—I even had a beau, a pupil from the male department. There was a male and a female department in the same school and most of my girl friends had beaux—we used to meet after school hours and walk home together. My beau's name was F. He was lanky and thin and the girls used to tease me about him. Whenever they saw him coming they said, "Belle here comes your chicken"—that was his nickname among the boys.'

"On being asked if she now understood who the chicken in the dream was she laughingly said: 'You don't mean to say that the chicken with the long neck was Mr. F.?' When asked if she still kept up her acquaintance with Mr. F. she stated that she had not seen him for the last few months, but prior to that she saw him quite often. On further analysis it was found that this early schoolday love was still kept up. He had proposed to her no less than three times, but she had never given him any definite answer. She only 'liked' him and her family opposed him on account of his financial position.

"The last time she met him was at a military ball. He was an officer of a military organization and 'he looked quite handsome in his smart uniform.' He danced with her and 'was very kind,' but he did not propose. She frankly admitted that she looked for a fourth proposal at this ball and that she was quite ready to accept him. She had heard only recently that he was paying attention to another young lady, a thing which caused her considerable annoyance—to put it in her own words, 'I can only blame myself and I will have to forget it.'

"We see that the most impossible and ludicrous part of the dream, that is, 'the talking of the chicken,' is now quite plain. The 'chicken' is simply the nickname of Mr. F., who is the hero of the dream. There were other chickens, but they were blurred, that is, there were other young suitors, but they were relegated to the background.

"The chicken said, 'Come with me into the dark.' The word 'dark' evoked the following associations: Indistinct—obscure—mystery—marriage. She recalled that after her father's death her mother once spoke sympathetically of Mr. F., saying 'Money is not all,' and philosophized on marriage in the following remarks: 'You will never know a man until you have eaten a peck of salt with him,' and 'Marriage is a mystery.' These words made a deep impression on her, and the last Biblical quotation frequently recurred to her. We then see that in her mind the word 'dark' was used synonymously with mystery and marriage, and hence we can understand its meaning in the chicken's speech. Briefly stated it was the fourth proposal of Mr. F.

"The first part of the dream reads, 'I was in a lonely country place,' &c. She stated that she recalled the beautiful country around H. Bay, where she had been the preceding Summer. She could not quite understand what Liconow or Liconor Bay meant, and gave the following associations: Liconow—Lucknow—meaning a painting representing the famous battle of Lucknow which she had recently seen. The soldiers recalled the military organization at whose ball she had met Mr. F. The word 'Liconor' suggested by sound association Lucarno and Lugano, two places which she had visited while abroad two years before. H. Bay often recalled the beautiful Italian lakes, Lucarno and Lugano, whither she hoped to go on her honeymoon.

"Finally, Liconor Bay resolved itself into Lik-onor Bay, which, by sound association, can be readily recognized as 'like, honor, and obey.' If 'like' is substituted by 'love' it gives the familiar formula well known to all maidens seriously contemplating matrimony. The dreamer used 'like,' because, as aforesaid, she thought she only 'liked.' Such condensations of words and ideas are not at all rare in dreams.

"If we now rewrite the first sentence it will read as follows: 'I was in a lonely country place and was anxious to reach my home in "LIKe (love), hONOR, and oBEY,"' that is, 'I was lonely and anxious to get married.'

"The next sentence reads, 'But could not,' &c. She stated that her legs were as heavy as lead, she was alone and was afraid that something might happen, but she was unable to make any headway. The sensation of inhibition experienced in dreams, like the inability to make any headway when one most desires to do so, signifies a marked mental conflict. Here, too, it merely shows the great mental conflict in our dreamer's mind. She is anxious to marry.

"She 'likes' Mr. F. Moreover, she is of an advanced age and, as the dream shows, she could walk only very slowly as if 'she were weak or very old,' that is, the difficulties on the road to matrimony increase with advancing age; she is weak and old, that is, she is an 'old maid,' an expression by which she often jocosely referred to herself in her waking state; all of these arguments are in favor of accepting Mr. F., but then her family is opposed to him. He is a nice enough young man, but he is unable to care for her in a manner befitting her station in life.

"The dream continues: 'Every time I made a move there was a wall in the way, it looked like a street full of walls,' &c. A street full of walls signifies Wall Street, hence money—that was the real obstacle. When told of the interpretation she laughingly remarked, 'That's it exactly. I even thought very seriously of helping him along, as Pa left me some money, but then everything is invested in Wall Street and there is a tacit understanding among ourselves that the whole estate shall be left intact until mother's death.'

"We now understand the latent thoughts of the dream. The first part can be translated as follows: I am 28 years old, an old maid, and I am anxious to marry Mr. F., but then he is not rich enough to take care of me. I perhaps can help him financially. In the second part we find the wish realization, as here Mr. F. actually proposes to her for the fourth time.

"These were the actual thoughts which had occupied our dreamer's mind for the past months and which, as she quite frankly admitted, she tried hard to forget. It is quite obvious that the dream deals here with the thoughts which a young lady would not consciously disclose even to her physician, and we can also understand why she was 'ashamed to tell it' because she understood it unconsciously, though not consciously. The dream never deals with trivialities, and, no matter how simple and innocent it may seem, the analysis invariably shows that the thoughts behind it belong to the inmost recesses of personality. This accounts for the many resistances encountered during the analysis. The psychic censor constantly inhibits the painful or disagreeable complexes from becoming conscious and is also responsible for the rapid forgetting of dreams on awakening."

Later in his book Dr. Brill discloses the outcome of this interesting case:

"These brief analyses distinctly show the connection between the dream and the neuroses. I am quite convinced that had we not analyzed the dream, the psychic conflicts underlying the neurosis of Miss G. could not have been discovered, as they were unconscious to the patient, and that she would have merged into a chronic neurosis. Very soon after the complexes were discovered and brought to her consciousness her symptoms began to disappear and within two months she was completely cured.

"It must be added that besides analyzing the dream her other symptoms had to be explained to her. Thus her abnormal attachment to her mother disappeared as soon as she became conscious of the fact that it was hiding a repressed wish that her mother might die so that she could use the estate to assist Mr. F. The insight and psychological education which she gained during the analysis also helped her to overcome some of her false pride and prudishness, and as a result she is now happily married to Mr. F. Thus her wish was realized."

Here are Dr. Brill's conclusions on the analysis of dreams:

"1. As Freud has shown, dreams are perfect psychological mechanisms. They have a definite meaning and contain a wish fulfillment.

"2. Every psychotic symptom is the expression of a former mental occurrence and symbolically represents a wish fulfillment.

"3. The repression of the unconscious is at the basis of both the dream and the psychotic symptom.

"4. Dreams are the product of the unconscious and hence afford the easiest access to the exploration of the neurosis."

In an absorbing chapter on the psychopathology of everyday life, the author gives several instances of forgetfulness and the astonishing results obtained by the application of psychanalysis. In this connection Dr. Brill relates this personal experience:

"While reading one day the text recalled to me a case which I had published years before. I desired to make a marginal note to that effect when I suddenly found that I could not recall the name of my patient. This patient was under my personal care for months and the features of the case were such that I had daily spent hours with him, so that it was the more remarkable that I could not recall the name. As usual I made a great effort to recall it and it was only after some time that I thought of Freud's theories and decided to test them by analyzing this lapse of memory. The case had presented so many unusual and interesting aspects that I was advised to publish it.

"After a painstaking preparation I was ready to send it to the publisher, when I was informed that my senior had decided to read a paper on this very subject before a medical society and that I was to have this paper ready for him on a certain date. My feelings on hearing this can readily be imagined. The thought of having labored for days and of some one else getting the credit for it caused me indignation and depression. My colleagues sympathized with me, but all they could do was to make merry over it. This continued until the day before the meeting, when I was informed that owing to unforeseen circumstances I was to attend this meeting myself and read the paper.

"I read this paper as directed, but very few of the members knew the true circumstances of the matter. Most of them thought that I was merely sent to read the paper. The reports of the meeting as given in the different medical journals gave the name of my senior as the reader of the paper. The reader will pardon my indulging in personalities. It is indispensable in psychanalysis and here it serves to show the marked displeasure and pain which caused the repression.

"When one attempts to follow Freud's method of 'free association' he soon finds himself in a maze. The longer he proceeds the more complicated the problem seems to become, and to the inexperienced it appears like an endless confusion. Now and then our thoughts, as it were, stop. We call this an 'obstruction' or a 'blocking' and experience teaches us that this phenomenon generally accompanies or precedes some important complex. In analyzing psychoneurotic symptoms the patients often stop and say 'That's all. I cannot think of anything else.' After considerable urging they finally, perhaps after blushing, laughing or stammering, do think of something else. Frequently the mind makes use of symbolic expressions and ambiguous terms which the physician must always be alive to. All these are due to the inhibitions of the psychic censor against the painful and disagreeable thoughts.

"On beginning to discover by analysis the name of my patient I soon found myself in a very complicated milieu. I distinctly saw his features in my mind. I reviewed all the circumstances connected with the case and noted all my associations. Page after page was filled and time flew faster than it seemed. I suddenly found that I had spent five hours of assiduous application and filled over two dozen pages, but was seemingly as far from getting the name as when I first started. Frequently my thoughts stopped only to start anew. I was most desirous not only of recalling the name but of testing Freud's theory, as it was my first attempt. It would be useless and impossible to recall the different associations, but the following will suffice to explain the analysis: On seeing the patient in my mind's eye the name Appenzeller presented itself to me. Appenzeller was the name of one of my patients in the psychiatrical clinic at Zurich where I was at the time of the analysis. There was no resemblance between the two patients except that my New York patient was a psychic epileptic and Appenzeller suffered from motor epilepsy, yet the latter name persistently emerged from the association mass.

"The scenes connected with my New York patient as well as numerous other hospital experiences continued to pass in a panoramic review. Some were especially persistent and vivid, recurring with greater frequency than the others. Thus, one scene, an actual occurrence, was especially vivid. It recalled a forest fire near the hospital. I stood watching the fire with my senior, Dr. Z., who played such a great part in the episode, and Dr. X. joined me. Many rabbits driven out by the fire were shot. While thus standing Dr. Z. turned to a hospital attendant and asked him for his shotgun, as a rabbit was seen running from the underbrush. He waited for the animal to come within range and then got ready to fire, remarking: 'Let me see whether I can get this rabbit.'

"A crack was heard, but the rabbit scampered away. Dr. X. and I looked at each other smilingly, but quickly changed countenance when Dr. Z. turned to us and said, 'My finger slipped on account of the rain.' This scene persistently recurred from time to time, but I attached no more weight to it than to the hundreds of others. Yet whenever my supply of associations seemed to be exhausted and I started over again, the name of Appenzeller and this scene continually reappeared. I finally tired of the whole process and thought of giving it up, but despite my willingness to do so I could not banish the numerous scenes from my mind. While thus contemplating I again saw the rabbit scene and heard Dr. Z. say, 'Let me see whether I can get this rabbit,' and just then the name of the patient suddenly came to me. It was 'Lapin,' which is the French for rabbit.

"It can readily be seen that had I been keen enough it would have saved me hours of labor, for during the analysis this scene occurred twenty-eight times more than any other. But owing to my inexperience at the time and my intense desire to get the name I overlooked the very thing Freud lays so much stress upon—that is, the symbolic expressions, &c. This whole rabbit scene symbolizes the Lapin episode. Dr. Z. attempted to get the rabbit (Lapin) but missed it.

"To be sure, it must be remembered that although I am conversant with French, in my mind Lapin was always translated into rabbit because I think in English. In fact I distinctly recall that I had frequently translated mentally the name Lapin into rabbit. If we now bear in mind the French pronunciation of Lapin we can understand why Appenzeller continued to substitute itself. The first part— Appen—phonetically resembles Lapin—Appen, Lapen. Furthermore, both patients suffered from epilepsy. The case clearly shows how a name may be repressed on account of a disagreeable experience."

*March 2, 1913*

# Surgery Used on the Soul-Sick; Relief of Obsessions Is Reported

By WILLIAM L. LAURENCE

A TLANTIC CITY, N.J.—A new surgical technique, known as "psycho-surgery," which, it is claimed, cuts away sick parts of the human personality, and transforms wild animals into gentle creatures in the course of a few hours, will be demonstrated here tomorrow at the Comprehensive Scientific Exhibit of the American Medical Association, which is holding its eighty-eighth annual assembly here this week.

The new "surgery of the soul" has been applied to twenty mentally ill human beings, 15 per cent of whom, it is claimed, were "greatly improved," with an additional 50 per cent "moderately improved." It is asserted the mental symptoms relieved by this new brain operation, often performed under local anaesthesia, include tension, apprehension, anxiety, depression, insomnia, suicidal ideas, delusions, hallucinations, crying spells, melancholia, obsessions, panic states, disorientation, psychalgesia (pains of psychic origin), nervous indigestion and hysterical paralysis.

When performed on wild monkeys, two of which were placed on exhibition here today, the brain operation changed the apprehensive, anxious and hostile creatures of the jungle into creatures as gentle as the organ grinder's monkey.

The new "soul surgery" was originally announced last year in a French scientific publication by Dr. Egas Moniz of Lisbon, Portugal. The results obtained by him appeared so startling that they were repeated in this country on cases in which every recognized form of treatment had been employed without improvement.

The exhibit is presented by Dr. James W. Watts, Dr. Walter Freeman and Dr. Ralph W. Barris of George Washington University Medical School. A supplementary paper will be presented by Drs. Watts and Freeman before the section on nervous and mental diseases on Wednesday. The title of the paper is "Psycho-Surgery: Effect on Certain Mental Symptoms of Surgical Interruption in the Pathways in the Frontal Lobe."

The new surgery consists in separating twelve small cores of the white matter in the brain, underlying the gray matter of the two frontal lobes, from the rest of the brain's white matter. The cores, each one centimeter in diameter, are not taken out of the brain, but are left in their places after the surgical instrument, known as the leucotome, has separated them from their original environment.

The twelve cores are separated in two groups of six each, one group below the gray matter of each of the two frontal lobes, which are regarded as the seat of intellectual integration. Only two holes, however, are drilled in the scalp, each hole being sufficient, by proper manipulation of the instrument, for the separation of six cores.

## Case Histories Are Cited

Here are a few of the cases to be described by Drs. Freeman and Watts before the meeting:

"Mrs. A. H., housewife, aged 63. Two previous nervous breakdowns. Always meticulous and exacting. Increasing apprehension, anxiety, insomnia, agitation and tension for one year, so that the patient was confined to her home with special day and night nurses.

"After the operation (prefrontal lobotomy), Sept. 14, 1936, the symptoms disappeared immediately. Now manages home and household accounts, enjoys people, attends theatre, drives her own car. Great improvement.

"Case 2. Mrs. E. A., bookkeeper, aged 59. In bed since nervous breakdown May, 1936. Complained of anxiety and agitation, fear of being poisoned, constant mourning and weeping. Disoriented. Confined to hospital with special day and night nurses. Immediate disappearance of anxiety, apprehension and pain after a prefrontal lobotomy Oct. 7, 1936. Has been working in old position as bookkeeper continuously since Jan. 1, 1937. Great improvement."

After citing a number of other cases, some of which were only moderately improved, while 35 per cent of the others showed no improvement, Drs. Freeman and Watts state:

"After cutting the pathways in the prefrontal area, there was a disappearance or a reduction of tension, apprehension, anxiety, depression and agitation in all but two cases. The relief of the symptoms has persisted to the present time in more than half of the patients. Ten of the twelve patients having ideas of suicide before operation no longer consider self-destruction. Crying spells have ceased in six of nine patients. Hallucinations have gradually cleared up in the seven patients who had them.

"More than half of the patients are unresponsive for a week or two after the operation. They answer questions, but speak only when spoken to. The change in behavior which persists is slight and may be described as emotional, flattening, diminished spontaneity, lack of attention and indifference.

"Seven patients, on the contrary, were very talkative and definitely euphoric for two or four weeks after operation. Transient perseveration of speech and disorientation have occurred a few times."

## Two Died After Operation

One patient died several months after the operation and another patient died on the sixth day after the operation, the physicians report.

On the other hand, some of the leading neurologists who viewed the exhibit today expressed themselves as being very skeptical about the new "psycho-surgery" and they predicted that the method would meet with considerable criticism.

In devising his new technique, Dr. Moniz worked on the assumption, Drs. Freeman and Watts said, "that while there are no detectable abnormalities of the brain in certain of the functional psychoses, the symptoms might be due to the development of stereotypy in cortical association centers, i.e., fixed patterns of response tending to perpetuate themselves to the detriment of the personality as a whole.

"By forcibly breaking up the connections over a large area, an opportunity would be given, Dr. Moniz argued, for reintegration of cortical activity along different lines."

## A Mysterious Cause of Tumor

A mysterious substance present in a crude preparation of wheat germ oil that produced a highly malignant form of abdominal tumor in ninety-three white rats to which it had been fed is reported in an exhibit by Drs. Leonard S. Rowntree, George M. Dorrance and E. F. Ciccone of the Philadelphia Institute for Medical Research. Four different strains of rats were used and every one developed the tumors.

"No spontaneous tumors have been encountered in approximately 20,000 rats utilized in the Philadelphia Institute during the past four years," Dr. Rowntree and his colleagues report.

That the tumors are due to a mysterious substance in the crude wheat germ oil extracted with ether and not to any substance so far known to be present in the oil, is indicated by the fact that the refined wheat germ oil intended for medicinal use for its content of vitamin E, the anti-sterility vitamin, failed to produce the tumors. Vitamin E concentrate, likewise, Dr. Rowntree reports, failed to produce the malignant growths.

The tumors appeared in from two weeks to six months, sometimes as single and again as multiple tumors. The tumor is always malignant, almost always a spindle cell sarcoma, which invariably kills. It is resistant to X-rays, which result in dissemination rather than amelioration or cure, the report states.

Transplantations have been successful in every one of the 300 instances tried, Dr. Rowntree added. In fact, he said, the cancer has been transplanted successfully fourteen times to successive recipients without loss of malignancy.

"This crude preparation of wheat germ oil," Dr. Rowntree said, "is the only vegetable product known at present capable of producing malignant neoplasms (cancer). Naturally our interest now centers on the source and nature of this sarcogenic (cancer-producing) agent and has led us to a study of the wheat germ itself. We are investigating the possibility that this malignant growth is directly or indirectly related to the growth impetus resident in the wheat germ."

A new hormone from the pancreas named lipocaic is described in an exhibit by Dr. Lester R. Dragstedt and Dr. John Van Prohaska of the University of Chicago. Without it animals die within two to three months of "extremely fatty infiltration of the liver," they report.

This fatty change may be corrected and life prolonged, they state, by the oral administration of this new hormone.

*June 7, 1937*

# Insanity Treated by Electric Shock

Physicians at the New York State Psychiatric Institute and Hospital of the Columbia-Presbyterian Medical Center are experimenting with a new method, introduced in Italy, of treating certain types of mental disorders by sending an electric shock through the brain, Dr. S. Eugene Barrera, principal research psychiatrist at the institute, reported yesterday.

Although Dr. Barrera emphasized that hope for any "miracle cure" must not be pinned on the new method, as the experiments have been in progress only a few months and findings are inconclusive, it was reported that "considerable success" had resulted in treatment of certain types of insanity.

Primarily, the treatment, if experiments prove it sound, is intended to produce the same results by an electric shock as are being obtained through injections of metrazol, a chemical that produces convulsions with beneficial effects in certain cases of insanity.

## Insulin Also Used

Insulin and camphor also are used by some physicians to produce therapeutic "shock" in treatment of some types of insanity, but the new electric method, it was explained, so far has been used in the treatment of "certain selected mental disease for which metrazol has been beneficial." It is hoped that experiments will prove the electric method to be safer, less disagreeable to the patient and less expensive for mass use in public clinics.

The electric shock is produced by a small portable electric box which was invented in Italy by Professor Ugo Cerletti of the Rome University Clinic. Dr. Lothar Kalinowsky, a Berlin scientist, now associated with the New York State Psychiatric Institute here, worked with Professor Cerletti and obtained his permission to introduce the treatment in other world centers. He used it in Paris and London and then brought it here, where he and Dr. Barrera have been using the machine at the institute.

As far as is known these are the first experiments with electric shock for insanity to be made at a public institution in New York, although physicians expressed the belief that some private psychiatrists might be interested in the method. Similar experiments also are said to be in progress at Johns Hopkins Hospital in Baltimore.

Although physicians were reluctant to earmark the new treatment as particularly beneficial for any specific type of insanity, it was said that it had been used successfully in treatment of schizophrenia, the "split-personality" type of mental disease.

## Electrodes Attached to Head

Attached to the electric box is an instrument resembling a large pair of calipers or forceps, to which electrodes are connected. This device is clamped to the patient's head above the ears. The patient is tested for electric resistance to determine how much voltage may be used. Then the current is turned on for one-tenth of a second, sending 70 to 100 volts—rarely more—through the brain.

The patient immediately becomes unconscious, and the shock produces a convulsion somewhat resembling a mild epileptic fit. Upon recovering consciousness within a few minutes, the patient is unable to remember what has happened from the time the treatment was administered.

The treatment is repeated three times a week until definite results are noted.

Adherents of the electric-shock method contend that metrazol sometimes is an uncertain treatment, and that the process of injection of the chemical into the veins has disagreeable features that sometimes instill fear in the patient. The electric treatment, they say, at least is not unpleasant, so the patient may be more inclined to cooperate with the physician in future treatments.

Statistics were not available on the number of patients treated and the results of the experiments here. A full report will be made through medical channels when the experiment is more advanced. However, it was said that "several hundred" cases wherein the electric-shock method has been used successfully have been reported in European centers.

*July 6, 1940*

# Pioneer Sees Peril in Brain Operation

By LUCY FREEMAN

D r. Walter Freeman, the neurologist who introduced brain surgery for the mentally ill to this country, announced today that he was giving up the very serious brain operations known as pre-frontal lobotomy and topectomy because of the complications that resulted from them, primarily epileptic seizures.

He will use these operations, he said, only on very disturbed children of the type who have to be "caged" to prevent them from destroying themselves.

He will continue, however, the brain operation known as the transorbital or "icepick" operation. This is a comparatively simple operation that severs fibers between the thalamus and the frontal lobes of the brain by means of inserting an icepick-like instrument through the eyelid and into the brain.

Dr. Freeman announced this in an interview at the American Psychiatric Association's one hundred and sixth annual convention, where he presented a paper tonight on "Psychosurgery."

## Operation Less Effective

Dr. Paul Hoch of New York City, who discussed Dr. Freeman's paper at the meeting, declared in an interview that from his own experience and from observation of the work of others, the transorbital operation was, statistically speaking, "less effective" than the other operations.

"Because of the minimal danger and relative safety to the patient, we feel that the transorbital would be the ideal procedure, psychiatrically speaking, but unfortunately, in our hands, it has not proved as successful as in Dr. Freeman's, even though we tried painstakingly to follow his technique," declared Dr. Hoch. He is in charge of the Department of Psychiatric Research at the New York State Psychiatric Institute and is Assistant Professor of Psychiatry at Columbia University.

"After the initial improvement many of our patients relapsed but have benefited later by more extensive operations," he said.

He urged further experimentation with more extensive frontal cuts in transorbital lobotomies, predicting that the results "will probably approximate the results obtained in the more serious lobotomies."

## "Cure" Questioned

Dr. Hoch said that in deteriorated patients, operations do not produce a "cure" but are only palliative. In non-deteriorated or chronic, neurotic patients who fail in all other treatments, the operation may produce "very good results which approximate a cure," he said.

Brain surgery should not be performed on patients in the early stages of schizophrenia when other treatments might work, but the operation should not be delayed too long or else the results will not be as successful, he said.

Dr. Freeman, who is Professor of Neurology at Georgetown University, in citing complications that occurred after the deeper operations, mentioned personality changes in the patients resulting in inertia, rudeness and inconsiderate and insensitive behavior, loss of control of the bladder and epilepsy.

Epileptic seizures occurred in 20 per cent of the cases that underwent the operations, he said. Breaking this down into the specific operations, he said that 47 per cent of the patients who had two brain operations followed by a lot of electro-shock therapy suffered the seizures; 15 per cent, following one operation and electro-shock treatment in quantity; 7 per cent following a single, simple operation without shock therapy, and one-half of 1 per cent following the transorbital operation.

"These epileptic convulsions are not disabling in themselves but they are embarrassing to the patient," he said.

Governor Luther W. Youngdahl of Minnesota, addressing the evening session of the association, declared that the care of the mentally ill should not be "a political issue."

*May 5, 1950*

# Child Psychiatry Found Advancing

By EMMA HARRISON

D r. Leo Kanner, one of the founders of child psychiatry in the United States, paused here last week to pick up an award and to talk briefly about progress in childhood mental illness.

Dr. Kanner, who founded the Johns Hopkins Children's Psychiatric Clinic, was optimistic, but wary of saying that any one of the present areas of research would bring the answer.

The most important thing to date, he said, is that many childhood disorders are being differentiated, where they were once generalized.

As an example he cited the disorder he first described: infantile autism.

Dr. Kanner termed the disorder an "innate inability of certain children to relate to other people."

At the time, he recalled, he was attacked for his theory. In those days, he said, it was always "cherchez la mère" when anything was wrong with the child.

## Term Discussed

Dr. Kanner, who was cited last week by the National Association for Mentally Ill Children, said he was almost sorry that he had invented the term "autistic," which he believes is characterized by two phenomena. They are an "extreme aloneness," not "withdrawal" as the symptom is often termed; and a desire to preserve the "sameness" of that condition.

"We are repeating things in all fields," said the 66-year-old emeritus professor at Johns Hopkins, who is this year visiting professor at the University of Minnesota.

"At first it was feeble-minded is feeble-minded, is feeble-minded, Gertrude Stein style," he said. Then gradually, he said mental deficiency was subdivided into groups and degrees. The same happened to the term "insanity" and the same is happening in childhood mental disorders, he explained.

"We are still struggling for a sufficient differentiation," he said.

The man who published the document "In Defense of Mothers" believes that childhood mental disorders are not caused by single factors. They are not all attitudinally, biochemically or genetically determined; hence, he believes, all factors must be minutely explored.

Dr. Kanner thinks it splendid progress that although scientists do not know the answers, they have reached the point where they can ask questions. And he cited the evidence of what has been done for many, including the autistic child.

A follow-up study of the first group of eleven children observed and treated at Johns Hopkins Hospital has shown positive results.

"With these extremely detached children you must give them the chance to relate to a limited number of people and to come into the world—to thaw out," he said. They do not always turn out to be the so-called "normal" people, he continued, and some never emerge, but when they do, it is particularly gratifying.

*May 22, 1960*

# New Antidepressant Is Acclaimed but Not Perfect

By NATALIE ANGIER

Buoyed by broad medical acclaim and exuberant patient testimonials since its debut less than three years ago, the drug Prozac has become the most widely prescribed antidepressant in the United States.

But while many doctors and therapists hail the new pill as an excellent and relatively safe treatment for severe depression, a growing number caution that its full spectrum of side effects is only now becoming clear.

Most experts concur that Prozac, the brand name for fluoxetine, is one of the best antidepressant drugs ever designed. It causes fewer adverse effects than the older generation of antidepressants, which means that physicians who might once have hesitated to treat their depressed patients with medications feel more confident about giving Prozac a try.

## Can Threaten Lives

Among the symptoms of clinical depression are dramatic changes in weight, sleep patterns, a prolonged period in which a person feels hopeless, racked with guilt and immune to stimulation by the outside world. Doctors say that when left untreated, depression can jeopardize marriages, careers and lives and that often the best remedies are antidepressants like Prozac.

Many people who failed to improve while on other antidepressants, or were unable to weather the side effects, have found in Prozac genuine relief. "Prozac helps a group of patients that wasn't able to be helped before," said Dr. Brian Doyle, a psychiatrist at Georgetown University in Washington. "I've seen patients respond to Prozac who never responded to antidepressants before. It's a very good and a very effective drug."

Prozac also looks as though it holds promise for treating bulimia, obsessive-compulsive disorders and other mental ailments that once seemed almost immune to intervention.

Nevertheless, experts say they are starting to see an increasing number of patients on Prozac who suffer from intense agitation, tremors and even mania or an apparently medication-induced preoccupation with suicide. Some researchers believe that the incidence of such side effects, in varying degrees, may be as high as 15 percent.

## Effects Can Wear Off

Experts say that instances of adverse reactions to Prozac did arise in clinical trials, but that the more extreme problems seemed to be confined to those patients who were the most profoundly disturbed, or who had failed to improve while on other antidepressants. Doctors now fear that as the use of Prozac soars, they will be seeing ever more people afflicted by severe hyperactivity, restlessness and mania.

Other doctors report that in some cases, the effectiveness of Prozac appears to wear off after a few weeks or months, and they find this disappointing and surprising.

"We're just beginning to hear anecdotal reports that Prozac may stop working after initially giving patients a boost out of their depression," said Dr. Husseini Manji, a researcher at the National Institute of Mental Health in Bethesda, Md.

A number of physicians and therapists also worry that the extraordinary popularity and visibility of the medication could spur people who suffer from milder forms of depression and anxiety to seek treatment with Prozac unnecessarily.

## Not for Everyone

"Some people are touting it as though it's a miracle cure for all problems, as though the key to happiness could be found in a pill," said Ellen McGrath, a clinical psychologist who heads the American Psychological Association's National Task Force on Women and Depression. "Prozac is a very good drug, but it must be kept in mind that it's a serious drug with serious side effects for a minority of people."

Dr. Martin Teicher, a psychiatrist at McLean Hospital in Belmont, Mass., said Prozac was "a selective, powerful drug" and the repercussions of using it were not completely understood. "Clinical research shows that Prozac is very sound, but it's still like diving off into the unknown without a good compass," he said. Because Prozac remains in the body for five to six weeks, he added, any negative effects that may arise will remain for some time.

Since receiving approval from the Food and Drug Administration in 1987, Prozac has been a spectacular success story, its use now far outstripping any of the other 20 or so antidepressants commonly prescribed. According to Pharmaceutical Data Services, doctors wrote or refilled about six million Prozac prescriptions last year, about double the number for Pamelor, the next most widely used antidepressant. The success is particularly impressive in light of Prozac's price: at about $1.50 per pill, it is several times as expensive as other antidepressants.

## Good Marketing Campaign

Doctors attribute part of Prozac's popularity to an exceptionally strong marketing campaign by Eli Lilly, the manufacturer. But they also say the drug is easier and safer to take than other antidepressants. They believe that for many of the estimated 15 million Americans who suffer from clinical depression during any given year, Prozac can be a revolutionary drug.

The traditional antidepressants, many of which were first introduced in the 1950s, can cause a constellation of unpleasant side effects, including dizziness, blurred vision, constipation, extreme dryness of mouth, sluggishness and a weight gain of as much as 15 percent. More seriously, some of the older drugs can on rare occasions provoke dangerously high blood pressure and can be lethal in overdose. About one in four people is unable to tolerate the side effects. For the remainder, however, traditional antidepressants help relieve the symptoms of depression 60 to 80 percent of the time.

Prozac's success rate in curing depression rivals that of the older drugs, but its common side effects are less severe—usually nothing more taxing than nausea and nervousness—and they often subside after the initial adjustment period of two or three weeks. In contrast to other antidepressants, Prozac can prompt a modest weight loss of three to five pounds, although the weight often returns over time.

## How It Works

The precise details remain cloudy, but much of the reason for Prozac's relative benignity is thought to lie in its novel biochemical nature. All antidepressants work by restoring the balance of neurotransmitter activity in the brain, correcting an abnormal excess or inhibition of the electrochemical signals that control mood, thoughts, appetite, pain and other sensations.

The traditional antidepressants fall into two chemical classes, known as the tricyclics and the monoamine oxidase inhibitors (MAOI's). Tricyclics are believed to affect two neurotransmitter pathways in the brain—those of serotonin and norepinephrine, a chemical cousin of adrenaline. The MAOI's are thought to

369

be more complicated still, acting on serotonin, norepinephrine and yet another neurotransmitter, dopamine. Each drug affects different steps in the neurotransmitter pathways, but their generally widespread and diverse impact on the brain partly explains why the older antidepressants spawn so many side effects.

By comparison, Prozac is the first of a new class of drugs known as serotonin reuptake inhibitors. It is believed to zero in on serotonin, blocking the removal of the important signal from the neurochemical loop in the brain and thus allowing serotonin to remain operative on neurons for a longer time. That blockage seems to restore overall serotonin activity to a more normal state, which somehow helps alleviate many cases of depression. Doctors suspect that it is because Prozac is more streamlined and specific than other antidepressants—at least initially—that its adverse effects are fewer.

However, some researchers believe that Prozac's specificity can occasionally backfire. Dr. Teicher recently reported six cases of patients who became dangerously obsessed with suicide after taking Prozac, and he has heard of five other cases.

He believes the profound influence of Prozac on serotonin may be a factor. "We're only starting to understand the role that serotonin plays in depression, aggression and suicide," he said. "It's possible that by prolonging the effect of serotonin in patients who are especially sensitive to it, you can tip the balance in the wrong direction, toward violence and aggression."

## Extreme Agitation Seen

Dr. Teicher also theorizes that Prozac's ability to foster hyper-serotonin activity in the brain may explain those cases of patients who flipped from being depressed to being manic, and others who became so agitated "that they wanted to crawl out of their skins," said Dr. Teicher.

Nor does the impact of Prozac on the brain necessarily remain specific. In studying mice, Dr. Ross Baldessarini of Massachusetts General Hospital has found that, by working so powerfully on serotonin, Prozac eventually begins to affect dopamine pathways as well. That secondary effect may explain why some users of the drug develop tremors and shakes not unlike those found in Parkinson's disease patients, who suffer from a lack of dopamine.

Despite the rare adverse effects, doctors say Prozac remains one of the best antidepressants available. They say depression must be carefully diagnosed by a trained physician, who is able to detect the clear signs of a biologically based illness.

But doctors warn that for those cases in which the apparent depression is transient, caused not by biochemical imbalances in the brain but by the usual vagaries of life, neither Prozac nor any other antidepressant will bring on happiness.

"Prozac is not like alcohol or valium," said Dr. Francis Mondimore, assistant medical director at Carolinas Medical Center in Charlotte, N.C. "It's like antibiotics. If you take penicillin but you don't have pneumonia, it won't do anything for you."

*March 29, 1990*

# Lifting the Veils of Autism, One by One by One

By ERICA GOODE

He is blond and 3 years old, 33 pounds of compressed energy wrapped in OshKosh overalls.

In an evaluation room at Yale's Child Study Center, he ignores Big Bird, pauses to watch the bubbles that a social worker blows through a wand, jumps up and down. But it is the two-way mirror that fascinates him, drawing him back to stare into the glass, to touch it, to lick it with his tongue.

At 17 months, after several ear infections and a bout of the flu, the toddler's budding language skills began to deteriorate, his parents tell the evaluators. In the playroom, he seems intent on his own activities and largely oblivious to the adults in the room. Only when the therapist bends down to tickle him does he give a blinding smile and meet her gaze with startling blue eyes.

Sixty years after it was first identified, autism remains one of the most puzzling of childhood disorders. Its cause or causes are still unknown. But in recent years, investigators have begun to dislodge some of its secrets.

Studies have offered clues to the brain mechanisms that may lie behind some features of autism—the tendency to focus on objects rather than human faces, for example—and geneticists have begun to home in on genes that may be involved. Scanning has provided glimpses of ways autism may affect brain development: the brains of autistic children, studies find, appear to be larger than normal for some time after birth.

In the future, experts say, such research may yield effective medical treatments to augment or even replace the intensive behavioral therapy that is the prescription most autistic children now receive.

In learning more about autism, a disorder that in some form affects at least 425,000 Americans under 18, scientists may also increase knowledge about language development, emotion, even friendship and love.

"Ultimately, research on autism may teach us a lot about what it means to be social," said Dr. Thomas Insel, the director of the National Institute of Mental Health.

Autistic children were once thought to have a form of childhood schizophrenia. Prone to repetitive, sometimes self-destructive behaviors and driven by "a powerful desire for aloneness and sameness," as Dr. Leo Kanner of Johns Hopkins put it in a now classic 1943 paper, they often spent their lives in institutions. Parents watched helplessly as their children disappeared into a world beyond their reach.

But much has changed. The notion that autism was caused by "refrigerator" mothers and absent fathers, promoted by psychoanalysts in the 1950s and 1960s, has yielded to the realization that the disorder is strongly rooted in genetics and abnormalities of brain development and function. Environmental influences early in life may also play a role.

At the same time, a sharp rise over the last decade in the number of autism cases diagnosed in the United States and other countries has raised public awareness and helped secure more government financing for research.

In the 2003 fiscal year, the National Institutes of Health spent an estimated $81.3 million on autism research, compared with $9.6 million in 1993.

The last two decades have brought a sea change in the way scientists view autism and those who suffer from it.

Researchers now recognize, for example, that autism is not synonymous with mental retardation: more than 80 percent of children with autism were once thought to be mentally retarded.

More recent estimates place the number at 70 percent, or lower if related disorders are included.

Dr. Kanner believed autism to be a product of upper-middle-class homes, a conclusion based on the children he examined, who were the progeny of doctors, lawyers and scientists. But it is now clear that autism crosses class boundaries.

Boys are four times as likely as girls to have the disorder. This sex ratio has led one researcher, Dr. Simon Baron-Cohen, director of the autism research center at Cambridge University in England, to speculate that autism is a form of "extreme maleness," but the theory has yet to be supported by research.

More rigorous studies have allowed clinicians to identify autism in children of younger and younger ages. In the past, the disorder often was not diagnosed until children were 4 or 5. But by studying home movies of birthday parties or first baths, investigators have found telltale signs of autism in children of 12 months or younger.

Dr. Geraldine Dawson, director of the University of Washington's autism center, for example, studied infants from 8 to 10 months old who were later identified as autistic. The infants, she said, often failed to respond when parents called their names.

"Even very young babies, when you call their name, will turn and look at you," Dr. Dawson said.

As toddlers, autistic children show other differences. For example, they make eye contact less frequently, and, unlike most 1-year-olds, do not point at objects or people.

Autism's hallmarks are a delay in language development, an inability to relate to other people and stereotyped or rigid behavior. But researchers have found that children vary greatly in the nature and the severity of their disabilities.

"If you put 100 people with autism in a room, the first thing that would strike you is how different they are," said Dr. Fred Volkmar, a professor of child psychiatry at Yale and an expert on autism. "The next thing that would strike you is the similarity."

Some children attend regular schools; others are so disabled they require institutional care. Some children speak fluently; others are mute. Some are completely withdrawn; others successfully navigate a path through the outer world.

In fact, studies show that many children with autism can improve with treatment, and some—from 15 to 20 percent, experts say—recover completely, holding jobs and living independent lives.

Yet the realization that autism takes many forms has also made its diagnosis more complicated. In 1994, psychiatrists added a new diagnostic category—Asperger's syndrome—to the psychiatric nomenclature, to take account of children who displayed some features of autism but did not meet the full diagnostic criteria.

Many researchers view Asperger's as distinct from autism. But the differences become blurred in cases where children have normal or above normal I.Q.'s. In such instances, experts say, whether Asperger's or autism is diagnosed is often arbitrary.

"I don't think anyone's got good evidence for a clear distinction between people with high-functioning autism and Asperger's," said Dr. Tony Charman, a researcher in neurodevelopmental disorders at University College London.

## The Disconnect: Calculations, Yes; Eye Contact, No

As a child, Donald Jensen lay in bed at night, tracing numbers in the air with his finger. He memorized lottery numbers. He was riveted by the pages of the calendar.

Now 19, his facility with mathematical calculation seems magical. Given any date—Jan. 7, 1988, for example—he can, in an instant, identify the day of the week it fell on. (It was a Thursday.) He virtually never makes mistakes.

Yet even in childhood, there were signs that Donald was exceptional in other ways. He was mesmerized by the washing machine, becoming upset if the laundry was finished before he got up in the morning. He started talking late. Once, when his grandmother slipped on some ice in the yard and fell, he continued to chatter about numbers, seemingly oblivious to her plight.

Problems in school led doctors to diagnose autism when Donald was 6, his uncle, Glen Jensen, said. As an adult, Donald's gifts—he is among the 1 to 10 percent of people with autism known as autistic savants—connect him to the world. "What day were you born?" he asks visitors.

But the things that Donald cannot do also separate him from other people. He rarely makes eye contact. Ask him how he calculates dates or what numbers mean to him and the inquiries are met with silence. His ability to empathize with other people has grown over the years—"John was angry today, and that was upsetting to me," he will say—but unexpected events disturb him, and his conversations sometimes take the form of asking questions over and over.

What lies at autism's core? Over the decades, researchers have come up with a variety of theories. But most were based on what clinicians observed, not on what might be going on in the brain. Only recently have sophisticated technologies allowed researchers to begin bridging the gap between the consulting room and the laboratory.

Dr. Ami Klin, an associate professor of child psychology and psychiatry at Yale, and his colleagues began with the observation that people with autism often have a great deal of intellectual knowledge, but lack "street smarts," and are unable to use what they know in social situations.

"Many of our clients know the currencies of all countries in the world, but they cannot go to McDonald's and buy a burger and count the change," Dr. Klin said. "They know all the bus ramps, but can't take a bus."

In a series of experiments to find out why it is so difficult for someone with autism to function in the world, the Yale team, including Warren Jones, a research associate, developed a device for tracking eye movements that could be mounted on the brim of a baseball cap. Then they had subjects, who either had autism or did not, watch a video clip from the 1967 film *Who's Afraid of Virginia Woolf?* and monitored their gaze.

The normal subjects closely tracked the social interactions among the actors in the films, focusing especially on the actors' eyes. In contrast, people with autism focused on objects in the room, on various parts of the actors' bodies and on the actors' mouths.

In one scene, Richard Burton and Elizabeth Taylor kiss. The subjects without autism looked at the actors' embrace; the autistic subjects' eyes went elsewhere: one man stared at a doorknob in the background.

Such research suggests that from birth, the brains of autistic children are wired differently, shaping their perception of the world and other people. "In normal development," he said, "being looked at, being in the presence of another, seeking another—most of what people consider important emerges from this mutually reinforcing choreography between child and adult."

If this duet cannot take place, Dr. Klin said, "development is going to be derailed."

Studies using brain scanning techniques like fast M.R.I. lend weight to the idea that for people with autism, perception molds behavior.

"There is a deep relationship between what we see and what we know," said Dr. Robert Schultz, an associate professor at Yale's Child Study Center.

Researchers have long known, for example, that people with autism have difficulty recognizing faces. In non-autistic subjects, a brain area called the fusiform gyrus is activated in response to the human face. But when pictures of unfamiliar faces are shown to children or adults with autism, studies show, the region is less active.

Dr. Schultz said that autistic people appear to identify faces the way other people identify objects, by piecing features together. While most people are better at recognizing images of faces when they are right-side up, autistic subjects identify them faster when they are upside-down.

A recent study, presented at the annual meeting of the American Association for the Advancement of Science in Seattle this month, illustrates this. Dr. Dawson, of the University of Washington, and a colleague reported that when autistic adolescents and adults were shown pictures of faces, another brain area involved with object recognition was activated, while the fusiform gyrus remained quiet. Yet when the researchers showed photos of the subjects' mothers, the fusiform brain did light up.

Work by Dr. Isabel Gauthier, an assistant professor of psychology at Vanderbilt University, suggests that, in fact, the fusiform gyrus is not programmed to react to faces per se but to things that people care about and learn to distinguish in detail.

Dr. Gauthier trained people to become experts on "greebles," a class of simply drawn imaginary beings. When the subjects became adept at telling one greeble from another, she found, the fusiform gyrus lighted up in response to pictures of the creatures. Similarly, when car experts were asked to identify different car models, the region was activated, Dr. Gauthier reported last year in the journal *Nature*.

The research suggests that children with autism can be trained to become better at face recognition—something that scientists at Yale and other universities are trying. But the seeming indifference to the human face that often accompanies autism has led the Yale researchers to propose that the fusiform gyrus may be a component of the social brain, intimately tied up with basic emotional responses like fear, anxiety and love.

In fact, some studies have found abnormalities in the amygdala, a brain region involved with emotion and social awareness. But the findings are inconclusive, and differences in autistic brains have been found in structure, including the temporal lobes and the cerebellum.

## The Physical: A Telling Find: Bigger Brains

In his early description of autism, Dr. Kanner noted that heads of the children were larger than normal. Modern researchers have confirmed this observation, finding that for some period of time during childhood, autistic children have bigger brains than their non-autistic counterparts. In 2001, Dr. Eric Courchesne, a professor of neuroscience at the University of California at San Diego, and his colleagues found that 4-year-olds with autism showed increases in the volume of the brain's gray matter, where the cell bodies of neurons are located, and white matter, which contains nerve fibers sheathed with an insulating substance called myelin.

In a 2003 study in the *Journal of the American Medical Association*, Dr. Courchesne reported that at birth, the heads of infants with autism were smaller than normal, but then showed "sudden and excessive" growth in size from 1 to 2 months and from 6 to 14 months. By adolescence, however, the children's brains were the same size as those of other children or slightly smaller.

Dr. Martha Herbert, an instructor in pediatric neurology at Harvard, has begun to zero in on precisely where this growth spurt occurs. At the annual meeting of the Society for Neuroscience in October, she reported that in autistic children, the outer zones of white matter became enlarged compared with normal brains beginning after age 6 months and continuing into the second year of life. Those outer zones, Dr. Herbert said, are insulated later in development than the areas of white matter deeper in the brain.

"It seems that something is going on that gets more intense," Dr. Herbert said.

In another study, Dr. Manuel Casanova, a professor of neurology and neuropathology at the University of Louisville, found an increase in autistic brains in the stacks of neurons known as mini-columns that extend through the layers of the neocortex. The brains of people with autism not only had more mini-columns, Dr. Casanova found, but the neurons that made up the columns were less variable in size than in normal brains.

Such findings are intriguing, but their meaning is not clear.

One possibility is that the enlargement in white matter reflects an overabundance of myelin, which could disrupt the timing of communication signals throughout the brain. But this growth in volume, Dr. Herbert said, could also represent an increase in nerve fibers, the migration of other types of cells or some type of inflammation.

Dr. Casanova, for his part, theorizes that the proliferation of mini-columns might result in a deluge of stimulation, or as he puts it, "way too much information."

"The sound of rain on a roof might seem like driving nails into a tin roof, a fluorescent light might become extremely perturbing," Dr. Casanova said.

Dr. Nancy Minshew, a professor of psychiatry and neurology at the University of Pittsburgh, argues that autism's core lies in higher brain areas, rather than in deeper structures that govern emotion.

"When I started about 20 years ago, I looked at autism and said this disorder is in the cortex of the brain," Dr. Minshew said. "It's the classical disorder of cognition."

## The Genetics: Child Rearing Not at Fault

In 1964, Bernard Rimland, a British psychologist with an autistic son, put forward the view, then controversial, that genes, not faulty child rearing, lay behind the disorder.

Most experts now agree that autism is strongly determined by heredity. Studies indicate, for example, that if parents have one child with autism, the chance that they will have a second autistic child is 2 to 6 percent—about 100 times the general risk.

Twin studies also argue for a large genetic component. Identical twins, the studies suggest, run a 60 to 85 percent chance of having autism or a similar disorder if their twins have it. For fraternal twins, the chances are 10 percent.

Two very rare forms of autism—one associated with the congenital disease known as tuberous sclerosis and the other with fragile X syndrome—are known to be caused by chromosomal defects.

But in most cases, autism is thought to have a more complex genetic origin, involving multiple genes acting together.

"The bulk of people with autism develop it because they have inherited a particular genetic predisposition," said Dr. Anthony Bailey, a professor of psychiatry at Cambridge.

Finding those genes, however, is a difficult task. The disorder is relatively uncommon, and most people with autism do not have children, making it difficult to track successive generations of a family.

To get around these obstacles, some researchers are studying families having two or more members with autism and searching for similarities in the genome that could provide the crucial link to the disorder.

Cure Autism Now, an advocacy group based in Los Angeles, has started a program to collect DNA samples from such families and use them for research.

Large-scale studies are in progress at a variety of institutions in the United States and other countries. DeCode Genetics, an Icelandic company that last year identified a gene that may contribute to schizophrenia, announced in January that it would use the Icelandic population to search for genes underlying autism and similar disorders like Asperger's.

Some researchers are also hunting for genes that may underlie specific aspects of autism.

Dr. Daniel Geschwind, director of the neurogenetics program at the University of California, Los Angeles is hoping, in a study of autistic children and their families, to find genes that contribute to the delayed development of language.

No specific gene for autism has yet been pinpointed. But promising areas have been identified on a variety of chromosomes, including the 2, 3, 7, 13, 15 and the X chromosome.

"My sense is that we are close to the tipping point in this illness," said Dr. Insel of the National Institute of Mental Health, "and that over the next couple of years we will have, not all of the genes, but many of the genes that contribute."

At the same time, the disorder is not entirely genetic, indicating that some environmental influences, either during a mother's pregnancy or in the first years of life, have roles in setting off the disorder, perhaps by changing the way genes function without actually altering DNA.

Over the years, many candidates have been proposed, including German measles during pregnancy; yeast infections; the sedative drug thalidomide; childhood vaccines; viruses; the labor-inducing drug Pitocin; and dietary, hormonal or immune system changes during pregnancy.

But so far, researchers say, solid evidence for any single factor has not emerged. Still, several research groups are trying to address the issue of environmental triggers. A study based at Columbia University, for example, will follow 100,000 pregnancies in Norway, examining a variety of environmental influences, including infections, vaccinations, mercury exposure and prenatal stresses.

Experts disagree about the importance of environmental influences. But there is a consensus that autism probably has more than one cause, its symptoms the common end point of different biological pathways.

Yet it may be some years, experts say, before scientists are able to link the findings from genetic studies and brain research with the outer signs of the perplexing world that people with autism inhabit.

When it comes to autism, said Dr. David Amaral, a professor of psychiatry at the University of California at Davis, "In many respects, we're still in the dark ages."

*February 24, 2004*

# Vaccine Cleared Again as Autism Culprit

By GARDINER HARRIS

Yet another panel of scientists has found no evidence that a popular vaccine causes autism. But despite the scientists' best efforts, their report is unlikely to have any impact on the frustrating debate about the safety of these crucial medicines.

"The M.M.R. vaccine doesn't cause autism, and the evidence is overwhelming that it doesn't," Dr. Ellen Wright Clayton, the chairwoman of the panel, assembled by the Institute of Medicine, said in an interview. She was referring to a combination against measles, mumps and rubella that has long been a focus of concern from some parents' groups.

The panel did conclude, however, that there are risks to getting the chickenpox vaccine that can arise years after vaccination. People who have had the vaccine can develop pneumonia, meningitis or hepatitis years later if the virus used in the vaccine reawakens because an unrelated health problem, like cancer, has compromised their immune systems.

The same problems are far more likely in patients who are infected naturally at some point in their lives with chickenpox, since varicella zoster, the virus that causes chickenpox, can live dormant in nerve cells for decades. Shingles, a painful eruption of skin blisters that usually affects the aged, is generally caused by this Lazarus-like ability of varicella zoster.

The government had asked the institute to review the known risks of vaccines to help guide decisions about compensation for those who claim to have been injured by vaccines. Legislation passed by Congress in 1986 largely absolved vaccine makers of the risks of being sued for vaccine injuries and forced those who suffer injury to petition the government for compensation.

The government generally restricts compensation to cases involving children who suffer injuries that scientists deem to have been plausibly caused by vaccination, including seizures, inflammation, fainting, allergic reactions and temporary joint pain. But battles have raged for years over whether to expand this list, with most of the fighting revolving around autism.

Many children injured by vaccination have an immune or metabolic problem that is simply made apparent by vaccines. "In some metabolically vulnerable children, receiving vaccines may be the largely nonspecific 'last straw' that leads these children to reveal their underlying" problems, the report stated.

For instance, recent studies have found that many of the children who suffered seizures and lifelong problems after receiving the whole-cell pertussis vaccine, which is no longer used but once routinely caused fevers in children, actually had Dravet syndrome, a severe form of epilepsy. The flood of lawsuits over the effects of the whole-cell pertussis vaccine was the reason Congress created the national vaccine injury compensation program in the first place, and children who suffered seizures after getting this vaccine have been among the most well-compensated.

In retrospect, the whole-cell pertussis vaccine may have played little role in the underlying illness in many of these children other than to serve as its first trigger.

The Institute of Medicine is the nation's most esteemed and authoritative adviser on issues of health and medicine, and its reports can transform medical thinking around the world. The government has asked the medicine institute to assess the safety of vaccines a dozen times in the past 25 years, hoping the institute's reputation would put to rest the concerns of some parents that vaccines cause a host of problems, including autism. It has not worked.

Sallie Bernard, president of SafeMinds, a group that contends there is a link between vaccines and autism, said the latest report from the Institute of Medicine excluded important research and found in many cases that not enough research had been done to answer important questions.

"I think this report says that the science is inadequate, and yet we're giving more and more vaccines to our kids, and we really don't know what their safety profile is," Ms. Bernard said. "I think that's alarming."

Dr. Clayton said: "We looked at more than a thousand peer-reviewed articles, and we didn't see many adverse effects caused by vaccines. That's pretty remarkable."

*August 25, 2011*

# The Autism Wars

### By AMY HARMON

The report by the Centers for Disease Control and Prevention that one in 88 American children have an autism spectrum disorder has stoked a debate about why the condition's prevalence continues to rise. The C.D.C. said it was possible that the increase could be entirely attributed to better detection by teachers and doctors, while holding out the possibility of unknown environmental factors.

But the report, released last month, also appears to be serving as a lightning rod for those who question the legitimacy of a diagnosis whose estimated prevalence has nearly doubled since 2007.

As one person commenting on *The New York Times*'s online article about it put it, parents "want an 'out' for why little Johnny is a little hard to control." Or, as another skeptic posted on a different Web site, "Just like how all of a sudden everyone had A.D.H.D. in the '90s, now everyone has autism."

The diagnosis criteria for autism spectrum disorders were broadened in the 1990s to encompass not just the most severely affected children, who might be intellectually disabled, nonverbal or prone to self-injury, but those with widely varying symptoms and intellectual abilities who shared a fundamental difficulty with social interaction. As a result, the makeup of the autism population has shifted: only about a third of those identified by the C.D.C. as autistic last month had an intellectual disability, compared with about half a decade ago.

Thomas Frazier, director of research at the Cleveland Clinic Center for Autism, has argued for diagnostic criteria that would continue to include individuals whose impairments might be considered milder. "Our world is such a social world," he said. "I don't care if you have a 150 I.Q., if you have a social problem, that's a real problem. You're going to have problems getting along with your boss, with your spouse, with friends."

But whether the diagnosis is now too broad is a subject of dispute even among mental health professionals. The group in charge of autism criteria for the new version of the *Diagnostic and Statistical Manual of Mental Disorders* has proposed changes that would exclude some who currently qualify, reducing the combination of behavioral traits through which the diagnosis can be reached from a mind-boggling 2,027 to 11, according to one estimate.

Biology, so far, does not hold the answers: there is no blood test or brain scan to diagnose autism. The condition has a large genetic component, and has been linked to new mutations that distinguish affected individuals even from their parents. But thousands of different combinations of gene variants could contribute to the atypical brain development believed to be at the root of the condition, and the process of cataloging them and understanding their function has just begun.

"When you think about that one in 88, those 'ones' are all so different," said Brett Abrahams, an autism researcher at Albert Einstein College of Medicine. "Two people can have the same mutation and be affected very differently in terms of severity. So it's not clear how to define these subsets."

Some parents bristle at the notion that their child's autism diagnosis is a reflection of the culture's tendency to pathologize natural variations in human behavior. Difficulty in reading facial expressions, or knowing when to stop talking, or how to regulate emotions or adapt to changes in routine, while less visible than more classic autism symptoms, can nonetheless be profoundly impairing, they argue. Children with what is sometimes called "high functioning" autism or Asperger's syndrome, for instance, are more likely to be bullied than those who are more visibly affected, a recent study found—precisely because they almost, but don't quite, fit in.

In a blog entry, Christa Dahlstrom wrote of the "eye-rolling response" she often gets when mentioning her son's autism by way of explaining his seeming rudeness: "The optimist in me wants to hear this as supportive (Let's not pathologize differences!) but the paranoid, parent-on-the-defensive in me hears it as dismissive."

There are, Ms. Dahlstrom acknowledges, parents of children with autism whose challenges are far greater. And perhaps it stands to reason that at a time when government-financed services for such children are stretched thin, the question of who qualifies as autistic is growing more pointed. "'You don't get it; your kid is actually toilet trained,'" another mother told her once, Ms. Dahlstrom recalled. "And of course she was right. That was the end of the conversation."

But Zoe Gross, 21, whose autism spectrum disorder was diagnosed at age 4, says masking it can take a steep toll. She has an elaborate flow chart to help herself leave her room in the morning ("Do you need a shower? If yes, do you have time for a shower?"). Already, she had to take a term off from Vassar, and without her diagnosis, she says, she would not be able to get the accommodations she needs to succeed when she goes back.

According to the C.D.C., what critics condemn as over-diagnosis is most likely the opposite. Twenty percent of the 8-year-olds the agency's reviewers identified as having the traits of autism by reviewing their school and medical records had not received an actual diagnosis. The sharpest increases appeared among Hispanic and black children, who historically have been less likely to receive an autism diagnosis. In South Korea, a recent study found a prevalence rate of one in 38 children, and a study in England found autism at roughly the same rate—1 percent—in adults as in children, implying that the condition had gone unidentified previously, rather than an actual increase in its incidence.

Those numbers are, of course, dependent on the definition of autism—and the view of a diagnosis as desirable. For John Elder Robison, whose memoir *Look Me in the Eye* describes his diagnosis in middle age, the realization that his social awkwardness was related to his brain wiring rather than a character flaw proved liberating. "There's a whole generation of people who grew up lonelier and more isolated and less able to function than they might have been if we had taken steps to integrate them into society," he said.

Yet even some parents who find the construct of autism useful in understanding and helping children others might call quirky say that in an ideal world, autism as a mental health diagnosis would not be necessary.

"The term has become so diffuse in the public mind that people start to see it as a fad," said Emily Willingham, who is a co-editor of *Thinking Person's Guide to Autism*. "If we could identify individual needs based on specific gaps, instead of considering autism itself as a disorder, that would be preferable. We all have our gaps that need work."

*April 7, 2012*

CHAPTER 17

# Public Health

# How We Poison Our Children

There is some prospect that the most disgraceful nuisance of the metropolis is about to be abated. The "Swill Milk," as it is most appropriately denominated—that bluish, white compound of true milk, pus and dirty water, which, on standing, deposits a yellowish, brown sediment, that is manufactured in the stables attached to large distilleries by running the refuse distillery slops through the udders of dying cows and over the unwashed hands of milkers—is at last becoming intolerable to civilized society, and there is a demand for its utter abolition. Why its sale has so long been permitted is one of the marvels that we shall all ponder hereafter.

Swill Milk is no new thing in our City. Wherever there is a distillery, there is a temptation to its manufacture. The grain, after maceration, and the alcohol that is extracted from it, still contains some nourishment, and the distillers early found that it increased the secretion of milk in the cows to which it was fed. Hence, a stable for cows became a necessary part of the economical arrangements of every distillery. That under the most favorable circumstances of cleanliness, exercise and air, the swill-fed cows soon contracted disease was obvious, and the unwholesome character of their milk early attracted the attention of the Temperance Societies, who, years ago, began a crusade against the whole system, and easily convinced the world that, inasmuch as the greater part of City milk was of this origin, milk in the cities was no longer a healthful, but a most noxious diet. But some years since it became known that the distillery-stabled cows of our vicinity contracted a strange disease—that their lungs rapidly ulcerated, and that with their disease the secretion of milk increased, from which it was natural to conclude that the impurities of the animal's body passed off with the milk, and an increased mortality among the children to whom the milk was fed gave double assurance that the article which had borne from the beginning of the world a reputation for wholesomeness was in reality a deadly poison.

The New-York Academy of Medicine some years since set one of its committees to examining the facts in the case; and its report, written by Dr. A. K. Gardner, and embodying several carefully prepared analyses of the Swill Milk, both distinctly showed the connection between it as a cause and the astounding infant mortality of the city, and, by means of an extensive publication, fixed the facts in the public mind. The public opinion was still more firmly grounded by the issue of a pamphlet written by a gentleman connected with the daily Press, rehearsing the medical facts, and exposing minutely the disgusting particulars of the milk manufacture.

So well assured were the people of the poisonous effects of the milk that it has long been told as a curiosity that one wealthy distiller of Brooklyn dissented from the catholic faith, and did not hesitate to admit the milk made in his own establishment to his own table!

It was hardly to be expected that the people of New-York, whose toleration of slipped veal, high beef and strychnined whisky is notorious the world over, would dream of interfering with any traffic in which men were engaged of large property, and who could command numerous votes. But the Brooklyn folks, in the borders of whose pleasant city several of the largest of these distillery stables are located, have felt impelled by all motives of economy, interest and decency to make strenuous war upon them for some years back. The unprecedented expansion of the city, encouraged by its lace work of railroads, has brought some of its most desirable suburbs into close and most annoying proximity to the nuisances, and an ordinance was passed which it was hoped, without doing unjust violence to any large interest, would gradually drive the stables out and abolish the business. Husted's establishment on Skillman Street, in the Seventh Ward, was perhaps the largest, the nastiest, the most offensive in every respect to the neighborhood it cursed, and the fountain of a wider spread mortality than any in the City. Besides the deaths it effected among the children of both cities—for the milk-carts it sent forth daily perambulated almost every street in New-York, and to which the community were easily reconciled (inasmuch as slaughtering innocents is always in Christian cities a very venial offence)—it offended the nostrils of every passer by, and sadly depreciated property in the vicinity. The liquid manure that was sent out in carts to the farmers from the establishment made the cleanest streets filthy and noisome, but far the larger portion of it was emptied by drains upon the Wallabout flats, which, in hot Summer days, gave out a horrible stench, that when the wind was westerly was wafted over Williamsburg, causing—we speak from personal observation—vomiting in many persons half a mile away from the Wallabout shore, and full a mile and a half from the distillery. No dozen other nuisances about which the Brooklyn indignation has been exercised, from time to time, ever amounted to a tithe of the offence of this one. But Mr. Husted was a man of wealth, character and influence, and his cows, whose number, from year to year, was rapidly increasing, all had votes. In this juncture—it was early last Summer—a kind Providence interposed to save life and stop the depreciation of property. By an accident, for which good men thanked God, his stables were burned down—and, according to the City ordinance, they could not be rebuilt. The Board of Aldermen, however, with a promptness which showed their appreciation of the strongest arguments of wealthy men—we never heard the Aldermanic intelligence insulted by the suggestion of any other motive—voted to waive the ordinance and permit the rebuilding of the stables on a larger scale than before. The Board of Health soon after pronounced them (the stables, not the Aldermen) a nuisance, but there was not back-bone enough left at the City Hall to abate it. It was hoped, at the late election in April, when to give citizens just the opportunity they professed to agonize after, the general and local elections were divorced, that citizens would recognize the issue that the Swill Milk men fairly opened, and make the cheap sacrifice of half an hour in the morning and a vote, for the salvation of their little ones. But their office business was pressing, and so except in the Nineteenth Ward, where Alderman Scholes, who had done more towards breaking up the nuisance than any dozen other men in the City, was triumphantly reelected, the City was again handed over to the filthy hands of the Swill people. In the Seventh Ward, the successful candidate for Alderman was a man who had been for years engaged as Swill Superintendent in Husted's establishment.

Thus unpromisingly matters stood, when Frank Leslie found left at his door as milk a disgusting dose of milk and pus, which fairly threw his illustrated paper into an emetic convulsion. Bound to know the worst of the horrible story, he ana-lyzed the specimen, and then dispatched his corps of reporters and artists to the head-quarters of the poison, and in two last numbers he has reproduced pictures that are true to the life, and so shocking that the very word *milk*, or the sight of the dainties into which it enters as an important component, turns the stomach. The whole town suffers nausea. Hundreds of families have turned the milkmen from the door, and until they can have time to reconnoitre and study out by Frank Leslie's lists of Swill Milk carts, and routes, and places served, whether the wagon that stops at their door boldly marked "Orange County Milk," "Westchester," or "Long Island" is milk or poison, forswear the article altogether.

So bold and thorough an attempt on the part of a widely circulated journal to arrest attention to an outrage that has lain patent to every thinking person for years could not fail of wholesome results. Mayor Tiemann has resolved to do his duty, and yesterday several drivers of milk wagons were arrested by his order and fined, under the just suspicion that a milk-cart which is not numbered and named according to law is engaged in the nefarious business. Unfortunately our City Inspector's Department, which ought, through its abundant Health Wardens, to be cooperating with the Mayor, is a sham and an impotent humbug. It never "has power" to aid in reforming abuses, all its energies being exhausted in operating on the Albany lobby to prevent wholesome sanitary enactments, and in seizing dead hogs to supply the Barren Island superphosphate-of-lime demand. If it should conclude to help in this effort to reduce the percentage of infant mortality, let the Health Wardens seize every can of Swill Milk that they can recognize, and empty it into the gutter. Let Grand Juries indict the manufacturers and the sellers of the stuff; let the Boards of Health declare it a nuisance, and with the abundant power vested in them for such purposes, abate it wherever found; for, last year, without much doubt, it fatally poisoned 8,000 infants in this City. But, seeing how like clay in the hands of the potter the public's salaried servants are apt to be, and how one wealthy distiller takes by the nose a whole Board of Health, it is obvious that with the people themselves lies the power to stop the Swill Milk trade. Every father of a family must for himself look into the milk-can and study its contents before trusting any of them on his table. If he is too busy, heaven help him when his little one wilts in Summer, however pure the air it breathes, and turning over in its agony, dies, to the consolation of a clean conscience and the assurance that the busy father did not poison his own babe. There is good milk to be had even in the City, though the Railroad Companies have a way of charging outrageous freights upon its transportation, and the innocent Orange County farmers have lately devised lactometers by which and by the aid of spring water they prevent its coming too rich and thick into market; but water, though it is a shave to charge us six cents a quart for it, is no poison, and the children's lives are probably well worth the added price of railroad tariffs.

*May 13, 1858*

# The Yellow Fever Plot

We find in the *Bermuda Advocate*, of April 26, a very full report of the examination of a confederate of Dr. Blackurn, a Mr. Swan, in the infamous conspiracy to introduce yellow fever into New-York and other Northern cities by means of infected clothing. Mr. Swan was cited before the magistrates at St. Georges, and after an examination of a large number of witnesses was committed for trial. The pressure on our columns is so great that we can give only the principal points of the testimony. The examination occupied several days.

## The Testimony

Mr. Thies, President of the Board of Health for the town of St. George, deposed substantially as follows: On the 10th instant I was informed by Charles M. Allen, United States Consul, that there was secret in the house of one Edward Swan, a resident of this town, three trunks said to contain clothing infected with yellow fever, and I was requested by Mr. Allen not to move immediately in the case and that he would convey to me additional information. On the 12th instant a meeting of the Board of Health was convened, and the circumstances of the case were made known to them by me. After considerable inquiry into the matter it was decided that two members of the said Board of Health, accompanied by the Town Inspector, should enter the premises of the said Swan, and obtain, if possible, the reported clothing; on arriving at the house of the said Swan I told him the object of our visit, and after some demur he acknowledged that he did have in his possession three trunks which answered the description given of them by me; I requested to see them, and he assented; I then told him I wished him to deliver the three trunks to me, and after some delay he agreed to do so on my promising to give him a receipt for them, and that in case the report was unfounded they would be returned to him; I asked him in presence of Mr. Fox, a member of the board, and Nathaniel Jackson, Town Inspector, of whom he obtained the package, and he said by or through one Dr. Blackburn; he also said there was certain remuneration due to him for storing and taking care of the package, and requested that I would also be responsible for the same; I then asked him if he had received any remuneration from any one, and if Mr. Blackburn had ever tendered any money or compensation to him; he said he had not; the trunks were then taken in charge by the inspector and placed in the custody of the police. On the 13th inst., an examination of the articles in the trunks was made at Nonsuch Island by the Health Officer, who can testify as to their condition, and which by his direction were destroyed. I make this complaint against the said Edward C. Swan, for harboring a nuisance, detrimental to the health of the community. The marks were as follows: On the Portmanteau, "St. Louis Hotel, Upper Town, Quebec"; another ticket on the same was "Clifton House, Niagara Falls, Canada Side." The green trunk was not quite full when I first saw it. There was no direction or address on either of the packages.

Mr. Edward C. Swan said—The three trunks were placed in my possession by the request of Dr. Blackburn, and he requested me to keep them until his return; he did not name any particular time for returning. He said in case he did not return I should receive compensation from Confederate Government officers; he said I could apply to Mr. Black, as Major Walker was not in the island at the time.

Benjamin Burland, sworn, said: I am Health Officer for the east end of these islands; on the 13th instant, I was called by the President of the Board of Health to inspect the contents of a green trunk, a leather portmanteau and a black trunk, and which I saw for the first time in the boat of the Health Officer; I proceeded to Nonsuch Island, by direction of the President of the Board of Health, with instructions that if on examining the three trunks said to contain clothing, I should be of the opinion that they contained infection, that I should have them buried; in the several trunks I found sundry articles of clothing, as follows: In the green trunk, which was open, I found shirts and guernseys, quite new and unwashed, in the top of the trunk; I directed the Inspector of Nuisances to take an inventory of the clean and unworn articles, while I made an inventory of the more suspicious articles; I next found a white blanket, nearly new, but covered with dark stains, some large, others small; they bore all the traces of having been used in a sick chamber; the stains resembled those from "black vomit," and which I have before frequently seen; the next thing was an old clothes-bag—then several guernseys, apparently new and unworn, and finally, at the bottom of the trunk, a sheet very extensively stained; some of the stains were of a dark color, others yellow, as if from mustard; there were marks on the trunk, but I did not regard them, and took no notice of them; the portmanteau was locked, and I had it broken open, and found on the top a woolen shawl, old, but free from stains; then a pair of drawers, very dirty, with yellow stains, as if from mustard; then socks, a pocket-handkerchief, coat and trowsers, all worn and dirty; next a quantity of guernseys, shirts, both flannel and cotton, all apparently new and unworn; then two pillow-slips, very much soiled, and a shirt, stained as if from port wine, and finally a sheet at the bottom, stained all over with some kind of a dark color; others lighter, also mustard stains. The black trunk was corded and locked; this I also ordered to be broken open. I found in it first shirts, both cotton and woolen, quite new; then a shirt and guernsey, stained and very dirty, then a white pocket-handkerchief, with dark-colored stains, and a few dark spots such as would the produced by black vomit; next a bandage of linen, deeply stained by mustard; then two blankets, quite free from stains, but not new blankets; next a pair of drawers and socks, much worn and dirty; and, lastly, two pillow-slips on the bottom, also stained as if from perspiration.

I considered the articles to be of a suspicious character, as many of them had been used in a sick-chamber, and I ordered them to be buried; there were addresses, I think, on all the trunks, but I took no notice of them; the green trunk was full, but it could have contained more. I noticed the lock had been broken or forced off, and that it adhered to the hasp. I considered the articles to be of a very suspicious character, particularly when I remembered the epidemic of last year; but whether they were removed from yellow fever patients or not, I cannot say. If infection existed, it must have pervaded all the articles in the trunks. I don't know where the articles came from, or yet the trunks. I certainly should have considered the articles as a nuisance in a sanitary sense to have been retained in the Town. Assuming the articles to have been taken from yellow fever patients, I consider them very prejudicial to the health of the community.

Another witness, Mr. G. P. Black, on being sworn, deposed as follows—On or about the 30th of September last, when the mail steamer was about leaving for Halifax, Dr. J. P. Blackburn told me that he had left some trunks with a man by the name of Edward C. Swan, who had been recommended to him an account of his fidelity; he asked my opinion of Swan and I told him as I had rarely seen the man, or heard anything about him, I could not give him any satisfaction as to his qualification as a faithful individual. He then told me that he had made a contract with the said Swan; that he had paid him $250 on account of it, and that the balance of the money—an additional $250—he was to pay the said Swan in the fulfillment of his contract; which was, to carry the trunks he alluded to New-York City during the present Spring—but that, as he had some doubts as to his fidelity, he might, after he arrived in Halifax, change his mind; if so, he would send me an order on Swan for the trunks, and requested me if he did so to send them to Halifax. How many trunks there were, or what were their contents I never knew or enquired. A few days after Doctor Blackburn left I stopped at Swan's as I was passing, and was shown the trunks. I have never seen them since.

Frederick Buckstaff, sworn, says: Some three or four months ago Mr. Swan told me that three or four trunks had been left in his possession by Dr. Blackburn, and frequent allusion has been made to me since both by Mr. Swan and his wife—and also by Mr. Alexander, employed in Mr. Walker's office, about them.

About a month ago Mr. Swan told me what the trunks contained, and repeated a conversation he had with Dr. Blackburn, and which was to the effect that the clothing in the trunks came from yellow fever patients, and that they were intended to be sent to New-York or Philadelphia, or it may have been to both places; he also told me that Dr. Blackburn had promised him a remuneration of $150 a month; during the time he had never received anything from either Dr. Blackburn or Maj. Walker's office; I saw a letter written by Mr. Swan to Mr. Black about the trunks, and also reminding him of the promised remuneration, and as he did not receive any answer during a space of two or three weeks, he wrote a second one threatening Mr. Black that if he did not receive an answer he would draw the remuneration from another source some two months or ten weeks since Mr. Black came to Swan's house and had an interview with Mrs. Swan in a room adjoining the one occupied by me, and without listening I heard him say that he would pay her a considerable sum of money if she could get the trunks out of the house without Mr. Swan's knowledge; I have seen Mr. Black several times at Swan's house, and Mrs. Swan has told me that he referred to the trunks several times. Mr. Swan told me that Dr. Blackburn had informed him that the intention of sending the clothing to New-York was for the destruction of the masses there. Swan told me he knew the contents of the trunks from what Dr. Blackburn had told him. He also spoke to me of his intention of going to the Magistrates about the trunks. Mr. Swan once told me that Dr. Blackburn was going to leave some five or six trunks of clothing from yellow fever patients at his house, but he afterward told me there were only three, and that Dr. Blackburn had told him he had changed his mind, that he had engaged the services of a colored man who would take the other three with him. He also told me he was afraid to expose the trunks as he had nothing but Dr. Blackburn's word about their contents and he would prefer waiting his return. Mr. Swan also expressed his suspicions that the other trunks taken by Dr. Blackburn were infected. He also said he was afraid if he exposed the trunks and the charge was not proved Dr. Blackburn might prosecute him.

Dinah Amory, sworn, said; I reside in the town of Hamilton, in Pembroke Parish; I am in the habit of nursing invalids; during the late epidemic I was engaged in that capacity; I attended some at the Hamilton Hotel, viz.: Mr. and Mrs. Crowell and a colored woman, one of the servants of the hotel. The two former suffered from yellow fever very severely, but the servant woman only had it about twenty-four hours; Dr. Rees attended Mr. and Miss Crowell, and Dr. Blackburn attended the housemaid; Dr. Blackburn boarded at the hotel. He attended her for the first time on Friday morning—I also nursed her on the Saturday following; Dr. Blackburn again visited her and said she must have more covering, and be sweated more; I requested a blanket from Miss Crowell, but she told me she did not wish any others used but those which had already been done with the fever patients; I did not think the woman required any extra clothing, as she was sweating profusely at the time; when Dr. Blackburn returned and found I had not put any extra blankets or covering over her he seemed annoyed, and told to me come to his room, and I did so; and I then helped him to lift down a trunk from which he took some guernsey coats, trousers and different things, all of them being woolen, and laid them over her and around her, as he said, to prevent the air getting to her; and he ordered me not to disturb them till he returned; he put the things on the top of the bedclothes; he took the trunk, with my assistance, into the room of the servant woman; during the night the woman was so exhausted by the sweating and the weight of the clothes, that I removed the things placed over her by Dr. Blackburn, down to her feet, and when he returned at four o'clock on Sunday morning, he scolded me for removing any of the things before he came. He then took all of the things and placed them back in his trunk. Dr. Blackburn said the woman was suffering from yellow fever which was broke in about twenty-four hours. After the doctor had repacked his trunk, I assisted him to take it back to his room; I don't know what became of it afterward; I can't say whether the articles were stained or not; but I don't think they could have been, as there were two blankets between them and the patient; she was not sick at the stomach; on Sunday night I again saw the doctor, and he told me that if I had not been so much of a doctor instead of a nurse, he would have liked for me to attend a Capt. Galloway, then sick with fever at Mrs. Slater's; Capt. Galloway died the following night; he was the pilot of the steamer *Mary Celeste*; a Mrs. Cameron nursed him; I never saw Capt. Galloway while he was sick; I don't know what doctor attended him; the trunk that I packed was not the one he took the clothes from and put over the sick woman; I don't know whether he had any more trunks; I don't remember what I packed in the top of the trunk; I don't remember a woolen shawl being in the trunk.

William Blackman, a cart-driver, deposed to carrying the trunks to Mr. Swan's house; Mr. Swan seemed to know that the trunks were coming.

Francis Cameron, sworn, said: I reside at Hamilton, and have lived there all my life; my time is principally engaged in nursing sick people; I nursed several patients with yellow fever during the epidemic of last year; I nursed one at the Hamilton Hotel and four at Mrs. Slater's; three of the cases were very bad, and two died out of the four at Mrs. Slater's; Dr. Blackburn attended one of the patients that I nursed—a Capt. Galloway, of the Confederate army, but who had lately been pilot of a steamer; he was one that died; I only attended him from eight o'clock on Sunday night, and he died at a quarter to one on Tuesday morning; Dr. Blackburn came to the house about twelve o'clock, and remained there until he died; after he was dead, Capt. Stevens—Mrs. Slater's son-in-law—asked what was to be done with the clothes; I supposed he meant the clothes he died in; and then Dr. Blackburn turned to me and said: "You go out of the room, for a little while," and I went out; Capt. Stevens immediately followed me, and gave me directions to go at once and see about his being buried; he then turned round and said: "I must go up and see what is to be done about the clothes;" when I returned, about an hour afterward, I found the dead body shrouded, but I saw nothing of the clothes that had been taken from him; I don't know what became of them; Mr. W. Stevens and Mrs. Slater deposed to substantially the same facts. Mrs. Slater said that many articles of bed-clothing which had been used about the patient were missing after his death. She suspected some of the servants of having taken them.

Joseph Headden Rainey, sworn, said: I reside at present in this town; during the epidemic of last year I was living at the Hamilton Hotel; I was bar-keeper and barber to the establishment for a portion of the time; there were several cases of yellow fever at the hotel; Dr. Rees and Dr. Tucker attended some of the patients, and Dr. Blackburn attended a woman, one of the chambermaids in the house; he was in the house about nine or ten days; after leaving the house he went to Halifax; I know he went to Halifax, because I went in the same boat with him; when he first came to the house he had one trunk, but when he left he had more; I know he had two, because I received one which he had bought at Hamilton; I don't know anything personally about Dr. Blackburn while at the hotel, but I heard some things from the nurse who attended the patient he was attending that I thought was strange; the nurse asked me if I did not think it strange, that Dr. Blackburn should put so much woolen clothing round Mary (the sick woman) and then have them all packed in his trunk with blankets, and I told her I thought it very strange; Dr. Blackburn's baggage was all sent to St. George the day before he left the hotel; I saw a portion of the baggage the next day at Mr. Swan's; it was behind the counter; I don't know whether it was all there or not; he took away one trunk from Swan's; I know he only took one, because he asked me to see after it, and I sent a dray and got it; I did not get the other portion because he instructed me only to bring one; Mr. Swan did not make any remark about the portion left behind that I remember; I saw Dr. Blackburn at Mr. Swan's the day he left for Halifax; I did not hear any conversation between Dr. Blackburn and Mr. Swan, but I saw them in conversation; I can't say that I heard any instructions given to Swan by the Doctor about the portion left behind. I am confident I heard Dr. Blackburn tell Swan to see that he attended to the shipping of the baggage left behind by the first opportunity. The reply Swan made as near as I can recollect, was "Very well, Sir."

## The Judgement

On considering the foregoing testimony, the magistrates deemed it advisable to send the case to the Attorney-General for prosecution before the Court of General Assizes or Quarter Sessions, at either of which he may see fit to indict E. C. Swan, who was remanded to the gaol in St. George, there to be kept until summoned to appear, unless he should enter into full and sufficient recognizance himself in the sum of £50, with two sureties of $25 each, for his appearance.

*May 16, 1865*

# The Code of Health—Practical Requirements of the Sanitary Law

"The Code of Health Ordinances," passed by the new Board of Health, took effect on Tuesday. In most respects it is but a re-enactment and simplification of existing City ordinances, but the latter have been so long utterly disregarded that, if now enforced, as we are assured they will be, we shall see a great change in New-York and Brooklyn. Besides being published in several of the newspapers, the Code has been printed in a pamphlet, and can be obtained at the office of the Board of Health. Among the provisions applicable to New-York and Brooklyn, we note the following:

Physicians, hotel-keepers, officers of vessels, and all other persons are required to report within twenty-four hours every case of smallpox or other contagious disease that comes to their knowledge. Persons or articles that have been exposed to any contagious disease, or persons sick with it, are not to be brought into or removed within the district without a permit from the Board. Vessels, persons and articles from Quarantine cannot be brought up or landed without a permit; nor can rags, hides, skins or similar articles from foreign ports, or ports south of Norfolk, be landed or stored without permission.

All butchers, vegetable and cattle dealers require a permit. Meat from calves less than four weeks old, from pigs less than five weeks old, and sheep less than eight weeks old is absolutely forbidden. No cattle can be driven in the built-up portions of the cities except between 9 o'clock at night and an hour after sunrise, and then not more than twenty cattle or one hundred hogs or sheep can be driven together. No meat, fish, vegetables or milk can be sold under a false name—in other words, "swill milk" cannot be represented as "Orange County." Butchers and marketmen must remove all offal and garbage every twenty-four hours, must not kill in the street or in a place exposed to view from it. Every slaughter-house must be connected with the street sewer, and after June 1 no slaughterhouse or cattle-yard can be carried on, nor can any be established after to-day, without a permit. This is preliminary to the final and proximate expulsion of all those establishments from the built-up portions of the cities. Provision is made by section 59 for the seizure of unfit articles of food. No meat, fish or vegetable dealer can occupy the street or sidewalk.

Careful provisions are made as to the removal of night-soil, garbage, offal, &c., to make it as little offensive as possible. Among other things all night-soil must be disinfected before removal, and all carts used for such purposes must be tight and proper, and of a form to be prescribed. Privies and sinks are to be constructed according to regulations. Persons building cannot occupy more than 100 square feet of the street, and that at one side.

A most important provision is contained in the 68th section, which requires that every owner, tenant, occupant and lessee of any building, or part of one, must within forty days provide "a suitable and sufficient box, barrel or tub (and several thereof if needful) for receiving and holding, without leakage and without being filled to within four inches of the top thereof, all the ashes, rubbish, garbage and liquid substances, of whatever kind, that may accumulate during thirty-six hours from any such building" or part thereof. The box, barrel or tub for ashes must be of metal; and "all ashes, rubbish, garbage and liquid substances that should be removed from such building shall be daily placed therein before nine o'clock in the forenoon," except that they may be retained and delivered to the proper carts as they pass. This provision alone, in connection with the recent law as to throwing garbage into the street, if enforced, will do a great deal to render our streets decent and to deprive the contractors of their last excuse for not keeping the streets clean.

A stop is to be put to the practice of allowing dirty water and filthy liquids to flow from yards and areas across the sidewalks. A passage under the sidewalk must be provided in all cases, and every stable must be connected with the sewer. The accumulation of manure and dirt upon any lot, dock, pier or bulkhead is forbidden. The inhabitants of the upper portion of the City will be glad to know that no swine can be kept "within the built up portions of any city, or within one thousand feet of any residence, or place of business, or street thereof," without a permit from the Board. If the Board is as chary of granting such permits as we hope they will be, pork will fall, noses will cease to be held on to, and real estate will rise. We beg the owners of the cattle-yards on Fifth Avenue to notice that no cattle, swine, sheep, geese, goats or horses can be yarded without a permit, nor can such animals be allowed to go at large. The goats of the Twelfth Ward will please take notice that their privileges are thus abated.

We trust the street-cleaning contractors will comply with the 114th section, which forbids them to sweep the dirt into heaps and leave it there more than four hours.

Some of the offensive trades seem likely to be driven out, for no establishment for tanning, or dressing hides, or carrying on any offensive or noisome trade can be opened without a permit, while the entire tribe of bone-boiling, offal-boiling, fat-boiling, bone-grinding, shell-burning and similar nuisances are specifically proscribed. The milkmen are interested in the provision that no person "shall bring or send to any city or village any unwholesome, watered or adulterated milk, or milk known as swill-milk, or milk from cows or other animals that for the most part lived in stables, or that fed on swill, garbage or other like substance." Not more than one cow to an ordinary city lot can be kept.

It is probably impossible to make our tenement and lodging houses, as now constructed, healthy, but the provisions of the Code will do much toward this desirable result. In the first place every owner and lessee of a tenement house, lodging house or factory is required to have it adequately lighted, ventilated and cleansed, and to provide adequate privies or water-closets, He must not allow it to be overcrowded, and what is meant by this is shown by the provision, "nor shall more persons than one for one thousand feet of cubic contents be allowed to sleep in any apartment of any such boarding house, tenement house or lodging-house, nor shall more than one person for every one thousand feet of cubic contents be allowed to dwell in any such last-mentioned house." In reckoning the space, halls, closets, &c. are excluded. The landlords of our cellars will please notice that no person shall "rent, let, hire out or allow to be used" for a sleeping room "any apartment which has not at least one-half of its height and space above the level of every part of the sidewalk and curbstone of any adjacent street." No tenement or lodging house can be used as a place of storage. Detailed provisions are made for the proper sanitary construction of all tenement houses hereafter built or rebuilt.

There are many provisions of general interest, besides those which are applicable only to particular classes, which we have not space to note here. The law establishing the Board of Health, after providing for a publication of the ordinances, says: "and every person, body or corporation that shall violate, or not conform to any ordinance, rule, sanitary regulation or special or general order of said Board, duly made, shall be liable to pay a penalty not exceeding fifty dollars for each offence, which may be sued for and recovered by and in the name of said Board." The law gives a concurrent criminal remedy, and, also, in certain cases, increases the penalty to two hundred and fifty dollars.

*May 20, 1866*

# Facts About the Cholera

No other disease known to the medical world has been the subject of such deep and exhaustive study during the past twenty-five years as cholera. Koch spent nearly ten years in constant search after the source and action of the disease, and the best minds of the medical world have grappled with the subject. But out of all this study and research very little absolute knowledge has come. Improved methods of treatment simply have resulted. They know, among other things, that cholera is produced by a germ. Koch discovered this, and the knowledge has materially aided in making up a course of treatment. But the great stumbling block in the way of perfect treatment is the ignorance regarding the character and nature of this germ. For several years Koch studied the disease at its root in India, enjoying the co-operation of the Government and a special staff of highly qualified experts. He made post-mortem examinations on hundreds of victims, often performing these operations within a few moments after death ensued. When he announced, therefore, that he had found the bacillus, every scientist supposed that the greatest fight against the terrible pest had at last been won. By cultivating the germs artificially in gelatine, it could readily be ascertained what condition was most favorable to their propagation, and what medicines were most effective in killing them without injury to the human system.

Koch's announcement that he had found what he considered was the true germ was hailed with delight in the medical world.

In every case where he had examined the bowels and alimentary canal of patients who had died of cholera while he remained in India, Dr. Koch found a form of bacteria that at first escaped his attention among the myriads of other bacilli that abound in the intestines. Gradually, however, he came to observe this peculiar form, and once his notice was attracted, he began to look for it closely, with the result that he found it in great numbers in every case on which he operated. The bacillus was of a peculiar curved shape and looked like a section of a circle, with just a suspicion of thickness or head at one end. From this shape he named it the "comma bacillus." In some instances he found two of the bacilli joined together, forming a shape something like the letter S.

He at once began to cultivate this germ artificially, but subsequent experiments with it were not very satisfactory. Though introducing it in every form into the organization of various animals with which he operated, he could not produce a case of genuine Asiatic cholera. After a long term of experimenting, a number of eminent scientists who opposed his theory offered to swallow any number of these bacilli.

Koch and his followers were not discouraged by these attacks, however, and a large portion of the medical world still adheres to the belief that the comma bacillus is the genuine bacteria of cholera.

One point, however, has certainly been gained by the Koch experiments. It has been shown that the treatment employed in cholera by the introduction of acids into the system is in all human probability the best that can be devised until the real bacillus is found. Acids have in every case destroyed the comma bacillus, which, if it is not the true source of cholera, is at least intimately connected with it. The acid treatment has been considerably strengthened, and the mortality of the disease has certainly been lowered. All that is positively known of the disease now has been embraced in the following propositions:

First—It is caused by the access of a specific organic poison to the alimentary canal.

Second—This poison is contained primarily in the ejections of persons afflicted with the disease.

Third—A process of incubation lasting from one to three days is required to make the poison active in a person into whose system it has entered.

Fourth—Water, decomposing animal or vegetable matter, and the alkaline contents of the alimentary canal furnish the most favorable conditions for this incubation.

The disease as observed in this country has been divided into four stages. The first stage or symptom is a painless diarrhea, lasting generally from one to five days, except in acute cases, when the disease at times attacks persons and carries them off inside of a few hours. The second symptom in the majority of cases is a nauseating sensation, followed by violent vomiting and an increase in the diarrhea. The ejections from both stomach and bowels are of a fluid character and the patient loses strength very rapidly, frequently sinking into a languor. The thirst of the afflicted person is incessant and cramps set in in the extremities, generally the fingers and toes. Abdominal pains are scarcely if at all perceptible. The voice grows husky, the skin begins to shrivel, and an intense perspiration breaks out in all parts of the body. The urine is suppressed, and the body in the region of the abdomen seems to be afire. This stage lasts generally from two to six hours, though there is a case on record where it lasted only twenty minutes.

After this comes the third stage, during which the patient either dies or, if an improvement comes, he enters on the fourth stage, or, "stage of reaction." The third stage is ushered in with a general collapse. The vomiting ceases somewhat and the diarrhea becomes involuntary. The pulse becomes more and more feeble and the heart beats are scarcely perceptible. The skin becomes livid and the lines of the face undergo a complete change. This stage lasts on an average from four to thirty-six hours, and if death ensues the patient generally loses consciousness just before dissolution. If a reaction takes place, the vomiting and cramping cease, the breathing becomes steadier, the heart begins action again, and the patient falls into a deep sleep, during which the face is restored to its original form and outline again.

Treatment, to be efficacious, must be begun at once, and it is well, in times when cholera is suspected, to have a remedy at hand which can be used even before the arrival of a physician, who should be immediately summoned in all cases that look at all like cholera. Opium and its salts are among the most beneficial remedial agents in the early stages of the attack. This drug may be given alone in very small and oft-repeated doses, or it may be combined with tannin, bismuth, nitrate of silver, and other astringents. The patient should be at once put to bed and kept perfectly quiet, and to satisfy the thirst beef tea, barley water, and other bland drinks should be given.

In the second stage the use of opium should be almost entirely discontinued or given in very small doses. Iced effervescing drinks will in a measure relieve the vomiting and purging, and reduce the terrible thirst. During this stage mustard plasters and heating liniments may be applied, and the body should be wrapped in flannels, and surrounded with hot-water bottles. Chloroform inhaled or chloral will aid in relieving the cramping. If under all this treatment the patient continues to sink, ammonia, brandy, and other stimulants should be applied.

The utmost care should be taken at all times to keep the sickroom clean, and all ejections should be thoroughly disinfected with carbolic acid. Only in this way can the spread of the disease be prevented. In this country it is never endemic. It must be introduced from abroad through the arrival of a person afflicted with the disease, or the germs may be carried in a dried form in the clothing or baggage, to be spread wherever these may be unpacked. It has not yet been settled how the germs enter the body and reach the alimentary canal. Some authorities assert that they are taken in through the stomach alive, while some others say that they are also taken into the body through the lungs, entering the blood and finally reaching the alimentary canal. On one thing, however, all are agreed, and that is that the germs are only given out by persons affected with the disease through the ejections from the body.

Hence, cleanliness is an almost certain preventative. Food or drink should never be carried to the mouth unless the hands have been thoroughly washed, and the vessels in which the food is served should always be thoroughly boiled and scoured. Only cooked food should be eaten, and fruit and raw vegetables should be avoided. Water is one of the most fruitful sources of spreading this disease, and the only safeguard in this direction lies in boiling all water before drinking. Heat is a positive destroyer of the cholera poison, and everything introduced into the stomach should first be subjected to it.

The household arrangement should be particularly looked after. Dirt is the great breeding place of cholera, and every dark, dirty corner is a nest where the seeds of the disease thrive and spread. Disinfectants should be freely and constantly used, carbolic acid being the best possible preventive. Frequent scrubbing with hot water is an excellent scheme.

All these precautions, however, only prevail in case the greatest care is exercised in dieting and mode of life. Unusual exertion should be avoided, and the system should be kept properly toned up. Alcoholic stimulants, especially in excessive quantities, should, however, be avoided, and purging substances should only be taken into the system with the utmost caution. Anything that tends to irritate or inflame the intestines furnishes a good lodgment for the disease germs.

*August 28, 1892*

# Women to Assure Healthy Homes

### By M. A. TAFT

They will look exceedingly well in uniform, the younger members of that brave party of seven new-fledged women Tenement House Inspectors, the first ever appointed in this city, who reported for duty to Commissioner De Forest at his office, 61 Irving Place, last Monday morning. They are young, the greater number of them, bright and vivacious, and they came from the Inspector's room, where they had received the first insight into their duties, with beaming eyes, flushed cheeks, and in a state of delighted excitement not to be seen in the most enthusiastic matinee girl after an afternoon spent with a favorite matinee idol.

And those girls had spent more than two and a half solid hours sitting at little desks provided for the purpose, with their backs to the windows and the other people in the room, that their attention might not be distracted, taking notes vigorously and listening with open eyes and ears to a technical discussion upon tenement house sanitary matters, with cheerful side lights thrown upon the idiosyncrasies of supply and waste pipes, and other equally exciting matters.

Not a word did they breathe about uniforms. It is doubtful if such a frivolous subject has entered their serious young heads.

"I am sure we are all very busy indeed," cried hurriedly the plumpest and prettiest Inspector, the girl with the pinkest cheeks, when a *New York Times* reporter approached to venture a question upon this seemingly momentous matter. And there was a flurry of skirts and every one of the new Inspectors had vanished from the building with a celerity which promises well for the work they have undertaken. As a matter of fact, it had been announced before the lecture began that the young women would be instructed not to talk.

"We prefer to do all the talking ourselves," said Deputy Commissioner Veiller, with a laugh.

## The Question of Uniforms

As for the uniforms, there is nothing definite decided upon that subject. Commissioner De Forest says that the matter is under consideration. It is necessary for many reasons for Inspectors to have something by which they may be distinguished: it is an aid in their work, vesting them with authority. For the time being the young women will wear the large badges of the commission on their coats.

Men Inspectors—there are now 177 of them—wear a neat dark-blue uniform. There are brass buttons of military design, bearing the name of the department in letters around the edge and the coat-of-arms of the city in the centre. These they wear on sack coat and vest, with a large metal badge, and the dark-blue soft felt hat, on the order of a Fedora, is lettered in front, and the word "Tenement" stands out distinctly, and may be read several feet away.

"But they could not put the women in uniform," said a young man Inspector who kindly allowed the buttons of his coat to be examined. "How could they?" he added, evidently with the idea that a uniform means bifurcated garments.

There are nine women Inspectors all told, and they are well fitted for their work. They are college educated as a rule, have taught or practiced medicine, and have had more or less experience along the line of work they are now undertaking. They are all unmarried.

## Candidates Accepted

Miss Mary B. Sayles is a graduate of Smith College, Northampton, Mass., a teacher by profession, and investigated tenement house conditions for the College Settlement Association of Jersey City. She has also worked for the Brooklyn Bureau of Charities.

Miss Margaret P. Brewster is a graduate of the medical college formerly connected with the New York Infirmary for Women and Children, and has practiced professionally, doing much work in the tenement house districts. Miss Gertrude W. Light, who is a graduate of the same college, has had a similar experience.

Miss Anna L. Nevins is a teacher by profession. She has studied at Columbia University and abroad, and speaks several languages. Miss Jeannette Moffett, who is a graduate of Barnard, took special courses at the college in history and economics and was in charge of the Department of Social Economics at the Paris Exposition in 1900. Miss Emily W. Dinwiddie, also a teacher, is a graduate of the University of Virginia. She has been investigator for the New Jersey State Board of Children's Guardians, and has been, until her present appointment, assistant agent and investigator of the New York Charity Organization. She compiled the present directory of charities. Miss Helen D. Thompson, a Vassar graduate, has been officially connected for some time with the Charity Organization Society, New York, and left a position of Sanitary Inspector for the Civic Sanitary Association of the Oranges. N.J., to take up her present work.

Miss Mildred H. Fairfield is a Normal School graduate, has been Principal of the city training schools at Lewiston, Me., and Manchester, N.H. Recently she has been Inspector and Supervisor of the People's University Extension Society of Greater New York. Miss Christine L. Kunz is a teacher and a graduate of the School of Philanthropy. She is a sister of George F. Kunz, the jewel expert.

## Duties of Inspectors

What is known as the new tenement house law, which makes no reference to sex and makes it possible for women to serve as Tenement House Inspectors, is the result of the work of a commission, of which Mr. De Forest was Chairman, appointed by President (then Governor) Roosevelt in 1900. In regard to the new Inspectors Mr. De Forest said last week:

"We believe that there are certain lines of this work in which the services of women will be valuable, and we are going to see if this will be the case. They will study the sanitary conditions of the tenements and see that the people are comfortable as well as healthy. There are many ways in which women are adapted for the work. There are points about the home which they will notice, they will be able to get information about the way people live, and will gain their confidence. No, they will never take the place of men; men will always be needed in the work."

It is not expected that the women will meet with trouble or opposition in their investigations. While there have been small annoyances, as there will be in all kinds of work, Commissioner De Forest says the men Inspectors have not had any trouble worth considering. The working hours of the Inspectors are from 9 to 5 daily, and the salary is $1,200 a year.

The examinations which the young women Inspectors passed were held on July 14, and the result of the competition was announced on Sept. 20. The nine young women were among 700 applicants who took the examination. Since then they have been waiting until their services were required.

Frequent comment is made upon the inapplicability of civil service examinations to the duties the applicants are to perform. This was not the case with the municipal civil service examination for Tenement House Inspectors. President Ogden of the Municipal Civil Service Commission says that the examinations should fit exactly the work those who take them will be called upon to perform, and make it impossible for any one not fitted to pass. The examination papers given this new lot of Inspectors bristled with technicalities. The woman who could pass the examination might build a house.

## Puzzlers on Paper

There are four sheets, the first given to general questions applicable to the work; the second showing a plan of a tenement house floor, upon whose conditions the contestants were obliged, to pass; the third given up to such arithmetical questions as will be likely to enter into the reports of the Inspectors; and the fourth devoted to personal matters, education and experience in this class of work, the name and residence of the applicant, and the age, for those who pass a civil service examination must tell how old they are, and that may be kept a secret or it may not.

Here are some of the puzzlers of the first page of the examination papers:

1. Enumerate the evils which are likely to arise from the overcrowding of tenement houses.

2. Suppose a fashionable apartment house, five stories high, with two apartments on each floor. There are no kitchens in any apartment, but the occupants take their meals in a restaurant on the ground floor. In the Summer the restaurant is closed for several months for repairs. Some of the tenants then prepare their own breakfasts in their apartments. Does this action make a tenement house of the place or not? Give reasons for your answer.

3. Explain the meaning of the following terms: "Gooseneck ladder," "winder," "string" in stairways, "Louvre."

4. Under what conditions may a cellar be used for living purposes?

5. If in making an inspection you should find tenants beating a carpet on a roof or hanging it out of a window, what would you do?

In the plan of an imaginary floor in a tenement house given in the second paper all the details are noted, with the height of building, width of street, &c., and would-be Inspectors are required to write a report upon violations of sanitary laws.

## Problems in Figures

There are only four questions on the page devoted to arithmetic, and here they are:

1. A corner lot extends 92 feet on one street and 45 on the other. The streets are at right angles with each other, and the side parallel to the 92-foot side measures 84 feet. How many square feet are there in a block which covers 87 feet of the above lot?

2. Multiply 300.75 by 9.2046.

3. Divide 12.885865 by 629.5.

4. A lot whose front is 240 feet and whose depth is 100 feet is bought by A, B, and C, paying respectively $3,000, $4,000, and $5,000. To how many feet front is each entitled if it is divided in proportion to their investments?

The lecture given the new women Inspectors on Monday was the first in a course of two weeks' education they will receive before they are assigned to their respective posts. Lectures are given by the Chief Inspector upon various topics, and technical information is combined with instructions as to terms to enable the workers thoroughly to understand their business and to make their reports in a concise and satisfactory manner. One week will be devoted to practical work among the tenements under the direction of other Inspectors. The size of the district each will cover will depend upon the population, Inspectors assigned to the more congested parts of the city being required to cover a smaller land area.

*October 12, 1902*

# Declares Raw Milk Worse Than a Plague

PARIS—The International Congress dealing with the philanthropic distribution of milk, which was opened yesterday at the Pasteur Institute here, closed its sessions to-day. There was a large and representative attendance of delegates from many countries.

Dr. A. P. Greene, director of the Straus milk depots in New York, read a paper written by Nathan Straus explaining the methods of the Straus system of distribution. In the course of the paper Mr. Straus said:

"Millions of dollars annually are spent to counteract the evils of popular ignorance. Why not treat physical ailments in the same manner? Prevent them. Prevent helpless infants developing from puny, sickly childhood into diseased, weakened, and helpless manhood and womanhood. The enormous sums paid annually to hospitals and like institutions should, as far as possible, be saved. And a great deal is possible.

"It is milk—raw milk, diseased milk—which is responsible for the largest percentage of sickness in the world. Milk is the one article of food in which disease and death may lurk without giving any suspicion from its taste, smell, or appearance. Why, then, use in its raw form? Why ever trust it without due precaution? I hold that the only safe rule is—Pasteurize the entire milk supply and make it a function of the municipality.

"The evils of impure milk, which, according to the United States Department of Agriculture, are the leading cause of a mortality of 33 per cent of children before 3 years old, and of many adults, are threefold. First—It is generally known that it causes diarrhoeal disturbances, which, especially during the hot months, are the most fruitful source of infant death. Second—A number of the most violent infectious diseases to which the human race is subject are communicated by milk. For milk may, and frequently has, become the carrier of disease not found in cattle, but occurring on the farm or dairy, in the person of human beings. Thus Prof. Kober traced 148 epidemics of typhoid to the dairy, and an incredible number of epidemics of scarlet fever and of diphtheria have been traced beyond the chance of doubt to the same source. Third—Contamination occurs through diseases of the cattle themselves, the most prevalent being tuberculosis. The extent to which tuberculosis exists in cows is shown by the following:

"Prof. Bang of Copenhagen says that in Denmark over 60 per cent of the animals are tuberculous in all herds of over fifty head. Macfadyen estimates that

30 per cent of all the cattle in England are tuberculous, and in tests made in various parts of the United States it was found that from 2 to 50 per cent of the cattle gave evidence of the disease. So appalling is this evidence that Prof. von Behring asserted categorically in 1903 that 'the milk fed to infants is the chief cause of consumption.'

"Let us stop and consider—that if the assertion of Behring reveals the truth, of which, though not a physician, I have long been convinced, its practical importance is appalling; at least 50 per cent of all the children who die have been infected with tuberculosis through their food and one-seventh of all deaths are due to tuberculosis."

Mr. Straus proceeded to give formulae for the Pasteurization of milk, and to describe the methods of distribution adopted by him in New York and the excellent effects which followed his efforts to supply the poor in that city with Pasteurized milk. In conclusion he said:

"I contemplate with dismay the time when any organization which I am able to provide will be inadequate to supply the demand—a demand constantly increasing as the people are becoming impressed with the saving of child life thus effected. I can only trust that before that time arrives the State itself may be prepared to enforce the obligation of making a supply of wholesome milk food for infants a municipal function, and so stamping out the seeds of a plague more destructive than any that is to be dreaded under conditions of our modern civilization. For no plague could yield so plentiful a crop of deaths as that which is reaped annually from the seed of contagion deposited in the human system by millions of noxious bacteria developed in milk."

*October 22, 1905*

# Alcohol's Appalling Effect on Infant Mortality

"The effect of alcohol upon infant mortality is appalling." That is the verdict of Dr. J. Wallace Beveridge of the Cornell Medical College—a verdict that he reached after years of close observation in hospitals, and one that has been affirmed by a long series of laboratory experiments.

Dr. Beveridge's verdict against alcohol is a sweeping one. As a medical man, he disapproves of its use by any one. Injurious in the cool seasons, it is trebly injurious in hot weather. The person who takes it lowers his mental and physical efficiency, his working capacity, and also reduces his power of resisting the inroads of disease.

In the hot weather the alcohol drinker invites sunstroke. At all seasons of the year (and this is a theory new to the medical science) the tippler increases the possibility that he or she will be afflicted by that scourge of the civilized world—cancer.

But it is on the effect of alcohol upon infant mortality that Dr. Beveridge dwells with particular emphasis.

"The mother of a young child," says Dr. Beveridge, "should not touch alcoholic liquor in any form. Alcohol is not a food. It does not supply to women the nourishment of which at certain periods of their lives they are in particular need.

"On the contrary, the mother of a young child who drinks alcoholic beverages even in their mildest forms—beer, ale, and stout, for instance—runs the risk of absolutely cutting off the supply of food that nature intended an infant to have.

"If the supply is not entirely cut off, the quality is so impoverished that the health of the infant is ruined.

"The bottle does not provide a means of avoiding the effects of a mother drinking alcohol. Bottle feeding does not produce children that develop into healthy men and women. Nature intended that infants should be fed in one way, and in one way only. If a mother voluntarily jeopardizes this one way, she is willingly jeopardizing the health, perhaps the life, of her child.

"Not only is this true, but I can go further and say that the father and mother who drink (for here the stricture perhaps applies equally to both sexes) are jeopardizing their possibilities of parentage.

"As an indication of what alcohol does in the human system, I may mention some recent laboratory experiments showing the action of alcohol directly on cell structures from the lower orders of life.

"With the cells of torula (the yeast plant) taking one cubic centimetre as the standard, there were found after seven hours 2,061 normal cells present. When a one-thousandth per cent alcohol solution was added, the normal cells were reduced to 1,091. "When a one-hundredth per cent solution was added, the cells numbered 992. With a one-tenth per cent solution, the figures dropped to 852. And when a five per cent solution was added, only 69 normal cells were found.

"Let us see what happens when a small amount of alcohol is added to a vigorous culture of byerincks. These are a phosphoric bacilli, which can be readily photographed if placed in a cup or other vessel, and a dark screen with one or more holes in it placed over the top. The phosphorescent light will show through the one or more holes in the screen and be indicated on the photographic negative.

"But add a seven to twelve per cent solution of alcohol, and no matter how long the exposure of the negative may last, no indication of the phosphorescent light will be found. This shows conclusively that the bacilli died.

"To come higher up in the scale of existence: add one-tenth of one per cent of alcohol to the water in an aquarium in which perch, crayfish and gold fish are swimming, and the fish will drop to the bottom. Unless removed to an aquarium containing unpolluted water, they will die.

"If a fertile egg of a chicken is immersed in a 5 per cent solution of alcohol for about two hours, or subjected to the fumes of alcohol, the embryonic chicken will die.

"By administering alcohol to a guinea pig in minute doses—about half a dram during every twenty-four hours while it is with young—the offspring if alive at time of birth will die within six hours thereafter.

"But we do not need to rely upon experimental analogy to show the evil effects of alcohol upon prenatal life. Statistics tell their own story.

"In countries like France, Russia, England, and America, where alcohol drinking has been on the increase, the birth rate has been steadily diminishing.

"In France the birth rate per capita is now only one-fifth of 1 per cent. In Russia a century ago the birth rate per family was five. Now it is only two. In this country during the past ten years the birth rate has diminished 11.4 per cent.

"So startling are these figures in France and Russia that the Governments have appointed investigating committees. In both cases the verdict has been alcohol. In France the Government for some years past has been contemplating radical action to reduce the amount of alcohol consumption.

"But suppose the baby is born. Now let us see the effect of alcohol drinking, skipping for the moment the tendency toward insanity and epilepsy that results from an alcoholic ancestry and confining myself to the malnutrition of the baby.

"Recently it has been proven by a number of our best physiological chemists, among whom I need only mention Prof. Chittenden, Dr. Berkley, and Prof. Ehrlich, that if a woman takes spirituous drinks during the period prior to her becoming a mother and afterwards, even though the alcohol be in very small quantities, it has a very deleterious effect upon the natural nourishment that she can offer her baby.

"The alcohol produces a chemical change in the proteids, carbohydrates, and the fats, which are the chief nutritive factors in the milk.

"For a practical, read-to-hand demonstration of the truth of this, we need only observe the success that Jewish and Mohammedan mothers have in raising their children. Both the Hebrew and Mohammedan religion forbid a nursing mother to drink spiritous liquors.

"But there is no such inhibition upon the Christian mother. And so we find many of these mothers unable to nurse their children, and if they can do it at all, the children are often ill-nourished.

"Wherefore we of the medical profession have been compelled to create foods such as modified milk, barley water and other diets acceptable to infants. But at best these are only a poor substitute for the natural diet.

"Every baby that is properly nourished during the first twelve to fourteen months of its life is far better able to withstand or combat the invasion of virulent disease in after life.

"The death rate to and including their third year of babies that have been properly nursed is 69.4 per cent, less than those brought up on artificial food.

"It has been found that babies brought up on the bottle—even if the food is properly adapted to their systems and they increase in weight and strength as a normal baby should—are the ones that in after life are most apt to be stricken with typhoid, pneumonia, and diseases of this character. The proper foundation of health has not been laid in infancy, their power of resistance is small.

"From the age of 7 to 11 years children that were bottle-raised often become involved with rheumatism. This is a term used to describe a distinct chemical change that has taken place in the system. It involves the tonsils and the heart, and often causes a great deal of damage unless remedied.

"In babies that have been fed by the natural method this rheumatic condition is rarely noticed.

"Alcohol taken by a nursing mother is also a great factor in producing rickets in children.

"Just glance at this report of the observations made by Dr. W. C. Sullivan of the General Hospital at Liverpool on female prisoners in the alcoholic ward. He took the history of 120 women to whom 600 children were born. Of this 600, 55 per cent were dead at birth, 22 per cent died before the third year, 11 per cent died before the fifteenth year, and the remaining 12 per cent may or may not have reached maturity, Dr. Sullivan not being able to collect the data.

"Or take the histories of 827 cases of marasmus, an infant disease due to inanition primarily caused by improper milk. These histories, gathered at the clinics of the Cornell Medical College, Bellevue, and Roosevelt Hospitals, were taken with especial regard to the fact that the mother had nursed her child. In 87.4 per cent of the cases the mother had used alcohol in some form, either as beer, gin or whisky. One should not need a more striking proof than this of the injurious effect of alcohol upon the natural food of babies.

"There have been a number of investigators who have made the positive assertion that the effect of alcohol on the human race is very slight. But this assertion is not borne out by the facts brought to light recently.

"The men in charge of our insane asylums and sanatoriums for the care of alcoholics have been gradually giving us a great deal of information that was lacking some years ago.

"Now, one of the principal causes of insanity, of mental deficiency, and of epilepsy is recognized as the consumption of alcoholic beverages. It may be that the victim of one of these forms of mental derangement has never touched a drop of intoxicating liquor in his life. The father or the mother, or perhaps one of the grandparents drank; and the old law—'unto the third and fourth generations'—is again scoring. Or it may be that only an alcoholic, a neurotic tendency is inherited and the victim's mental unbalance has been brought about by his or her own drinking.

"In no country of the world is the consumption of alcoholic beverages increasing at so rapid a pace as it is in Russia. And what's the result? Fifty years ago sanitariums and public institutions for the care of the insane, the feeble-minded, the mentally unbalanced, and incapables were very rare. To-day we find them springing up in every centre of population throughout European Russia.

"In America we have caught an echo of this condition. The increase of insane emigrants from Russia and of neurotics from other foreign countries has been brought to public attention by Gov. Dix in one of his messages and legislation suggested to prevent these undesirable aliens from entering our State and becoming public charges.

"With so many counts in the indictment of alcohol—and there are more to come—it is interesting to ask one's self why one drinks. As a joy-giver alcohol is only a temporary and a most uncertain expedient. As the man who drinks knows to his cost, alcohol is both a stimulant and a depressant. Depending on various causes, it may act one way and it may act the other.

"I think that the great majority of people who drink alcohol take it as a 'bracer.' There are those who take it in Winter 'to warm' them up, and who take it in Summer for the opposite reason.

"Now, as a matter of well-established scientific fact, alcohol does not 'brace' a man for his work, it does not warm him in Winter, and in Summer it increases the possibility of his being a victim of sunstroke.

"Just let us glance for a moment at the physiological action of alcohol. It causes a lowering of the body temperature of from one to three degrees. At first it increases the heart action, but lowers the blood pressure through the dilation of the blood vessels. It affects the nervous system directly through the blood. It has been found present in the blood stream fifteen minutes after taking. It causes a tremendous flow of blood to the capillaries and small blood vessels that supply the stomach. At the same time there is a corresponding lessening of the blood supply in the brain.

"After alcohol has been taken for some time either in small or greater amounts the muscle cells degenerate through a fatty degeneration or through direct starvation. The small blood vessels of the brain often are ruptured and minute clots form.

"This breaking down of the cell structures of the body, of the lessening of the oxidation, creates a distinct toxic condition which is very difficult to eliminate. In time various portions of the body, such as the liver, stomach, and kidneys, become seriously damaged.

"One very interesting fact which I have noticed is that in the majority of cases when the patient is suffering from malignant growths, such as cancer of the abdominal organs, there is usually an alcoholic history.

"It is reasonable to presume that where a vital organ like the stomach has its delicate tissues constantly irritated, as is done by the steady use of alcohol, that the way is opened for whatever pathological change may take place wherein cancer is given a chance to manifest itself.

"In reference to immunity from disease, it is an established fact that the individual subject to alcoholism is always open to the invasion of hostile bacilli, particularly those of typhoid and of pneumonia.

"This has been shown by laboratory tests made on rabbits, dogs, and guinea pigs. In these tests half the number of animals were subjected to a course of alcohol, and the other half kept normal. Then all were injected with an equal amount of typhoid, pneumonia or tubercle bacilli.

"All those animals which had been subjected to alcohol became infected, while only 2 per cent of the animals that were free of alcohol became infected. The normal, healthy systems of the latter threw off the hostile bacilli, showing conclusively that alcohol reduces immunity from disease.

"Now, as for the use of alcohol," concluded Dr. Beveridge, "as a drink in cold and hot weather.

"I have already mentioned the fact that alcohol causes a lowering of the body temperature of from one to three degrees. This is so well established as a physiological fact that I do not need to dwell on it here.

"But now that the hot weather is with us what is of immediate interest is the effect of alcohol as a Summer drink.

"During the heat waves many prostrations are reported and they show grave mortality. With the exception of infants and elderly people and those directly occupied as stokers or similar tasks, over 85 per cent of the heat prostrations are directly due to the use of spirituous liquors.

"In the tropics, where malt and spirituous liquors are seldom used, heat cases are comparatively rare.

"In Sweden Dr. Mernetsch, the staff surgeon of the army, in his report made in 1905 called special attention to the fact that only those men, whether officers or privates, who drank alcoholic beverages were affected by the heat during the Summer manoeuvres of that year.

"Why does alcohol induce sunstroke? To put the matter as simply as possible, I may say that the heat centre is located in the fourth ventricle in the brain. By artificially stimulating this we can lower or raise an animal's temperature. Alcohol, through the blood, by virtue of its toxic effect, has a direct action on this centre."

*July 7, 1912*

# Dr. Noguchi Is Dead, Martyr of Science

A CCRA, GOLD COAST COLONY, AFRICA—Professor Hideyo Noguchi, bacteriologist of the Rockefeller Institute for Medical Research, died here today from yellow fever, which he contracted during a laboratory experiment. Professor Noguchi arrived at Accra in November to investigate this disease.

## His Research Problem Solved

His research problem solved—the relationship between South American and African yellow fever and the source of the latter—Dr. Hideyo Noguchi died just two days after the date set for his sailing back to New York.

Dr. Noguchi had used his own illness to bring his studies to completion. Monkeys were inoculated with blood from his own body, developing the symptoms of the disease. Dr. Noguchi had written to friends here telling of his success in identifying the carrier of the disease. The Rockefeller Foundation in its report, made public recently, told of the progress made in the fight on yellow fever and said, "The Rockefeller Foundation could not ask men to volunteer."

But Dr. Noguchi, a patient in the hospital in West Africa from Dec. 28, 1927, to Jan. 9, 1928, as he wrote to friends, had used his own illness to further his scientific study. A monkey inoculated with his blood was the first animal ever to develop the disease and provided the answer to the scientists' first problem, the discovery of an animal that reacted to the disease similarly to man.

Dr. Noguchi had a long record of achievement behind him when, against the advice of friends and in spite of advancing age, he went on the arduous trip to Africa. At the institute at Avenue A and Sixty-sixth Street, where so much of his time had been spent, flags flew at half staff yesterday, and on the bulletin board on a small white card with a fine black border was the simple announcement: "Dr. Noguchi died at Accra, midday, Monday."

No announcement was made concerning plans for his burial. He leaves a wife, Mrs. Mary Dardis Noguchi, whom he married in 1911. She lives in this city.

## Ranked With Greatest Scientists

Dr. Hideyo Noguchi ranked with such scientists as Metchnikoff and Pasteur in the work of alleviating the ills of the human body. His tireless efforts in the fields of medical and bacteriological research were invaluable in combating trachoma, infantile paralysis, rabies and yellow fever, and he did much toward identifying the causes of paresis and locomotor ataxia. No other member of his race was so distinguished in pathology.

Born Nov. 24, 1876, at Inawashiro, Yala, Fukushima, Japan, the son of Shika and Sayoske (Kobiyama) Noguchi, he was educated in Japanese public schools supplemented by private instructions in German, French and English and in Chinese literature. He received a medical degree from Tokyo Medical College when 23 years old and later attended the University of Pennsylvania and the Statens Serum Institute of Copenhagen, Denmark.

Dr. Noguchi was the discoverer of many serums which have influenced the treatment of various diseases, notably rabies, rattlesnake bite and infantile paralysis. With Dr. Simon Flexner of the Rockefeller Institute he isolated the germ of the latter disease, and later produced a smallpox vaccine said to be free from bacterial impurity, and identified paresis as a manifestation of a dreaded blood disease germ.

In 1911 he was appointed to a titular professorship by the Imperial Government of Japan, where from 1897 to 1898, prior to entering the University of Pennsylvania, he had been Assistant Superintendent of the Government Institute for Infectious Diseases.

Dr. Noguchi had held professorships in pathology at the Tokyo Dental College, the University of Pennsylvania and the Carnegie Institute. In 1904, the year of its founding, he became one of the original members of the staff of the Rockefeller Institute, where immediately his discoveries were of vast aid to the work of Dr. Heinrich Ehrlich.

## Cultivated the Rabic Virus

In the early part of 1912 Dr. Noguchi undertook to cultivate the rabic virus and obtained results. About fifty series of cultivations were made with the brain or medulla aseptically removed from rabbits, guinea pigs and dogs infected with "street" virus, "passage" virus or "fixed" virus. Usually the animals were etherized just before spontaneous death occurred.

The method which yielded the isolation of the rabic germ was similar to that employed successfully for the cultivation of the spirochaete of relapsing fever.

While he was on his way to Vienna in September, 1913, Dr. Noguchi decided to have his discovery verified at the Pasteur Institute in Paris. Professor Metchnikoff's laboratories were thronged with physicians on the day appointed for the test, and Dr. Noguchi demonstrated the facts as he described before leaving this country.

During the latter part of his career he was affiliated with the Rockefeller Institute for Medical Research, of which he had been a member since 1914. At various times during his connection with the Rockefeller Institute Dr. Noguchi came into conflict with the Vivisection Investigation League, which had for its officers some of the most prominent men and women of the city. In 1912 a charge that Dr. Noguchi had inoculated 146 persons of pure blood with the poison of an ancient and virulent blood disease was proved baseless by District Attorney Whitman.

Wild rats in this country had been found to be carriers of the germs of yellow jaundice, or Weil's disease, an infectious ailment from which many soldiers on the battlefields have suffered, according to an investigation into the disease conducted by Dr. Noguchi. He found that the disease is communicated to man even by wild rats which were apparently healthy.

The success of Dr. Noguchi's experiments was made possible by the importation from Japan and from Flanders of guinea pigs and rats which had been inoculated with the causative organism in those two countries.

Dr. Noguchi's experiments showed that wild rats in America carried the same causative agencies in their kidneys as are to be found in Asia and Europe. Thus was revealed a latent danger to which this country has been exposed, but which we had thus far escaped through improved conditions.

In 1915 the Emperor of Japan sent word to the Rockefeller Institute that he had conferred an imperial prize on Dr. Noguchi for his researches regarding the germs of a dreaded blood disease, rabies and infantile paralysis. In 1914 the Emperor had conferred on Dr. Noguchi the highest medical degree in Japan. He had been also knighted by the King of Denmark, the King of Sweden and the King of Spain.

In waging his battle against yellow fever, Dr. Noguchi went to Guayaquil, Ecuador, in 1919, where he directed efforts to subdue an outbreak of the dread disease, which was exacting a toll of many lives yearly in Latin America. His efforts were successful, and it was largely due to his work and the example set by it that yellow fever has been virtually curbed in Central and South America.

One of his most important achievements, isolation of the germ that causes trachoma, he announced in 1927 after two years of patient research. In his investigation he had inoculated monkeys with cultures obtained from Indians affected with the disease. Leading physicians asserted that his work might result in prevention of trachoma.

Just last Saturday the award to Dr. Noguchi of the silver medal of the American Medical Association for his discovery of the organism causing trachoma was announced.

Following his work in this field, he went to Lagos, Nigeria, probably one of the most unhealthy localities in Africa, to carry on further warfare against yellow fever. Upon his departure he said that he hoped to pursue further his studies of trachoma while in Africa.

## A Hero to Countrymen

The great bacteriologist was something of a hero to his countrymen, who looked upon him as one who had done more than any other for the advancement of his nation in the realm of science. Not only to the Japanese public but to his associates in this country he was an extraordinary character. He was often referred to as a "human dynamo," forgetting the world entirely and working day and night for weeks on end when on the path of a new discovery.

He was a slight man, of nervous manner, with drawn features and dark eyes that seemed to snap with intelligence. He took his relaxation at the Nippon Club, where his chief diversion was a game of chess with one or another of his countrymen.

Dr. Noguchi was honored by institutions and Governments throughout the world, and belonged to organizations in many parts of the globe. His native land gave him a titular professorship early in his career. The University of Pennsylvania awarded him an honorary degree of Master of Science two years after completion of his course there. In 1915 the Japanese Emperor awarded him the Order of Merit. The City of Philadelphia gave him the John Scott medal.

He was a member of the Association of American Physicians, the Association of American Pathologists and Bacteriologists, the American Society for Experimental Pathology, the Harvey Society, the American Philosophical Society, the American Medical Association, the American Association for the Advancement of Science, the American Society of Immunologists, the Society for Experimental Biology and Medicine and honorary or corresponding member of many foreign organizations.

*May 22, 1928*

# "Typhoid Mary" Dies of a Stroke at 68

Mary Mallon, the first carrier of typhoid bacilli identified in America and consequently known as Typhoid Mary, died yesterday in Riverside Hospital on North Brother Island.

With the exception of a five-year period from 1910 to 1915, this isolated spot in the East River had been her home since 1907 when she was committed after it had been discovered that she was a veritable peripatetic breeding ground for the bacilli. Fifty-one original cases and three deaths had been attributed to her although she was held immune.

While her system was loaded with typhoid germs to such an extent that some physicians referred to her as the human culture tube, it was not typhoid that caused her death. She died, according to authorities, as a result of the effects of a paralytic stroke dating back to Christmas day, 1932.

## Services This Morning

Funeral services will be held this morning in St. Luke's Roman Catholic Church, 623 East 138th Street, where a mass of requiem will be offered for the repose of her soul. For years her religious and spiritual needs had been administered by the priests of St. Luke's, who visited her often.

Typhoid Mary's known history goes back to 1904, when an epidemic of typhoid spread through Oyster Bay and adjacent towns. It was discovered that the source of the trouble was in a household where Mary had been a cook. But when this became known Mary had gone. It was not until 1907 that she was discovered working as a cook in a Park Avenue home. Again she fled when the authorities sought her. She was finally overtaken after considerable difficulty.

Health Department officials rushed her to the Willard Parker Hospital, where it was discovered that she was a typhoid carrier. That year she was committed to North Brother Island, where she stayed, despite an appeal to the Supreme Court, until 1910, when the Health Department released her after she had promised to accept employment only where the handling of food was not involved.

## Epidemic Is Traced

Four years later the authorities started looking for Mary again when an epidemic broke out in a sanitarium at Newfoundland, N.J. Investigation disclosed that Mary had been the cook there. Shortly afterward twenty-five employees were stricken with typhoid at the Sloane Maternity Hospital and two of them died. Again it was found that Mary had been in the kitchen there and left just ahead of the investigating agents.

She was found in a suburban home and once more sent to the island, this time to stay. She admitted to be 68 years, but most persons thought her to be older. She said she had been born in the United States, but this was never confirmed. Although she fought isolation for many years, she finally adopted a philosophic attitude and tried to make the best of her cloistered existence.

*November 12, 1938*

# The Vaccination Effect: 100 Million Cases of Contagious Disease Prevented

By STEVE LOHR

Vaccination programs for children have prevented more than 100 million cases of serious contagious disease in the United States since 1924, according to a new study published in the *New England Journal of Medicine*.

The research, led by scientists at the University of Pittsburgh's graduate school of public health, analyzed public health reports going back to the 19th century. The reports covered 56 diseases, but the article in the journal focused on seven: polio, measles, rubella, mumps, hepatitis A, diphtheria and pertussis, or whooping cough.

Researchers analyzed disease reports before and after the times when vaccines became commercially available. Put simply, the estimates for prevented cases came from the falloff in disease reports after vaccines were licensed and widely available. The researchers projected the number of cases that would have occurred had the pre-vaccination patterns continued as the nation's population increased.

The journal article is one example of the kind of analysis that can be done when enormous data sets are built and mined. The project, which started in 2009, required assembling 88 million reports of individual cases of disease, much of it from the weekly morbidity reports in the library of the Centers for Disease Control and Prevention. Then the reports had to be converted to digital formats.

Most of the data entry—200 million keystrokes—was done by Digital Divide Data, a social enterprise that provides jobs and technology training to young people in Cambodia, Laos and Kenya.

Still, data entry was just a start. The information was put into spreadsheets for making tables, but was later sorted and standardized so it could be searched, manipulated and queried on the project's website.

"Collecting all this data is one thing, but making the data computable is where the big payoff should be," said Dr. Irene Eckstrand, a program director and science officer for the N.I.H.'s Models of Infectious Disease Agent Study.

The University of Pittsburgh researchers also looked at death rates, but decided against including an estimate in the journal article, largely because death certificate data became more reliable and consistent only in the 1960s, the researchers said.

But Dr. Donald S. Burke, the dean of Pittsburgh's graduate school of public health and an author of the medical journal article, said that a reasonable projection of prevented deaths based on known mortality rates in the disease categories would be three million to four million.

The scientists said their research should help inform the debate on the risks and benefits of vaccinating American children.

Pointing to the research results, Dr. Burke said, "If you're anti-vaccine, that's the price you pay."

The medical journal article notes the recent resurgence of some diseases as some parents have resisted vaccinating their children. For example, the worst whooping cough epidemic since 1959 occurred last year, with more than 38,000 reported cases nationwide.

The disease data is on the project's website, available for use by other researchers, students, the news media and members of the public who may be curious about the outbreak and spread of a particular disease. Much of the data is searchable by disease, year and location. The project was funded by the National Institutes of Health and the Bill and Melinda Gates Foundation.

"I'm very excited to see what people will find in this data, what patterns and insights are there waiting to be discovered," said Dr. Willem G. van Panhuis, an epidemiologist at Pittsburgh and lead author of the journal article.

The project's name itself is a nod to the notion that data is a powerful tool for scientific discovery. It is called Project Tycho, after the 16th century Danish nobleman Tycho Brahe, whose careful, detailed astronomical observations were the foundation on which Johannes Kepler made the creative leap to devise his laws of planetary motion.

The open-access model for the project at Pittsburgh is increasingly the pattern with government data. The United States government has opened up thousands of data sets to the public.

Just how these assets will be exploited commercially is still in the experimental stage, other than a few well-known applications like using government weather data for forecasting services and insurance products.

But the potential seems to be considerable. Last month, the McKinsey Global Institute, the research arm of the consulting firm, projected that the total economic benefit to companies and consumers of open data could reach $3 trillion worldwide.

*November 27, 2013*

# Ebola Virus Is Outpacing Efforts to Control It, World Health Body Warns

## By ADAM NOSSITER AND ALAN COWELL

A BUJA, NIGERIA—In an ominous warning as fatalities mounted in West Africa from the worst known outbreak of the Ebola virus, the head of the World Health Organization said on Friday that the disease was moving faster than efforts to curb it, with potentially catastrophic consequences, including a "high risk" that it will spread.

The assessment was among the most dire since the outbreak was identified in March. The outbreak has been blamed for the deaths of 729 people, according to W.H.O. figures, and has left over 1,300 people with confirmed or suspected infections.

Dr. Margaret Chan, the W.H.O. director general, was speaking as she met with the leaders of the three most affected countries—Guinea, Liberia and Sierra Leone—in Conakry, the Guinean capital, for the introduction of a $100 million plan to deploy hundreds more medical professionals in support of overstretched regional and international health workers.

"This meeting must mark a turning point in the outbreak response," Dr. Chan said, according to a W.H.O. transcript of her remarks. "If the situation continues to deteriorate, the consequences can be catastrophic in terms of lost lives but also severe socioeconomic disruption and a high risk of spread to other countries."

She said the outbreak was "caused by the most lethal strain in the family of Ebola viruses."

The gathering in Conakry came a day after West African leaders seemed to quicken the pace of efforts to combat the disease, in what some analysts depicted as a belated acknowledgment that the response so far had been inadequate.

Before the meeting started, there were indications of discord. The leader of Guinea's Ebola task force said that emergency measures in Liberia, where schools have been closed, and Sierra Leone could set back efforts to control the worst outbreak of the virus since it was identified almost four decades ago.

"Currently, some measures taken by our neighbors could make the fight against Ebola even harder," Aboubacar Sidiki Diakité, the Ebola task force leader, told Reuters. "When children are not supervised, they can go anywhere and make the problem worse. It is part of what we will be talking about."

Sierra Leone's emergency measures include house-to-house searches for infected people and the deployment of the army and the police.

One person, traveling from Liberia, died in Nigeria, Africa's most populous nation, which introduced airport screening of travelers from the stricken region on Thursday.

Dr. Chan said that the virus seemed to be spreading in ways never seen before.

"It is taking place in areas with fluid population movements over porous borders, and it has demonstrated its ability to spread via air travel," she said.

Making matters worse, health workers have been hit particularly hard. Top doctors in Sierra Leone and Liberia have died, and two American aid workers have contracted Ebola and were due to be flown back to the United States for further treatment at Emory University in Atlanta.

The two Americans will be flown in a private air ambulance specially equipped to isolate patients with infectious diseases. The first patient is expected to arrive as soon as Saturday, an Emory spokeswoman said.

"We feel that we have the environment and expertise to safely care for these patients and offer them the maximum opportunity for recovery from these infections," said Dr. Bruce S. Ribner, an infectious disease specialist at Emory, in a news conference on Friday.

According to the W.H.O., the $100 million plan "identifies the need for several hundred more personnel to be deployed in affected countries to supplement over-stretched treatment facilities."

Hundreds of international aid workers and W.H.O. specialists "are already supporting national and regional response efforts," the statement said. "But more are urgently required. Of greatest need are clinical doctors and nurses, epidemiologists, social mobilization experts, logisticians and data managers."

As the alarm about the outbreak has grown, so, too, have concerns that the disease will be carried farther afield by travelers from the stricken countries, despite official efforts to tamp down such fears. The African Union, for instance, announced on Friday that it was postponing a routine rotation of its peacekeeping force in Somalia for fear that new soldiers arriving from Sierra Leone could be infected.

The Philippines said Friday that it would screen travelers from Guinea, Sierra Leone and Liberia when they arrived and monitor them for a month. Lebanon was reported to have suspended work permits for residents of the same three countries, news reports said. Emirates, an airline based in Dubai, said it was suspending flights to Conakry as of Saturday.

At the Commonwealth Games in Glasgow, Moses Sesay, a cyclist from Sierra Leone, told the British tabloid the *Daily Mirror* that he had been quarantined for four days and tested for Ebola after feeling ill. He has since been pronounced healthy.

"I was sick. I felt tired and listless," he said. "All the doctors were in special suits to treat me—they dressed like I had Ebola. I was very scared."

Jackie Brock-Doyle, a spokeswoman for the games, told reporters on Friday: "Just to be really clear, there is no Ebola in the athletes' village. There is no Ebola virus in Scotland."

Only weeks after the beginning of the outbreak, the Italian authorities tightened health checks at airports and on ships from West Africa. But epidemiologists in Italy suggested there was little risk that the hundreds of unauthorized migrants who reach southern Italy every day were carrying the virus.

"Migrants cross the desert in journeys that take weeks, if not months, before getting on a boat to Europe," Dr. Massimo Galli, a specialist in infectious diseases at the University of Milan, said in a telephone interview. "They would manifest the disease long before arriving."

*August 1, 2014*

# U.S. Patient Aided Pregnant Liberian, Then Took Ill

## Liberian Officials Identify Ebola Victim in Texas as Thomas Eric Duncan

By NORIMITSU ONISHI

MONROVIA, LIBERIA—A man who flew to Dallas and was later found to have the Ebola virus was identified by senior Liberian government officials on Wednesday as Thomas Eric Duncan, a resident of Monrovia in his mid-40s.

Mr. Duncan, the first person to develop symptoms outside Africa during the current epidemic, had direct contact with a woman stricken by Ebola on Sept. 15, just four days before he left Liberia for the United States, the woman's parents and Mr. Duncan's neighbors said.

In a pattern often seen here in Monrovia, the Liberian capital, the family of the woman, Marthalene Williams, 19, took her by taxi to a hospital with Mr. Duncan's help on Sept. 15 after failing to get an ambulance, said her parents, Emmanuel and Amie Williams. She was convulsing and seven months pregnant, they said.

Turned away from a hospital for lack of space in its Ebola treatment ward, the family said it took Ms. Williams back home in the evening, and that she died hours later, around 3 a.m.

Mr. Duncan, who was a family friend and also a tenant in a house owned by the Williams family, rode in the taxi in the front passenger seat while Ms. Williams, her father and her brother, Sonny Boy, shared the back seat, her parents said. Mr. Duncan then helped carry Ms. Williams, who was no longer able to walk, back to the family home that evening, neighbors said.

"He was holding her by the legs, the pa was holding her arms and Sonny Boy was holding her back," said Arren Seyou, 31, who witnessed the scene and occupies the room next to Mr. Duncan's.

Sonny Boy, 21, also started getting sick about a week ago, his family said, around the same time that Mr. Duncan first started showing symptoms.

In a sign of how furiously the disease can spread, an ambulance had come to their house on Wednesday to pick up Sonny Boy. Another ambulance picked up a woman and her daughter from the same area, and a team of body collectors came to retrieve the body of yet another woman—all four appeared to have been infected in a chain reaction started by Marthalene Williams.

A few minutes after the ambulance left, the parents got a call telling them that Sonny Boy had died on the way to the hospital.

Mr. Duncan had lived in the neighborhood, called 72nd SKD Boulevard, for the past two years, living by himself in a small room that he rented from the Williams couple. He had told that them and his neighbors that his son lived in the United States, played baseball, and was trying to get him to come to America.

For the past year, Mr. Duncan had worked as a driver at Safeway Cargo, the Liberian customs clearance agent for FedEx, said Henry Brunson, the company's manager. In a statement, FedEx said that Mr. Duncan was employed as a personal driver for the company's general manager, not to work for FedEx's global operations.

In an office with a large FedEx sign outside the building in downtown Monrovia, Mr. Brunson said that Mr. Duncan quit abruptly on Sept. 4, giving no reason. But Mr. Brunson said he knew that Mr. Duncan had family members in the United States as well.

"His sister came from the United States and he asked for a day off so that he could go meet her at the Mamba Point Hotel," Mr. Brunson said, mentioning a hotel popular among foreigners. "He quit a few weeks after that."

*October 1, 2014*

CHAPTER 18

# Reproductive Medicine

# The Caesarean Operation

The Caesarean operation was performed at the New-York Post Graduate Medical School and Hospital yesterday for the first time in the history of that institution. This is a dangerous and a rare operation, and it is never resorted to unless the birth of a child cannot be effected by natural means. During the last year there were only eight recorded operations of this kind in the United States.

How many of these were successful there are no available statistics to show, but it is rare that both mother and child survive. It is an operation which has been performed only in desperate cases, although the recent advances in surgery have done much to decrease the danger.

Yesterday's operation was entirely successful, in that both mother and child survived.

*February 8, 1893*

# Birth Made Easy by the Use of Gas

By EMANIE N. SACHS

The doctor sat in a big chair back of a mahogany desk, and his nervous fingers fretted with a bronze paperweight.

"You want to know about the use of laughing gas during childbirth?" he asked, "and you've promised that my name will not be printed?

"Well, it is not new, you know, the use of so-called laughing gas, or nitrous oxide, during labor. As a matter of fact, Klikowitsh of Petrograd used it in twenty-five cases in 1880. It has been used in dentistry for some time, but it has only gradually come into general use in obstetrics. I am not at all certain that it is in general usage even now. Twilight sleep came along with its poetical name and its alluring promises. Eager women seized upon it. In some cases it seized upon them and their infants. It is a potent, dangerous drug. Successful under ideal conditions, but ideal conditions are dismally rare. However, women began to clamor for relief. The use of anesthetics increased and is increasing."

## Complete Anesthesia Harmful

"Ether is not evanescent enough. It has unpleasant after-effects, and should not be given for a prolonged period. Of course, an operative case creates a different situation. There ether may be necessary. Chloroform sends the patient into complete unconsciousness. Labor pains are diminished and the function stopped. The entire enterprise is delayed. Not only is that the physical effect of both ether and chloroform, but there is a psychic effect. The patient's morale is lowered. She is not so inclined to help the physician. Laughing gas is immeasurably superior. It is evanescent. Kemp found that 20 per cent remaining in the blood after administration was reduced in two minutes to 6.09 per cent. The pains are not stopped nor are the uterine contractions which are the motor power for the birth of the child lessened. The woman has her intelligence left, but the edge of the pain is removed. I can say more than that. It is exactly comparable to having a tooth pulled under gas. The woman has no more consciousness of pain than the person in a dentist's chair who may know that there are instruments in his vicinity, but who sinks almost into oblivion when the yank comes. I can conservatively say that the use of laughing gas renders childbirth practically painless."

"This sounds like a cruel question, but I want to get your answer. Does the bearing of intense pain such as women have endured for so long have a bad effect on the woman physiologically?"

"Yes and no," he answered. "The modern woman, of course, is much more highly organized nervously than her mother and her grandmother. Worry destroys some of her resistance.

"It is said that labor pains are soon forgotten. The average woman does not forget them. If she has more children it is under protest. However, I cannot say that there is any definite ill effect from the pain attendant on a normal delivery. I cannot say it definitely, but there are statistics showing that maternal mortality increases in ratio with the longer duration of the woman's sufferings. I have a colleague who goes further than I. He says that the use of nitrous oxide, or laughing gas, not only brings relief to the patient, but that it shortens the duration of labor, permits the doctor to manipulate the child more satisfactorily, saves the tissues of the mother and hastens convalescence."

## Patient Can Give Herself Gas

"Must there be an expert anesthetist on hand during the administration of laughing gas?"

"There is a question for which there are several answers. With an expert anesthetist the birth can be absolutely painless. But there is the problem of the increased liability to use instruments, because the mother being completely unconscious is of no help. The expert mixes the gas with oxygen, which makes it more pleasant. Personally, if my patient is fairly intelligent I let her give it to herself.

"But it is necessary for a doctor to be on the premises at least. Some of my colleagues differ there, believing that the presence of a trained nurse is sufficient. Others even permit a member of the family to turn the plug on the gas tank.

"Have you ever seen a gas tank? Usually one to four tanks are provided on a portable platform about the size of a standard weighing scale. A flexible rubber pipe leads into a rubber bag resembling a football, and a smaller tube empties into an almond-shaped mask which fits over the nose and mouth. The patient feels the pain coming before it really hurts. She places the mask over her face, takes four or five deep respirations and escapes the suffering. It works automatically. She doesn't get too much, because as soon as she is under the influence of the gas her hand relaxes and the mask drops. You know that labor pains usually come more or less rhythmically. One-half hour apart at first, increasing to every five minutes, every two minutes, and so on. For the last stage, the actual birth of the child, we all use a few whiffs of ether, a complete anesthesia."

"Then the patient anesthetizes herself for each pain, with a lapse to consciousness in between?"

"Yes, she begins to come to as soon as the mask drops. The relief has an excellent effect on her morale. She feels that something is being done for her, that she is, in fact, helping herself. She is often willing to stand a few pains in between. You have no idea of the frenzy of pain into which women have at times been plunged. They don't know what they are doing."

"Well, if it's a benevolent agent, why is it not used always?"

"There's a question. The first answer is that the medical profession is the most conservative of bodies. The second answer is concerned with economics. I told you that I believe that a doctor must be present while the gas is in use, which is for the duration of ten or twelve hours possibly—used periodically, remember. And remember also that some of my colleagues do not agree with me on that point. I have a wife and four children to support. I am an attending physician at three hospitals. If I stayed ten or twelve hours with each patient I could not make a living for my family unless I charged a fee far beyond the means of the average person. The presence of a professional anesthetist would, of course, make my presence unnecessary until the very last stage, but it would add materially to the cost as far as the patient was concerned."

"But in the hospitals and in the free wards?"

"If the hospitals are organized to give this service, it can be practically managed there, both for private patients and in the free wards. There are always resident anesthetics who give far more dangerous drugs, ether and chloroform. There are nurses on duty to watch the hearts, in any case. The only additional cost to the hospital would be the actual cost of the gas itself.

"The point, of course, is the time element. The gas is given intermittently for four or ten hours sometimes. I think a rough estimate might indicate that it would cost about $10 for each patient if given nine or ten hours. This means the actual cost of the laughing gas. Of course, if we gave it to each woman in a hospital I know, where we confine about 2,000 women a year, that would add $25,000 to our annual budget.

"A twenty-five-thousand-dollar addition to an annual hospital budget is not to be lightly undertaken, I am afraid," he said gravely, "but when women clamor more and more for relief I am in hopes that the time will come eventually when relief will be freely offered them."

*February 5, 1922*

# Painless Method Is Devised for Childbirth; California Doctor Blocks Spinal Nerves

A method of providing painless childbirth by anesthetizing the nerves carrying pain fibers as they emerge from the spinal cord was reported today by the University of California.

Dr. Herbert F. Traut, chairman of the department of gynecology in the university's Medical School, said that it had been used successfully in about 100 selected cases at the university hospital but he cautioned that it was still experimental. The principle was "very sound," he asserted, adding, "this is why we have such hopes for it." He said, however, that it required expert handling and might never be widely employed by the general practitioner.

Credit for the development of the method was given to Dr. Shiras M. Jarvis, former assistant resident physician at the hospital, who is serving with the Navy in the South Pacific. A news release from the university declared that blocking the pain by means of spinal anesthesia was dangerous to the patient and frequently stopped the progress of labor.

As for caudal anesthesia, which was developed some years ago, the statement quoted Dr. Jarvis as saying that this affected the nerve pathways but "anesthetizes the skin and lowers the muscle tone of the lower body" so that "spontaneous delivery is not the rule."

"The new method, known as paravertebral sympathetic nerve block, affects the nerves that carry the pain to the brain, and at the same time accelerates the first stage of labor," the announcement went on. "It is accomplished by one or more injections into the nerve chains near the spinal vertebrae in the lumbar area of the back.

"Complete safety for mother and baby is maintained at all times and the patient is free to move about in bed, and can sleep or read, as she wishes."

No harmful after-effects have been observed in the experimental cases, it was stated.

*June 3, 1944*

# Birth Control Pills Reported a Success

Successful human use of pills as a method of birth control was reported today by Dr. Benjamin Sieve, who, while asserting he had preliminary success with them, declared further extensive studies must be made "before the general use of this anti-fertility factor is warranted."

The Boston doctor, in a paper in the technical journal *Science*, said 298 married couples had experienced complete lack of fertility during periods ranging from three to thirty months while taking the pills.

He emphasized that the anti-fertility action of the chemical prevailed only while it was being taken. He said 220 of the women have had a baby and had become pregnant since terminating a period of control.

He said that the chemical was first shown to have anti-fertility action in animals by other researchers, and later confirmed in such use by himself. It is called "phosphorylated hesperidin," and Dr. Sieve said it had previously been employed as a chemical to counteract hemorrhage.

The substance "promises safe and controllable anti-fertility," Dr. Sieve said, adding, it "can be taken indefinitely without toxic (harmful) effects or permanent inhibition of fertility."

The pills are taken at breakfast, lunch and dinner in dosages regulated for particular persons—and are taken by both the husband and wife. The pills must be taken for ten consecutive days before their action becomes effective, must be taken continuously thereafter to insure lack of fertility but "fertility can be restored merely by omitting the drug for a forty-eight-hour period."

*October 10, 1952*

# Wider Detection of Prenatal Flaws Expected to Spur Abortions

By WALTER SULLIVAN

Prenatal identification of birth defects has reached the stage where an increasing number of mothers are expected to take advantage of liberalized abortion laws to avoid the birth of children with severe disabilities.

In the long run, mass screening and weeding out of defective fetuses may become possible, but troublesome ethical questions have already arisen.

Where birth defects are suspected, or identified, in a fetus, what are the rights and obligations of the mother, the father, the physician, and the society that may have to render lifelong support to the infant?

What are the rights of the unborn child?

For example it is already possible to identify before birth (and abort) any fetus that will be mongoloid. Since half of all mongoloid children are born to mothers of 35 or older, by screening all such mothers in early pregnancy it should be possible to halve the birth rate of such infants.

It has been estimated by public health specialists that by 1975, if present birth rates continue, the yearly cost of maintaining mongoloids in the United States will have reached $1.75 billion.

## Parley on Problems

Last weekend a conference of specialists in law, genetic screening, obstetrics, abortion, public health and related subjects was held at Columbia University Law School to explore these problems. The subject was "The legal, social, and biological significance of prenatal genetic diagnosis."

The meeting was organized by the Council for Biology in Human Affairs of the Salk Institute in La Jolla, Calif. The participants, many of them distinguished university professors, spoke freely on these delicate subjects since their remarks were "off the record."

The extent of scientific concern in this area was also reflected in the testimony of Dr. Joshua Lederberg, winner of a Nobel Prize for his genetics research. Appearing before a House appropriations subcommittee on Wednesday, he urged formation of a national task force to identify and coordinate research in critical areas of genetics, particularly as they apply to genetic disease.

Prenatal screening depends on a procedure known as amniocentesis. A needle is inserted through the abdomen of the mother and a small amount of amniotic fluid is withdrawn from the sac in which the fetus is floating.

This fluid has special analytical value because it is normally swallowed by the fetus, which also discharges urine into it. The fluid thus contains cells washed from the interior of the fetus, plus cells from its exterior and from the sac.

## Amniotic Fluid Test

All of these cells are genetically part of the baby. About one cell in a thousand is still alive in the withdrawn fluid and can be cultured in the laboratory. During cell division the genetic material forms into chromosomes that can be photographed and sorted to see if the fetus has the proper quota of 23 chromosome pairs, or 46 in all.

If it has 47, with three, instead of two, "No. 21" chromosomes, it will be mongoloid. If it has an abnormal quota of the sex-determining chromosomes, it may either be mentally retarded, prone to violence, stunted, very tall—or normal and even of above-average intelligence.

By allowing the cultured cells to multiply until they number in the millions (they double roughly once every 24 hours), it is possible to test their chemistry for inherited disorders such as those where a particular enzyme is missing and the body chemistry goes awry.

However, while there are some 1,200 genetic diseases—as noted by Dr. Lederberg, a number far larger than most physicians realize—only eight of those involving biochemical defects have been identified so far by prenatal screening.

According to participants in last weekend's conference another 20 or 30 such defects seem within reach, including the enzyme deficiency known as phenylketonuria, or PKU, but the great majority will be difficult to identify in this way.

The reason is that cells found in the amniotic fluid tend to be of the type that evolve into connective tissue, rather than into more specialized organs. The chemical functions within such connective cells, by and large, are not those that figure in inherited disorders.

## Challenge to Researcher

However, like other body cells, those found in the amniotic fluid carry instructions for all body chemistry, even though most of the instructions are latent. Some optimists hope the cells can somehow be coaxed into performing enough of this latent chemistry to show whether or not the person-to-be is destined for trouble.

Another approach is to identify latent genetic defects in the parents. If both parents, although healthy, carry the same latent defect, there is a one-in-four chance that it will appear as a disease in their offspring.

Such latent, or "recessive," genes can now be identified in some cases by a series of chemical tricks. Each individual carries two genes, or bits of genetic instruction, for every human characteristic: one from each parent.

A recessive gene is thought often to be an inoperative part of the genetic code. If it is mated with a normal, or dominant, gene, the latter does the necessary job (such as making a certain enzyme) although usually at only half the rate, had there been two active genes of this type. However if both genes for the process are recessive, the function is not performed, and the person may be seriously affected.

## Radioactive Tagging

Ways have now been found—for example at the University of Colorado—to look into the chemistry of a person's cells and see if a particular recessive gene is there.

This is done in a sample of his body cells by tagging a starting substance with radioactive atoms and seeing if each step of the chemistry runs at full speed. If one step runs at half-speed, a hidden recessive is suspected.

This has already been done, for example, in the case of galactosemia, an inherited disorder in which the body lacks an enzyme needed to process sugars. Death or mental deficiency can result. If both parents carry the recessive gene for this disease, they can be warned of the danger to their offspring.

A major difficulty in performing abortions, once a defect has been identified, is the length of time required for the identification. While attempts to remove amniotic fluid have been reported in pregnancies only eight weeks old, the risk of injury to the tiny fetus at such an early stage is considered too great.

## Time Running Out

By 14 weeks, with the fetus in a cupful of fluid, a skilled specialist can do the job, being careful to locate and avoid both fetus and placenta. By 18 weeks, according to specialists, "any experienced obstetrician" should ultimately be able to carry out the procedure.

However it then takes a week or more to culture the cells and identify their chromosomes. Furthermore in 10 per cent of the cases the procedure may have to be repeated. By then it is close to the 20th week, beyond which time many physicians are reluctant to abort.

The fetus may have begun to move at the 15th week and so the mother, too, may shrink from the procedure.

During the first 13 weeks an abortion is relatively simple, particularly using the suction method devised by the Chinese in the 1950s. Until recently the standard method was to dilate the cervix and scrape the uterus, being careful to remove the tiny placenta, lest prolonged bleeding ensue.

Many physicians now consider the suction method simpler, and kinder to the uterus. A small device inserted by way of the cervix sucks out all that needs to be removed without need for scraping.

A fetus more than 13 weeks old must be removed surgically or "salted out." In the latter procedure some amniotic fluid is withdrawn and replaced with highly saline water. This causes death of the fetus and usually induces labor.

An experimental method, using a slow drip of prostaglandin into the bloodstream, is said to have induced labor in about 90 per cent of women less than 20 weeks pregnant. Prostaglandin is a product of both male and female reproductive systems. The process has to be closely watched, as it may induce vomiting and other side effects.

However, some physicians see it as an early step toward what might become a "do-it-yourself" method for early abortion.

The cost of prenatal genetic screening now exceeds $100, largely because of the laborious process of chromosome isolation. Furthermore, it has only been carried out in early pregnancy on a few hundred women and so recently (largely within the last 18 months) that latent ill-effects have not had much chance to appear.

Nevertheless the results reported so far have spurred optimism. At least partial automation of the analysis and economies from large-scale operation should bring down the cost, leading to forecasts that, at least with women over 35, such tests will become routine.

Should they be made mandatory, like vaccinations? What if a fetus is found to have a defect of the sex chromosomes that does not necessarily lead to an abnormal life? Who decides on abortion, the mother alone or she and the father?

Could an older mother who bears a mongoloid child sue her obstetrician for the cost of supporting such a child, if he did not perform a prenatal test? And to what extent should the Government take advantage of the new capabilities for preventing the birth of individuals destined to a life of misery and dependence?

The conferees last weekend examined these questions, but they were far from agreed on the answers.

*June 13, 1970*

# Woman Gives Birth to Baby Conceived Outside the Body

### By WALTER SULLIVAN

The first authenticated birth of a baby conceived in laboratory glassware and then placed in the uterus of an otherwise infertile mother occurred last night, apparently without complications.

Reports from Oldham General and District Hospital in Lancashire said the baby, a girl, was delivered by Caesarian section, appeared normal and weighed 5 pounds 12 ounces.

The birth culminated more than a dozen years of research and experimentation by Dr. Patrick C. Steptoe, a gynecologist, and Dr. Robert G. Edwards, a Cambridge University specialist in reproductive physiology.

## Unable to Conceive

The parents are Mrs. Lesley Brown, 31 years old, and her husband, John, 38, a railway truck driver from Bristol.

Mrs. Brown in more than 10 years of marriage had been unable to conceive a child because of a defect in the oviducts, or Fallopian tubes, which each month carry egg cells from the ovaries to the uterus. It is during this passage that the egg cells are fertilized.

In the procedure that culminated in last night's birth, an egg cell was removed surgically from Mrs. Brown's ovaries last Nov. 10 and fertilized with sperm from her husband in a petri dish. After two or more days in a laboratory culture, the fertilized embryo was injected into Mrs. Brown's uterus.

More conventional methods had been attempted in an effort to get Mrs. Brown to conceive, including surgical reconstruction of her oviducts. But the efforts failed, and about two years ago she turned to Dr. Steptoe and Dr. Edwards for treatment.

There have been previous reports of so-called "test-tube babies" but none have been authenticated. The Steptoe-Edwards efforts, which failed a number of times, have been followed closely by the medical profession.

While the experimenters have often been frowned upon, they also are highly regarded by many in the field of obstetrics.

443

Working with a succession of patients, Dr. Edwards has gradually improved his ability to manipulate the hormones that control the reproductive cycle.

## Perfection of Technique

Dr. Steptoe has used a surgical procedure known as laparoscopy to enter a woman's abdomen at the appropriate moment in her monthly cycle to retrieve one or more egg cells. The device, placed through a small incision near the navel, illuminates the target area and allows the surgeon to identify and withdraw by suction early mature egg cells.

Once the egg cells have been exposed to sperm, and once microscopic examination after a few days has shown that an embryo is developing normally, the embryo is placed in the uterus with a tube inserted through the cervix.

It is estimated that one-fifth of one-half of women who are sterile are unable to bear children because of absent, defective or blocked oviducts. Because of that, it can be assumed that there will be considerable pressure on physicians to repeat the performance of Drs. Steptoe and Edwards, even though their work is still at a very experimental stage.

The chief problem encountered by the two doctors has been obtaining a satisfactory implant of the embryo in the wall of the uterus.

## Problems with Hormones

In normal reproduction, the embryo lingers a day or more in the oviducts after fertilization and does not implant itself until, through cellular division, it has reached a multi-celled stage.

This process is controlled by hormones issued from various organs, including the ovaries, and from the embryo itself. The early efforts of Drs. Steptoe and Edwards were frustrated because their performing part of this process outside the body upset the hormonal signaling system.

Furthermore, the woman in many of the attempts was given added hormones to induce multiple egg production. The doctors hoped that this would give them more egg cells, improving their chances of success, but the added hormones seemed to throw the normal reproductive system off-balance.

Another fear was that culturing the embryo in glassware for four and a half days, as had been done, might place too severe a strain on it.

## Experiments on Monkeys

Shortly before their removal of one or more egg cells from Mrs. Brown last Nov. 10, it was learned from experiments at the University of Birmingham Medical School that rhesus monkey embryos inserted into the uterus after only one or two cell divisions could survive.

This suggested that the embryos of primates, including man, might differ from other mammals in being able to withstand implantation into the uterus at so early a stage.

Some specialists therefore suspect that Drs. Steptoe and Edwards may have decided to implant Mrs. Brown's embryo after only two days, allowing it to enter the uterus well before its normal implantation stage.

Reports from the hospital, this morning said that the baby was born just before midnight and that its condition was "excellent." Mrs. Brown and her husband were reported to be jubilant.

Once the fetus began developing, its own hormonal signals generated all the effects of a normal pregnancy. Mrs. Brown is reported to have experienced the sort of cravings often reported by pregnant women—in this case, a yearning for mints!

*July 26, 1978*

# Scientists Study Freezing and Storing of Embryos

## By WALTER SULLIVAN

The freezing and storing of embryos, already routine with cattle, could provide an infertile woman with "a whole family" of children after a single egg-harvesting procedure, according to the two doctors who brought such a patient to the successful delivery of a baby girl late last night.

As Drs. Robert G. Edwards and Patrick C. Steptoe have done in previous attempts to overcome infertility over the last 12 years, a doctor would use hormones to stimulate "superovulation," or the simultaneous production of many mature egg cells instead of the usual single cell. The eggs would be surgically removed, exposed to the husband's sperm and cultured briefly in the laboratory.

Then—and this has never been done with humans, as far as is known— the egg cells that showed signs of normal development as fertilized embryos could be frozen.

A month or two later, and at intervals of a year or more, the embryos could be implanted one by one in the woman's uterus and allowed to mature into babies in the normal manner. In this way, according to Drs. Edwards and Steptoe "a whole family could be established."

In the case of Lesley Brown, whose daughter was born last night, only one egg was removed and it was implanted two days later, according to an article on Monday in the *Daily Mail*. This implied that the superovulation technique was not used. The London newspaper and its parent organization, Associated Newspapers, have bought the exclusive rights to personal accounts by those involved.

Mrs. Brown, who will be 31 years old on Monday, and her husband, John, 38, a railway truck driver from Bristol, had been trying for more than a decade to have a child. The difficulty was diagnosed as a defect in the oviducts, where egg cells are fertilized and through which they descend to the uterus.

After various unsuccessful attempts, including surgery, to correct the condition, the Browns turned to Drs. Edwards and Steptoe. Over a two-year period, Mrs. Brown made a number of visits to Dr. Steptoe's clinic in Oldham, a Lancashire mill town, and there may have been several implantation attempts before the successful one, last Nov. 10.

While Drs. Steptoe and Edwards have shunned interviews on the Brown case, they have spelled out to colleagues their idea of producing a number of embryos from one egg-cell harvest. They described the procedure, for example, in a published account of a symposium on embryo freezing that was organized last year by the Ciba Foundation.

Many similar procedures, except for laboratory fertilization, have been used with livestock for some time. Breeders have no reason to produce offspring from an infertile female, so fertilization is achieved in the normal manner, with the embryos flushed out of the uterus.

## Survival for Years

Scientists working with the freezing of animal embryos believe that once an embryo has been chilled to the temperature of liquid nitrogen (minus 321 degrees Fahrenheit), it will survive indefinitely. Lambs have been developed from embryos frozen for two and a half years.

However, the optimum cooling rate and stage of embryo development for freezing varies from one species to another and can be learned only through experimentation.

The freezing technique has already led to extraordinary juggling of generations, including a case in which a lamb was born to its sister. After both embryos were flushed from the uterus of a ewe that had been stimulated to superovulate, one was implanted in a foster mother. The other was frozen until its sister was full grown, whereupon it was thawed and implanted in the sister. It developed into a healthy lamb.

Experiments with freezing livestock embryos have been intended primarily to facilitate shipment of new, highly productive strains. Another goal, however, is establishing deep-frozen "embryo banks" that would preserve the genetic diversity of domestic animals, laboratory mice and endangered wildlife.

Establishing such banks is a goal of Dr. Christopher Polge of the Animal Research Station of Britain's Agricultural Research Council near Cambridge, England. In a recent interview, he said that normal young had developed from once-frozen embryos of cows, sheep, goats, rabbits, rats, and mice.

## Concerns Over New Strains

Embryo banks could be the answer to fears that new livestock strains, while highly productive, may be more vulnerable to new diseases or environmental changes than those being allowed to pass out of existence. Similar fears have led to the creation of international repositories for grain seeds.

In the freezing experiments with animals, variations have been shown in the procedures required for successful freezing and thawing of embryos. For example, early experiments with mice by Drs. Peter Mazur and S. P. Leibo of the Oak Ridge National Laboratory in Tennessee, working with Dr. David G. Whittingham of Britain, showed that survival rates are high only when the embryos are cooled and thawed very slowly.

Routine implantations of thawed cattle embryos have been initiated in recent months by a Lincolnshire company, T. H. Saul Embryos of East Heckington, working with a veterinary group. According to Dr. Polge's colleagues, the concern has already done 200 implants; most of which involved an exceptionally productive strain of Friesian dairy cattle, the embryos are inserted through the foster mother's flank, with a 50 percent success rate.

This is said to be the first commercial application of the method, although some efforts have also been reported from New Zealand. Researchers hope to develop nonsurgical insertion, which has been done with humans—in Dr. Steptoe's method, the embryo is placed into the uterus through a tube inserted in the cervix.

The shipping of frozen embryos has largely supplanted an earlier practice, in which rabbits were used to transport cattle embryos. The chemistry of the rabbit uterus is sufficiently similar to that of a cow to sustain such an embryo for four or five days, long enough to fly samples of exotic strains as far as Australia.

Today, however, such shipments are ruled out by quarantine regulations against such ailments as foot and mouth disease. Only frozen embryos can be stored long enough to demonstrate that its parents were disease-free.

Freezing human embryos, as Drs. Steptoe and Edwards have proposed, would provide enough time before implantation to screen the embryo for genetic defects.

Such screening could also be used to determine the sex of the embryo. This, according to Dr. Polge, has already been done in cattle, sheep and rabbits. Only embryos of the desired sex would be implanted.

As noted by Dr. Polge, efforts have been made to "determine" the sex of an embryo by exposing an egg cell only to male sperm. Segregating sperm that carry the male and female "signals," however, has proved difficult.

*July 26, 1978*

CHAPTER 19

# Surgery

# Transfusion of Blood: Revival of the Operation in Modern Surgery

As a matter of curious information, it was noted some weeks ago, in the course of a brief description of a new instrument for the transfusion of blood, devised by Dr. A. Clendinen, of Fort Lee, that the operation has been increasing in popularity among physicians in general practice during the last few months, and is now favorably discussed by surgeons of high reputation. Dr. Clendinen, as a surgeon in the Confederate service, practiced it with success as a life-saving measure in cases of threatened collapse from hemorrhage, during the war, and has since perfected a method of operating with the instrument, immersed in water heated a little above tissue temperature, which has been favorably spoken of in the Medical Society of the State of New-Jersey. The experiments of Prof. T. Gaillard Thomas, whose surgical rank is undisputed, in transfusing moribund patients with milk rendered alkaline by forms of ammonia or soda, or injected without previous preparation other than attention to temperature, have been fully discussed in the medical and secular journals. Their successful issue was undoubted, and tended to raise the question—settled by recent experiments with albumen—of the capacity of such vital albuminous compounds as animal blood to digest and appropriate food, independent of gastric action. The digestive action of fresh blood on milk has been carefully observed by micro-physiologists, by adding traces of the latter to small quantities of the former placed in microscopic cells and maintained at an even temperature of 90° Fahrenheit during the examination. Blood, then, according to these observations, being capable of digesting milk, there is, to use the words of an eminent practitioner, "no good reason why it should not digest beef-juice, nor why that efficient nutrition should not be injected directly into the circulation in cases of extreme and persistent nausea, whether arising from gastric cancer, from simple gastritis, or from causes less intimately understood than these diseases."

A very full and careful exposition of the present standing of transfusion was recently given by Dr. Joseph W. Howe, Clinical Professor of Surgery in Bellevue Hospital Medical College, before the Brooklyn Anatomical and Surgical Society,* without, however, raising the fundamental question whether the blood of the inferior animals, as, for instance, the lamb or the calf, when injected into the venous system of man, passes into the circulation unaltered, and becomes a part of the life-basis of the patient without metamorphosis, or whether it is transformed and appropriated by a process akin to digestion. There is also the question whether, when the blood has

450

become deficient in corpuscular elements by long-continued and wasting disease, the restoration of the normal specific gravity brought about by transfusion is a factor in the recovery. Or is the increase of volume important? Or, finally, is the disturbance of the equilibrium, together with the stimulant to heart action thus furnished, a primary factor in the amendment? These are among the points which the resuscitated popularity of the operation has raised with experimental physiologists, and their solution will no doubt be forthcoming in a few months, unless, as has frequently occurred before after a brief notoriety, the subject drops into oblivion in consequence of some untoward accident.

Ovid, in his *Metamorphoses*, speaks of Medea as renewing the youth and vitality of aged men by transfusing them with blood medicated with vegetable extracts; but it is not until the times of Savonarola that any authentic record of the operation as a life-saving measure occurs. The story is a familiar one. Pope Innocent VIII, as he verged upon senility, became subject to attacks of coma, which menaced his life, and which his physician thought he could avert by resort to transfusion with the blood of a younger and more vigorous manhood. As he who supplied the Papal circulation would be essentially Pope, the physician did not find it very difficult to obtain the services of two healthy young men. His method of procedure was first to bleed his Holiness, and then to inject the blood taken from the Papal circulation into the veins of one of the young men. When it had been sufficiently renovated and imbued with vigor by circulating in the system of the self-sacrificing youth, the lad was bled profusely, and the supposedly rejuvenated life-current transferred to the circulation of the Pontiff. The experiment was repeated with the second candidate, but the result was unsuccessful.

This was a case of venous transfusion. Libavio, in 1615, resuscitated the idea by connecting the arteries of the giver and receiver with silver tubes, and 50 years later Lower, of Oxford, performed the series of experiments on dogs described in his work *De Corde item Motu, Colore et Transfusione Sanguinis, et de Venae Sectione,*" a copy of which (Leyden edition of 1708) was recently presented to the Anatomical and Surgical Society by Dr. E. H. Hartley, with a short disquisition on the book and the impulse given by Lower's successful operations—as described in the *Philosophical Transactions* for 1660, and in his letter to Robert Boyle—to the practice of transfusion in Europe. Lower's process was to bleed a small dog until the animal was moribund, then to connect the venous system of the dying creature with the cervical artery of a larger animal, with a heavier vascular pressure. When the smaller dog began to evince symptoms of plethora, the supplying artery was tied, and the bleeding was repeated until vital exhaustion supervened. Lower continued the experiment until he had exhausted the circulation of two large dogs in repeatedly reviving the small one. He then closed the jugular vein, after, as he says, removing a quantity of blood equal to the weight of the animal's body, and replacing it from the circulation of the two animals killed during the experiment. When released from the straps of the experiment table, the little fellow jumped down in the liveliest possible manner, wagged his tail in token of satisfaction, rolled on the grass, and trotted off, sustained evidently by the consciousness of having done something for science. At least, such is a fair version of Lower's not over-classical Latin. The rubber tubing, which plays such an important part in Clendinen's instrument, Lower compensated with a section of the cervical artery of the horse, in order to connect his canulae with a flexible conductor, and to prevent the spasmodic struggles of the two animals from vitiating the experiment.

Denis, of Paris, seized the idea as a remedial measure, and injected 10 ounces of lamb's blood into the veins of a young man who had been bled for fever until demise was imminent. The patient recovered. Denis's next exploit was to transfuse an insane patient with 9 ounces of calf's blood. The man recovered his mental balance, but was again attacked with aberration after a few months of sanity, and died in a few days. The death of this patient created a determined opposition to transfusion, although it had once restored the man's disordered wits; and the operation was forbidden by law, except under circumstances that rendered it impracticable.

From the date of Denis's operation until 1825, when Dr. James Blondell, of London, repeated Lower's experiments, and demonstrated that dogs could be resuscitated by transfusion after respiration and action of the heart had been suspended for four minutes, and they were virtually dead—as general death, in distinction from local or tissue death, is now understood by physiologists. Blondell also proved experimentally that animal life could be maintained without food for three weeks by occasionally injecting fresh blood into the circulatory system, and was successful in a number of cases in averting death from hemorrhage.

Prof. Howe cites Morton's statistics, showing 58 per cent of recoveries in the performance of the operation for hemorrhage, and then reverts to his own experience, which covers three successful cases in hemorrhage; one for malignant syphilitic ulceration, with pigmentation of the skin and ecthymatous pustules; four of less marked vital degeneration than the preceding, but from the same cause; and a large number of cases of pulmonary consumption, in all of which temporary improvement has followed. The most remarkable benefits were obtained, however, in the cases of the incurable ulceration and decay of tertiary disease, the sores healing as if by magic, the pigmentation disappearing, and the pustular eruption yielding readily, where iodide of potassium, tonics, and all the usual remedies had signally failed. Prof. Van Buren made one of these cases the topic of a clinical dissertation not long ago. After the ulcers healed, the man, whose case was complicated with pulmonary phthisis, had a severe attack of hemorrhage from the lungs, for which he was again transfused. A third transfusion finished the treatment; and when last reported the tuberculous deposits in the pulmonary system were gradually breaking down, and there was a good prospect of recovery for a man who had been an inmate of a pauper hospital for years. The case suggests that transfusion in leprosy might possibly eventuate in recovery, particularly if the blood introduced were to be previously treated with the hyposulphite of ammonia or of soda. Prof. Howe defibrinates the blood to be injected and mixes it usually with ammonia.

The advance in method of operating calls for a running review. The old practice was to open a vein in the arm of the donor, remove about seven fluid ounces of blood, whip it with glass rods to defibrinate it, then strain it, and perform the injection with a syringe of the common pattern. According to the statement of his paper, Prof. Howe's original practice was to use Dieulafoy's aspirator—a familiar instrument in the surgical shops—mixing the blood taken from the donor's arm with a solution of ammonia, previously introduced into the cylinder of the instrument. This proved a very satisfactory mode of operating, and in all, the Professor performed 13 transfusions with it before Collin's instrument attracted his attention. The latter consists of a basin-shaped reservoir, from the bottom of which an opening feeds the cylinder of an ordinary syringe placed at right angles to its perpendicular axis. A rubber tube terminating in a canula completes the instrument, with the exception of a ball valve guarding the entrance to the tube and excluding the passage of air, while permitting that of a fluid of such high specific gravity as blood or milk. The point of the canula fits hermetically, by simple pressure, into the opening of a second canula containing a probe-pointed stylet, which Prof. Howe prefers to the trocar for puncturing the walls of the vein. The instrument is warmed in a basin of water of finely graduated temperature.

Aveling's instrument, which that devised by Dr. Clendinen, although guarding more carefully against clots and air-bubbles, closely resembles in principle and mode of operation; differs from the Collin in transferring the blood directly from the giver to the receiver; but the risk of forming and introducing coagula, with blood not deprived of its fibrin, is, Prof. Howe thinks, a decidedly objectionable feature. The instrument employed by Prof. Thomas, in his recent transfusions of milk (*Medical Record* for 1879) was a simple glass funnel, over the point of which was drawn a rubber tube, furnished with a canula, to be introduced into the vein.

In operating, the general rule with expert surgeons is to select the cephalic vein just above the end of the elbow, first cutting down upon it by a longitudinal incision with the scalpel or the curved bistoury, then separating it from the surrounding cellular tissue with the director. This done, lift the vessel from its bed, very gently, with the forceps, and make a transverse incision sufficiently large to introduce the canula. Ligation below the opening, and over the canula, involving the use of two ligatures in all—formerly regarded as indispensable to the operation—has been abandoned by such expert operators as Prof. Howe, whose transverse incision acts like a valve, and enables the assistant to retain the canula in place by a gentle pressure of the finger. The incision in the cephalic vein of the donor should always be an ample one, in order to obviate the danger of coagulation while the operator is defibrinating. The current is received in a cold vessel and beaten rapidly with the glass rods tor four or five minutes, then strained through a piece of white satin into a glass vessel, whipped again with glass rods for two minutes, finally strained again through a second piece of white satin, and the dish set in a basin of water at a temperature of 110° Fahrenheit, where it remains for about five minutes, with the instrument and all its connections, to insure perfect uniformity. During these five minutes the operator exposes the cephalic vein of the patient, inserts the canula, closed by its stylet, and prepares for the work. The further successive steps are to pour the seven or eight ounces of blood into the receptacle of the instrument, which now contains the required quantity of ammoniac solution; draw the handle of the syringe, fill the cylinder, expel the air, withdraw the stylet, which the blood follows, connect the two canula, and work the piston slowly and steadily, observing carefully the pulse and respiratory movements of the patient, taking care to obtain the earliest notice of any pain in head or back, dizziness, momentary loss of vision, or sense of pulmonary oppression. The perils to avoid are possible paralysis of the heart by altering the vascular pressure too rapidly, introduction of clot, or infection of air, which, although usually supposed to be death, is not necessarily fatal, unless the bubble is a very large one.

While it is not very probable that Dr. Howe's enthusiasm will draw after him a large concourse of surgical disciples, it will perhaps lead to a thorough reinvestigation, when the Fall season opens, of the physiological relations of transfusion. With the sphygmoscope, devised by Prof. Stephens, an instrument better adapted than the sphygmograph to the study of the pulse of the lower animals, and the instrumental and clinical facilities furnished by veterinary colleges, one may expect to see questions of this class settled by carefully registered experimentation, in place of Lower's fantastic guesswork and Blondell's vague generalizing statements.

*Annals of the Anatomical and Surgical Society*, May, 1880. Edited by Charles Jewett, M.D.

*June 19, 1880*

# The Healing Knife: A Revolution in Surgery

By LEONARD ENGEL

Not long ago a 96-year-old woman was brought into a New York hospital with a broken hip. Fifteen years ago she would immediately have been put in a cast and immobilized in bed. And—since old people tolerate immobility poorly—the odds were that she would have been dead in two weeks.

Instead, she was taken to the operating room. There the hip was pinned together with a long nail driven down through the center of the bone. She was out of bed the next day and out of the hospital twelve days later, her hip usable and well on the mend.

This saving of a life was surely wonderful. But it is not unusual. During the past twenty-five years revolutionary advances have taken place in surgery. Surgeons can now even perform the spectacular feat of opening the heart at will—and even stopping it if necessary in order to make repairs deep inside.

Today, literally no part of the human body is beyond the reach of the healing knife. Segments of major arteries, blocked or weakened by disease, can be replaced nearly at will. Removing diseased sections of lung to prevent recurrence of tuberculosis and for other purposes is commonplace. Surgery has developed high skill in treating multiple injuries of appalling severity, as well as the major burns from gasoline that the automobile age has so sharply increased. Even the liver and pancreas, two organs that have been particularly resistant to surgery, can now be operated on successfully.

Surgeons have not only mastered new operative procedures. The benefits of life-saving surgery have also been extended to three great categories of patients largely excluded from this treatment a generation ago—the very old, the very young and the very sick.

Currently the United States is served by about 30,000 surgeons, of whom over 20,000 have met the stringent requirements for admission to the American College of Surgeons. (Of the others, several thousand are young men who have completed their training as specialists but who have not practiced surgery long enough to be admitted to the college.) They work in some 17,000 operating rooms in more than 6,500 hospitals. They perform well over 10,000,000 operations a year (not counting minor surgery on ambulatory clinic patients).

A far larger proportion of patients than ever before come safely through their operations. An example is the operation for closing a *patent ductus*, a serious and fairly frequent inborn defect of the great blood vessels from the heart. When this operation—one of the first successful heart operations—was first done, as many as one patient in ten failed to make it; now, 199 of 200 come through. In more routine surgery, such as removal of the appendix, deaths are almost wholly confined to patients with severe complications.

But operative mortality rates do not accurately measure progress in surgery. For, when operations—such as those on the heart—are first performed, they are often accompanied by deaths, both because there are some things that surgeons cannot learn in the animal laboratory and because the first candidates for a hazardous new operation are generally individuals already at death's door.

A truer reflection of surgical progress is given by patients like the 96-year-old lady with the broken hip, or those of Dr. Robert E. Gross of Children's Hospital in Boston. Dr. Gross, although he is even better known for his work in heart surgery, has been a pioneer in surgery upon the newborn. He has even performed major operations upon hundreds of premature infants (usually to correct birth defects incompatible with life). One of Dr. Gross's diminutive patients was a baby girl who weighed but 2 lbs. 6 ozs. at the time he saved her life with a major abdominal operation. Such patients are, in the language of the operating room, poor risks. They have little or no reserve strength. More deaths are to be expected among them than among older children or adults in good general health except for the illness or injury that brings them to the surgeon. It is a great achievement that the overwhelming majority of even very poor risk patients nowadays recover.

What has made possible the dramatic extension of surgery to new parts of the body and new classes of patients? It isn't greater manual dexterity. For the surgeons of today do not have more dexterous hands than the Theodor Billroths or other great surgeons of the past, any more than modern painters have better hands than Rembrandt.

The striking advances are primarily the result of a tremendously intensified application of the simple principle underlying all modern surgery. This is to design the operation and conduct both it and associated treatment so as to hold disturbance of the patient and his internal machinery to an absolute minimum.

Surgeons call this the "conservative" approach to surgery. Paradoxically, it is astonishing what radical operations are possible if the operation is designed and executed conservatively.

Rudiments of this concept of surgery are to be found in the work of individual surgeons of many eras. But the real architect of the conservative approach as a systematic method of surgery was William Stewart Halsted, the fastidious genius who came to Johns Hopkins Medical School as teacher of surgery in 1889. Dr. Halsted drank only coffee brewed from beans he himself had selected, one by one; for years he sent his shirts to Paris to be laundered because he could find in Baltimore no laundry that did them to his taste. He exhibited the same fussiness in his surgery.

In a day when surgeons still worked fast (a hangover from the pre-anesthetic era, when slashing speed was essential), Halsted operated with exasperating deliberation and care. In making an incision, he spent hours tying off blood vessels, one at a time, in order to keep blood loss as low as possible; in closing the wound, he matched layer on layer of muscle, connective tissue and skin with painstaking precision. Where others took an hour for an operation, Halsted took four or six. To the astonishment of his contemporaries, his patients not only survived, they did much better than the patients of other surgeons.

Since Halsted, meticulous care to minimize injury to the patient has been the watchword in the operating room. Thanks to modern research, however, the surgeon today has far greater knowledge than Halsted and his colleagues—or the surgeons of 1930—of what must be done to protect the patient. So the present-day surgeon can do more kinds of surgery on more patients.

The new ways in which the patient is safeguarded may be summarized under seven main headings. They are:

- Advances in diagnosis.

- Attention to nutrition.

- Safer anesthetics and methods of administering them.

- Use of antibiotics and other new antibacterial drugs.

- Making up losses of blood and other body fluids and preventing changes in the chemical composition of the blood.

- Application of sound physiological principles to the surgery itself, that is, to what the surgeon is trying to do as well as the procedure for carrying it out.

- Better post-operative care, especially the development of the recovery room.

When the patient arrives in a hospital for surgery, the surgeon knows, or quickly learns, a good deal more about his illness than the surgeon of a generation ago. Most of the basic tools of diagnosis, such as X-ray, were in existence by 1930. But there has since been a remarkable multiplication of techniques for using them. Almost any region of the body, from the chambers of the heart and the lobes of the brain to blood vessels in the toes, can be studied and troubles diagnosed with precision in advance of surgery. So the surgeon knows far better what he will find when the patient is on the operating table.

Many patients, especially those needing abdominal surgery, are likely to be extremely undernourished as a result of their illness. Experience has shown that patients weakened by malnutrition are poor surgical risks. So every artifice of nutritional science, from special diets to intravenous feeding, is employed nowadays to build them up before operation. The practice has saved the lives of thousands who at one time could scarcely be considered for surgery.

When the patient entered the operating room twenty-five years ago, he was apt to be deeply anesthetized. Deep anesthesia was the only means by which the muscular relaxation necessary in many operations could be achieved. Today, anesthesia is held to the bare minimum necessary to avoid pain; and such drugs as curare provide muscular relaxation.

The muscle-relaxants are but one of numerous innovations that have strikingly altered anesthesia. In the first place, it's recognized now that all anesthetics are more or less noxious and potentially dangerous to anyone sick or injured enough to need surgery. So anesthetics are used sparingly, and their use is hedged about by special precautions, special instruments and supplementary drugs to offset any possible adverse effects of the anesthetics and to make sure the patient is getting enough oxygen. In the second place, with its ever-widening armory of agents and methods, anesthesia can now be shaped to the requirements of almost any patient or any operation whatever. Thus, there are special procedures for diabetics (who tolerate ether poorly), for such new operative departures as surgery within the chest, and so on.

In operating rooms today, as in Dr. Halsted's operating room, blood vessels are painstakingly shut off to minimize blood loss. But the present-day surgeon and his aides also keep track of all blood lost (by drawing it into a measuring glass with a suction machine) and replace it by transfusion, literally as it is lost. Fluid lost by perspiration and evaporation from the wound is carefully replaced, too. Even the chemical composition of the blood is checked—illness, surgery, anesthesia, all may make it more acid than normal or bring about other chemical changes—and immediate steps are taken to correct any alterations detected. As a consequence, surgical shock—once a terror of the operating room—is now uncommon, though desperately sick patients prone to shock are operated on every day.

In well-run operating rooms, the first line of defense against infection remains the traditional aseptic procedure—rigorous sterilization of everything that may come into contact with the patient's wound.

Antibiotics and other antibacterial drugs are, of course, a powerful modern defense. Curiously, one of their effects has been to do away with much surgery. Operations like mastoidectomy (which once filled children's surgical wards every winter) are now uncommon; penicillin and its partners halt the ear infections that give rise to mastoiditis.

The antibiotics have also greatly simplified some operations (for bone infections, for instance) and made possible others that could not have been done before at all. An example is the removal of tuberculous tissue from the lung—a procedure that has dramatically speeded the restoration of thousands of TB patients to health. Such operations would be too hazardous to be widely attempted without streptomycin and isoniazid to prevent the spread of TB germs to other parts of the body. In addition, antibiotics have proved an invaluable backstop against infection in general surgery; for some wound infections do occur despite the most scrupulous sterile precautions.

The numerous advances we have been discussing have all, of course, had a part in the most spectacular recent development in surgery—open-heart surgery, an achievement all the world has marveled at in the last few years. As with other important new operations, though, success has come because the operations are based on an ever-growing understanding of the workings of the human machine.

To make repairs inside the heart, Drs. C. Walton Lillehei and Richard L. Varco of the University of Minnesota and Dr. John W. Kirklin of the Mayo Clinic lay the heart open for periods of from ten or fifteen minutes to an hour or more. This can be done because a heart-lung machine oxygenates and pumps blood for the patient meanwhile. The Minnesota surgeons have a heart-lung machine devised at Minnesota; Dr. Kirklin uses a machine developed by Dr. J. H. Gibbon of Jefferson Medical College in Philadelphia.

The heart-lung machines are a product of the physiology laboratory. They are an example—one of the great ones in medical history—of the basic interrelationship of physiology, medicine and surgery. They were developed successfully because Dr.

Lillehei and his colleagues and Dr. Gibbon had a thorough understanding of the heart and circulatory system, and saw clearly what a heart-lung machine must do.

Last but not least, surgery has been significantly advanced by improvements in post-operative care. There have been many of these, but the single most important has been the introduction of the recovery room, a small ward near the operating rooms under the direction of an anesthesiologist or surgeon equipped to deal in seconds with every conceivable emergency that might arise during the first critical hours after an operation.

In nearly all large U.S. hospitals and in many small ones, it is now routine for patients who have undergone general anesthesia (except for those it would be hazardous to move) to spend twenty-four hours or even longer in the recovery room. At first—back in the early 1940s—hospitals grumbled at the necessity for finding space for such rooms and funds to equip them. They have paid such handsome dividends in lives saved, however, that medical reports glow with satisfaction on the subject.

Conspicuously, surgery in recent years has been steadily transformed into a group undertaking. As many as a dozen-and-a-half people may take part in a long, complex operation. A score of others will be involved in the care of the patient before or after the operation.

The great increase in operating room and surgical-care personnel is chiefly a reflection of the growth of conservative practices in surgery; there are simply too many ways in which the patient must be safeguarded for the surgeon and a nurse or two to do the job. Burdensome as in some ways they are, the new means of protecting the patient have brought surgery to new heights of daring in saving life and health.

*September 8, 1957*

CHAPTER 20

# Transplants

# The Marvels Wrought by Plastic Surgery

Immured within the walls of the Rockefeller Institute for Medical Research as in a fortress, inaccessible and assailed in vain by the most bitter of the anti-vivisectionists, Dr. Alexis Carrel is carrying on wonderful experimental work in plastic surgery, which, in the view of many of the foremost men in the medical world to-day, is destined to entitle him to rank forever with the great pioneers of medicine and surgery.

Shrinking from publicity and appearing only at rare intervals before some ultra-scientific body to tell of the successful transplantation of organs and tissues from a dead or living animal to another living animal, the world hears but little of him and his work. Distinguished surgeons, admitting their inability to do the things that Dr. Carrel does with ease, speak of his achievements as marvelous.

Lest it be thought that Dr. Carrel's theories and experimental work have as yet no practical application in regard to the conservation of human life, let us consider the following case:

On March 4 last a daughter was born to a well-known surgeon of this city and his wife. The child weighed 8 pounds and 12 ounces at birth and appeared to be strong and healthy. In a few hours, however, it developed melaena neonatorum, which signifies "hemorrhage of the new born," a disease of the first two weeks of life and whose prognosis is extremely grave, the mortality ranging from 50 to 80 per cent. The child bled from the mouth, nose and intestines, and vomited blood. On March 8 the baby was near death.

In this extremity the surgeon-father invoked the aid of Dr. Carrel, with whose skill and theories he was familiar. Dr. Carrel, assisted by Dr. George E. Brewer, Surgeon to Roosevelt Hospital, proceeded as follows.

## Case of Blood Transfusion

The right leg of the child was held firmly and an incision was made in the hollow back of the knee, exposing a large vein which was severed. An incision was then made in the left wrist of the child's father and the radial artery, or pulse, exposed. This artery likewise was cut, and Dr. Carrel, whose technique in this line of work is described as amazing by his confreres, then proceeded to sew an end of the father's severed artery to an end of the child's severed vein.

Here was direct transfusion of blood. For some time the father's blood was allowed to flow into the anaemic and impoverished system of the child. In a few moments the baby's skin took on a healthy glow. As if by magic the vomiting and hemorrhage ceased, not to recur. In a word, the child was dying one minute, the next minute was a strong, healthy child. To-day this child weighs 6 pounds more than another born within a few days of it.

Dr. S. W. Lambert, commenting upon the foregoing case, said:

"The striking thing in the case is that the disease ceased suddenly and the child was cured from the moment of the transfusion of blood."

One of the most distinguished surgeons in America declared that this daring procedure demonstrated the fact that whereas, if the child had died, it would have been believed that the hemorrhages were the result of deficiencies in the walls of the blood vessels, yet the method of curing the baby proved absolutely that the disease was due to some deficiency in the blood itself. The healthy blood of the father, he declared, had brought about the required chemical change in the child's blood. He added that Dr. Carrel's method of direct transfusion was a distinct improvement over the old method of using a glass tune as an intermediary. The old method he characterized as dangerous, explaining that a clot might be formed in the tube and that this might be carried through the patient's lungs and to the heart, causing instant death.

But what of the transplantation of organs in the human being? The substitution of a healthy kidney for a diseased one? Are these miracles about to be accomplished? Dr. Carrel says so, and points out that he is accomplishing such things almost daily in his laboratory in the Rockefeller Institute in the cases of lower animals.

## Some Possibilities Expected

The possibility of such physical regenerations in man is predicted by Dr. Simon Flexner, Director of the Rockefeller Institute. He does not promise that it will be possible right away to give a man a new heart or stomach or kidneys in place of the ones that may be ready to fail him, but be holds out hope that some day medical science will be able to do that very thing. He declares that these substitutions will be made possible through the new experimental surgery and vivisection, and will revolutionize modern medicine.

The successful transplanting of arteries from one animal to another, he says, was the first step toward this end.

"The technical surgical operations involved in this kind of experimentation, on account of the necessity of maintaining unimpaired the circulation of the blood, are great," says Dr. Flexner, "but no effort should be spared to reach this goal."

"It is a matter of no small significance that arteries can be transplanted successfully from dog to cat, and vice versa, and from man to dog, and that keeping extirpated arteries under sterile conditions at refrigerator temperature for twenty or thirty days, or even longer, does not interfere with the results of transplantation."

Dr. Carrel is a native of France. He is a young man, still in the thirties, and was graduated from the University of Lyons. Immediately after graduation he took up original research work involving laboratory experimentation similar to that he is now engaged in. After spending a considerable period in Lyons he was induced to continue his researches in the laboratories of McGill University in Montreal. Then he was sought out by the University of Chicago, and he carried on his work there for two years. By this time his work as an original investigator had become widely known in scientific circles, and two years ago Dr. Flexner induced him to pursue his researches in the Rockefeller Institute.

The latest of Dr. Carrel's rare semi-public appearances was made before the American Philosophical Society in Philadelphia, of which Dr. W. W. Keen, the distinguished surgeon, is President. This society, founded by Benjamin Franklin, who was also its first President, in 1743, has the distinction of being the oldest scientific society in America. Thomas Jefferson was its second President. The transactions of this society reach similar organizations all over the world, and it was to disseminate more generally a knowledge of Dr. Carrel's work that he was urged to appear before it. He gave an illustrated lecture, showing some of the remarkable things he has accomplished. It is notable, however, that the word vivisection was not mentioned by Dr. Carrel at the meeting.

One experiment described by him indicates in itself the tremendous significance of his work and foreshadows its value in the relief of human suffering when the methods of procedure shall have been perfected. Following is an experiment which Dr. Carrel described as a "simple transplantation":

Having anaesthetized a cat so that the subsequent operation was absolutely painless, Dr. Carrel removed the kidneys, together with their blood vessels, the aorta (the largest artery in the body), the vena cava (the largest vein in the body), the nerves, the nervous ganglia (or centres), the urethers (the tubes running from the kidneys to the bladder), and part of the bladder. These organs were replaced by similar organs from another cat. The cat with the new organs recovered and the organs resumed their functions.

"No therapeutic value can be expected from a graft of kidneys," said Dr. Carrel, in commenting on this particular experiment, "unless the secretions of the new organs should be practically normal." Dr. Carrel performed somewhat similar experiments, though not on as extensive a scale as the foregoing, on dogs at the University of Lyons as early as 1902, and again in Chicago in 1905. The first transplantation in mass was made by Dr. Carrel, assisted by Dr. Guthrie, at the University of Chicago, in 1906. He modified and improved his methods of procedure in the Rockefeller Institute last year.

"All resources of modern surgery must be used," said Dr. Carrel, "to prevent infection and shock after such an operation."

Up to Jan. 1, 1908, Dr. Carrel said he had effected fourteen such transplantations in mass. Five of the animals died and nine recovered, a most encouraging ratio. In all nine cases the functions of the kidneys were re-established.

These and many other experiments were described by Dr. Carrel in his Philadelphia lecture. He told how the leg of one dog had been grafted on another dog, and of how the glands of an animal were kept in cold storage for sixty days and then successfully transplanted.

At the conclusion of the lecture Dr. Keen said:

"While it may seem rather a dream, it is quite possible from what we have heard to-night that the time may come when it will be possible for a human being who is possessed of defective kidneys, for instance, to go to some hospital and have a fresh, healthy set taken out of the refrigerator for his benefit."

Dr. Carrel was asked if such a thing could be done.

"Most assuredly it could be done," he replied. "I could do it now, and it would be an easier operation to perform on a man than on a dog or cat. The great trouble is, who is going to supply the fresh, healthy kidneys?"

### Transplanting Arteries

Dr. Carrel explained that in these transplantation operations—for instance, in the case of arteries—the first thing for the surgeon to accomplish was the immediate establishment of blood circulation. In this act the tissue must needs be kept alive outside of the body of the animal. The skill and technique of the work lay in the suture or sewing together of the two parts.

Dr. Carrel showed enlarged photographs of arteries which had been joined and through which blood had been coursing for months, which showed to the lay eye no sign of even a scar, only an experienced surgeon being able to distinguish the exact spot of the jointure.

The animals subjected to these experiments, Dr. Carrel said, were etherized in a room which had been thoroughly sterilized. The physicians were encased in sterilized masks and coverings, as the slightest infection would ruin the experiments. The animals suffered no pain and received as good, if not better, care than human beings would in the best equipped hospitals. He proved this by showing photographs of animals before and in the course of operations, compared with photographs of the same animals months and years afterward, in which they were seen to be jumping and skipping about in apparently complete health.

"Some time ago," Dr. Carrel said, "I received a human leg from a New York hospital. I removed some of the arteries and put them in a dog, which easily survived the operation and remained healthy. I opened the dog later and found that it was doing beautifully. The important thing is whether the tissue from animals can be used in man."

It was explained after the lecture that this had been done in minor ways.

Dr. Carrel showed pictures on the screen of the operation of grafting the leg of a dog which had just died on the stump of a leg of a fox terrier. The bones knit and the tissues healed and grew and remained healthy. Kidneys, glands, and veins were shifted between animals with success.

In response to the attacks of the anti-vivisectionists, Dr. Flexner already has answered them through *The Times*. He said:

"The people who oppose the use of animals in scientific research may be sincere enough—I do not doubt that. But they are ignorant, misguided, or misinformed. Their efforts are based, as often as not, purely on sentiment.

"To pass a law restricting or preventing vivisection on such a basis would be a grave injustice. Let these people inform themselves of the facts. Let them know what the use of these animals means to medicine and to mankind. Then let the law be offered only after full investigation.

"Birds and animals are being constantly put to death to supply mankind with adornments or for no reason at all. Birds are killed that their feathers may be used for women's hats—killed in the mating season, for only when birds are mating is their plumage at its best. Animals are killed for their furs. They are caught in traps and thereby subjected to pain greater than that of any animal used for science, for their pain lasts for many days.

"The animals used for medical science suffer, but no more than a human being suffers under an operation. Men and women permit operations upon themselves to save life and relieve pain. Yet those who oppose vivisection would not have science operate on animals to cure men of their ills."

Yet, while the opponents of vivisection scoff the majority of them are unaware that through the agency of animal experimentation there are men and women going about their daily tasks in the full enjoyment of health, using the healthy bones, joints, and tissues taken from others in place of their own diseased and useless joints and necrosed bones. Such, however, is the case. These substitutions have been made with the most gratifying results along lines and in accordance with theories similar to those entertained by Dr. Carrel.

## Operating on Bones and Joints

Prof. Erich Lexer, Director of the Royal Surgical University Clinic and Polyclinic of Königsberg, Prussia, has described some remarkable operations on bones and joints, and his description has been translated for *Surgery, Gynecology, and Obstetrics* by Dr. E. C. Riebel of Chicago.

After reviewing the history of attempts to restore motion to joints stiffened by bony anchylosis, Dr. Lexer says:

"Bony anchylosis can be removed by operation only."

Dr. Lexer had intended, he says, when he operated for a stiff joint again, to cover the surfaces of the joints with plates of joint cartilage from amputated extremities. In the meantime an article by Weglowski appeared which showed that the plan could be successfully carried out. Weglowski implanted cartilage between the bony surfaces of a stiff elbow joint after removal of superfluous bone and fashioning the ends so that they approximated the contour of a normal healthy joint. He took two pieces of cartilage from the sixth and seventh ribs and laid them side by side in the newly formed joint.

Unfortunately this patient died of pneumonia at the expiration of five weeks. It was possible then, however, to show that the transplantation had been successful. One side of the cartilages had grown firmly to the end of the upper arm bone.

"At the margins the cartilage decreased, to merge, without distinct boundaries with the surface of the bone. This proved the advantage of cartilage interposition: the transplanted pieces grew not only to the one bone surface, but flattened out and covered the other as well. The functional result was likewise satisfactory. At the end of a month the patient could flex and extend his joint within a range of 60 degrees to 70 degrees.

The operation was successful despite the fact that only one articular surface had been covered with cartilage."

"My intentions from the beginning," says Dr. Lexer, "were to transplant upon both articular surfaces and I have done this."

Dr. Lexer then operated upon a stiff elbow joint in a young woman. He transplanted thin disks of cartilage.

"After four weeks the dressing was changed and the elbow put up now in extension and then in slight flexion. Healing was perfect. Mobility began to become more extensive in the fifth week, when the patient left the clinic. She was extremely sensitive and afraid of pain during motion. The final result is not known.

"At the next occasion I proceeded another step forward and the desire to produce normal and normally covered joint surfaces led me to transplantation of an entire knee joint from a newly amputated lower extremity. The patient, an 18-year-old girl, suffered from bony anchylosis of the knee joint. The joint was fixed in acute flexion.

"A flap incision was made on the lower leg and the muscles and other tissues, together with a knee cap, were turned back so that the affected joint could be sawed out.

"The new joint was fitted into the defect," says Dr. Lexer, "amounting in the extended extremity to the width of three fingers. It was obtained from a limb amputated simultaneously for senile gangrene, and consisted of both epiphyses with crucial ligaments and semilunar cartilages. Each epiphyseal portion measured about one and one-half fingers. Both projected laterally beyond the margins of the leg and thigh bones, and required trimming. Each was fastened with a nail."

Following the readjustment of the soft tissues and the closing of the surgical wound, the leg was fixed in a plaster cast from the toes to the body.

"The cast," continues Dr. Lexer, was interrupted from the middle of the leg to the middle of the thigh and bridged over by several iron bands. This allowed complete immobilization, combined with ready accessibility. The wound healed smoothly and the cast was removed after seven weeks and active movements begun cautiously. Extensive movements were opposed by renewed union between the knee cap and the femur. I decided upon a complete removal of the former, and for this purpose detached the lower half of the flap, about three months after the transplantation. All expectations were realized. The epiphyses were in firm union with the corresponding sawed surfaces of tibia and femur. The union was so complete that it did not offer even a trace of motion. The epiphyses were firmly healed beyond a doubt."

## Some Successful Cases

Dr. Lexer easily established the fact that the interposed joint was living and connected with the general circulation.

"A second transplantation for bony anchylosis of a tubercular knee joint was likewise successful," says Dr. Lexer. "The entire knee joint was again taken from a freshly amputated limb. Technically the second case differs, inasmuch as the epiphyseal portions were not as wide as in the previous one, and wire was used for fixation instead of nails.

"Both cases show now (the first five months, the second nine weeks after transplantation) upon X-ray pictures excellent positions of articular surfaces and transplanted epiphysis. The operated extremities are somewhat shorter than the sound ones. The knee joint is usually in a position of normal extension. Lateral motion is present to a very slight degree in the second case; in the first one it has entirely disappeared. The patients can bear their weight upon the extremity during standing or walking without lateral deviation of the joint to either side. There is no pain while bearing weight.

"Operative improvement of unction could not be hastened, as liberal time allowance must be made for the healing of such extensive bone and cartilage transplantations. Frequent exercises within the limits of active mobility were ordered to strengthen the muscles and keep the joint active. Active motion is still considerably less than passive, on account of the contracted muscles.

"The possibility of organic incorporation of a transplanted joint taken freshly from man is proved. This promises well for the future.

"Other cases show that substitution of half a joint can be as easily accomplished as that of an entire joint. Tumors of bone are the causes for these operations."

Dr. Lexer then describes the removal of the upper end of the chief leg bone for a cancerous affection and the substitution of a corresponding portion of a newly amputated leg.

"Here, again," says the surgeon, "complete healing followed. The Roentgen picture shows at this date, five months after transplantation, that the articular surface of the tibial substitute fits well to that of the femur. Flexion as well as extension is nearly normal. On walking the patient finds support upon the operated leg. A thick callus has produced firm union of the substituted piece. At the end of two months the X-ray picture showed activity of the transplanted bone covering by production of new bone deposits in various places. In consequence there can be no doubt that the function of the knee joint will improve further and the endurance in walking will increase. The fact that the transplanted tibia was taken from the right leg to be placed into a left one led us to fear that the joint surfaces might fit badly and lateral mobility might ensue. This, strange to say, did not occur, perhaps on account of rapid rounding off after movements.

"In similar manner and with like success I substituted the upper two-thirds of the left upper arm bone. The lower portion of the thigh bone of an amputated limb was taken, as a disarticulated arm was not at hand. Here, also, uninterrupted healing took place. The patient is now commencing with active motion. Passive motion in the joint is extensive."

In the same way Dr. Lexer substituted part of a man's toe for part of a girl's finger. Healing was perfect. The joints are movable.

"These operations enabled us," says Dr. Lexer in conclusion, "by substitution of articular portions removed to preserve for the patients movable joints. In former times the result in the first case would have been a materially shortened limb with stiff joint by fitting the stump of the tibia into an opening in the articular surface of the femur."

The claim of the world's foremost surgeons and physicians is that by far the most important method of advance in medicine is by experiment. This in the human being, of course, is out of the question. Clinical observation, while very valuable, and indeed indispensable, never can be so exact as experimental investigation, because surgeons cannot open arteries and put tubes into them and conduct the experiments that they can on animals with the greatest accuracy as to blood pressure, study the effect of section of nerves, and so on.

All of this is done without the slightest pain to animals, and they receive the most antiseptic care, quite as much as any human being.

In this connection the investigations of Dr. George Crile of Cleveland and Dr. Cushing in reference to the prevention of shock are of great value. When surgeons have to amputate an arm or leg near the trunk, or when they have to extirpate tumors, for example, in the neck, large nerves have to be severed, and the cutting of these nerves produces very severe shock. This has been determined much more accurately by experiments on animals than by clinical observation on man, because the operator can accurately measure the fall in blood pressure and the irregularity of the heart's action in animals which cannot be done in man.

Crile and Cushing then tried the effect of injecting a few drops of cocaine into the nerves just above the point where they were to be divided. It was then found that dividing these nerves after the injection of cocaine produced no shock whatever.

The elimination of this element in shock in a critical case very easily makes the difference between recovery or death.

Dr. Crile also has achieved some remarkable results in the direct transfusion of blood, similar to the method employed by Dr. Carrel. A woman suffering from cancer, which demanded operation, was in a very impoverished condition physically. When Dr. Crile was ready to operate he sutured the severed artery in the arm of the patient's husband to a severed vein in the patient's leg. Blood was allowed to flow during the progress of the operation. When the operation was finished the patient was found to be in a much better physical condition than when it was begun.

Dr. Crile has reported several more similar cases, and soon will publish a book on the subject.

## Changing Heads of Dogs

Dr. C. C. Guthrie of St. Louis, who has been associated with Dr. Carrel in many of his experiments, describes in yesterday's issue of the *Journal of the American Medical Association* some of the physiologic aspects of blood-vessel surgery. In this article Dr. Guthrie says:

"Briefly, the results so far have demonstrated the feasibility of transplanting limbs. That the restored circulation is adequate is demonstrated by the absence of gangrene or other symptoms attributable to this factor, both in the case of a hind leg replanted on a dog by Carrel and myself, and also by both fore and hind legs which I have transplanted from dogs to dogs of other breeds. In addition, I have transplanted dogs' heads with preservation of cerebral and bulbar function. Even in a case in which the circulation was interrupted for twenty-nine minutes, good return of function was observed in the transplanted head. This demonstrated conclusively the adequacy of the restored circulation.

"Since I have found no evidence of serious derangement of metabilism (tissue change) in dogs' thighs up to eleven days after transplantation, nor in a dog's foreleg in six days after transplantation, and since there are no physiologic or other reasons known why such tissues as those found in the limb may not live and again function under such conditions, it seems justifiable to conclude that it is possible to transplant such a member with permanent success.

"It is now known that it is possible to transplant the legs or heads of dogs so quickly that perfusion (of blood) is unnecessary, coagulation not occurring under forty minutes to one hour or more, and the period of occlusion (shutting off of the circulation) requiring not over thirty minutes."

The same publication of yesterday contains the following conclusions by Dr. I Carrel:

"It is proved that the remote results of the transplantation of fresh vessels can be perfect, and that arteries, kept for several days or weeks outside of the body, can be transplanted successfully, and that after more than one year the results remain excellent. It has been shown, also, for the first time, that transplanted kidneys functionate, that an animal, having undergone a double nephrectomy and the transplantation of both kidneys from another animal, can live normally for a few weeks, and that an animal which has undergone a double nephrectomy and the graft of one of his own kidneys can recover completely and live in perfect health for eight months, at least.

"Finally, it has been demonstrated that a leg extirpated from a dog and substituted for the corresponding leg of another dog heals normally."

*November 15, 1908*

# Doctor Describes Grafting of Cornea

It has already been announced by cable that Prof. Dastre had witnessed the successful experiment of grafting a cornea on the human eye, and now Dr. Magitot, who performed the operation, has made a communication on the subject to the Academy of Science. The communication is in the form of an essay which is entitled "The Possibility of Preserving in a State of Slackened Vitality for an Indeterminate Period the Transparent Cornea of the Human Eye." The essay, which is a remarkable document, fully explains how the operation was performed and makes it clear that certain persons stricken with blindness may, by a similar operation, be able to see:

"The object of the present communication concerns the possibility of preserving the human cornea, and maintaining it outside the organism during an indeterminate period, and in certain conditions, with a sufficient vitality to allow of its being transferred to the cornea of the eye, one of the most delicate of tissues. It becomes glazed, and its epithelium is liable to desquamation very rapidly after life disappears, or after the eye has been removed. However, the experiments, which had already been published in the *Annales d'Oculistique* of 1911, enabled me to preserve its optical properties—that is transparency—and after a preservation of fifteen days to transplant it to another animal of the same species.

"My experiments on a human patient have been conducted in the same manner. A glaucomatose eye had to be removed on account of the intolerable pain which it caused. Sight in this organ had, moreover, been definitely lost for several months, but there had been such a hypertension that the cornea, in consequence of the interior pressure, had become insensible, and even opalescent. The entire eye immediately after its enucleation was bathed in a solution of Locke (a complex artificial serum) and then rapidly immersed in a flask containing sanguineous human serum procured from another person. The receptacle was without delay transferred to a freezing chamber, at a temperature of 22 degrees or 23 degrees Fahrenheit. In a few hours the internal pressure of the eye globe had fallen, and the cornea had recovered its transparency.

"This eye was preserved in excellent condition for eight days. At the end of that time a rectangular piece comprising half the thickness of this cornea was carefully cut out and transferred to a cavity of corresponding dimensions cut out of the cornea of another patient. This patient had some years before been accidentally burned in the face and in the right eye by quicklime. The consequence of this accident was that corrosive lesions of the eye were produced, and the cornea became opaque over almost its entire surface. The graft of the tissue, which had been preserved eight days, was put in place without any suture to the right of the pupil. The result was a little window of five by four millimeters, like a lookout opening pierced in a thick wall. The adhesion and the transparency of the transplanted tissue were perfect after forty-eight hours. It is now seven months since this transplanting was done, and not only has the foreign tissue been tolerated, but it has preserved its transparency, enabling the patient to have a visual acuity of one-tenth of the normal, which is more than sufficient for guiding one's steps. Better still, the grafted tissue has manifested vitality in a more perfect manner by resisting the tissue of the cicatrice which formed around it, and which limits it without encroaching on its border. From this it results that the survival of the cornea is possible in man as well as in animals.

"Two conditions are necessary to obtain its maintenance in the state of slackened vitality. First of all, an appropriate medium is required, which is constituted by a hemolized serum of an individual of the same species. The hemolization should be obtained by purely physical means (such as a sudden fall of temperature by shaking warm blood in a receptacle cooled with ice). Secondly a feeble temperature is required, but not too low. The best temperature is comprised between 4 degrees and 7 degrees Centigrade. It should be a constant temperature, and variations, especially above 7 degrees, are detrimental. "We may find, therefore, that to the biological interest as regards the suspended vitality of a tissue so delicate as that of a cornea is added the practical interest for human patients. The transplanting of corneas, however, between different species, such as from dogs, rabbits, &c., is not successful. The piece so grafted is not long without losing its transparency. But we can preserve the material necessary for the transplanting and keep it in reserve for an opportune moment chosen for an operation. It is, therefore, to this extent possible to restore sight in a certain proportion of cases to patients stricken with blindness."

*January 28, 1912*

# Man's Life Saved by Twin's Kidney

By ROBERT K. PLUMB

The first known case in medical history in which a man's life was saved because he happened to be one of a set of identical twins was reported here today.

At the annual meeting of the American College of Surgeons it was disclosed that a human kidney transplanted into a young man in Massachusetts last Christmas is still alive and appears to be functioning normally. The donor of the kidney was the victim's identical twin brother.

Never before has such a feat of organ transplanting in man been accomplished. In no other known case in the history of medicine has a human kidney transplant "taken" and lasted so long. Attempts at transplanting other organs have not succeeded, either.

The report was made by Dr. Joseph E. Murray, Dr. John P. Merrill and Dr. J. Hartwell Harrison, all of the department of medicine and surgery, Peter Bent Brigham Hospital, Harvard Medical School.

## Former Attempts Failed

In the past failure of kidney transplantings has been attributed to an "antigen-antibodylike" reaction. That is, the tissues of the host pour out disease-fighting antibodies. The antibodies attack the transplanted kidney just as they would any other germ material or "antigen." Dr. Murray reported that recent microscopic studies of kidneys suggest that the kidneys themselves react strongly against the host.

Last December, Dr. Murray reported, one of the twins entered the hospital in a desperately sick condition. A kidney inflammation called glomerulonephritis had severely damaged both kidneys. He suffered high blood pressure, convulsions and other symptoms of profound kidney infection.

The patient, a 24-year-old single male, had an identical twin brother. Identical twins grow from one fertilized ovum, in distinction to ordinary twins, who, in most cases, are different individuals from different eggs, merely born at the same time.

## 3 Operations Performed

The evidence suggested that a kidney transplanting between identical twins might "take," Dr. Murray said. Skin grafts between identical twins are successful whereas skin grafts between other individuals are not successful.

The ailing twin's brother had two healthy normal kidneys. Many individuals who have lost one kidney lead normal lives because the other organ takes over the entire kidney burden.

The twins were placed in adjoining operating rooms last Dec. 23. The first operation took five and one-half hours. The left kidney was removed from one twin. It was sutured into the lower right side of the other. The kidney graft was without blood during the operation for an hour and twenty-two minutes. Arteries were sewn in place and the tube leading into the bladder was put in position. After it seemed that the kidney was going to do well, two other operations were performed to remove the damaged kidneys. The patient is reported now to be without symptoms, carrying on unlimited activity with no apparent disability.

*November 3, 1955*

# Harvard Panel Asks Definition of Death Be Based on Brain

## By ROBERT REINHOLD

A special faculty committee at Harvard University has recommended that the definition of death be based on "brain death" even though the heart may continue to beat. The committee offered a set of guidelines for physicians to determine when such death occurs.

The 13-man panel was drawn from the university's faculties of medicine, public health, law, divinity and arts and sciences.

The panel said its action was prompted by the possibility that "obsolete criteria" for death might lead to controversy in organ transplants and in modern resuscitative methods, which can maintain heartbeat in comatose patients with irreversible brain damage.

In a report, to be published today in the *Journal of the American Medical Association* under the title "A Definition of Irreversible Coma," the committee urges physicians to accept new standards for determining the moment of death as a prelude to a change in the legal definition.

"We suggest that responsible medical opinion is ready to adopt new criteria for pronouncing death to have occurred in an individual sustaining irreversible coma as a result of permanent brain damage," the report states. "If this position is adopted by the medical community, it can form the basis for change in the current legal concept of death."

The committee was headed by Dr. Henry K. Beecher, the Henry Isaiah Dorr Professor of Research in Anesthesia at Harvard Medical School, who has written and spoken widely on medical ethics. In a telephone interview, Dr. Beecher said he did not believe that use of the committee's criteria of brain death would cause physicians legal difficulties.

"Only the physician can pronounce death," he said. "We think he can do it accurately on the basis of our criteria."

Legally, in most states, death occurs when the individual is declared dead by a licensed physician. Basically, the criteria are irreversible cessation of respiration and circulation. However, the development of heart stimulators, respirators and other supportive devices have enabled physicians to keep the heart beating in persons in coma for two years or more.

As a result, a number of complex questions with ethical and moral overtones have arisen. Is it worth $30,000 a year to keep alive indefinitely a person with irreparable brain damage? Can society afford to discard the organs of such patients if they can be used to restore health to salvageable patients?

To facilitate solutions to problems like these, the Harvard professors set forth the following criteria to determine the characteristics of a permanently nonfunctioning brain:

- Unreceptivity and unresponsivity—total unawareness of external stimuli and inner need; no vocal or other response to even the most intensely painful stimuli.

- No movements or breathing—one hour of observation is adequate to satisfy the criteria of no spontaneous muscular movements or breathing.

- No reflexes—the pupil of the eye will not respond to direct bright light; no eye movement or blinking; no swallowing, yawning or vocalization; tendon reflexes cannot be elicited as a rule.

The report said that a flat brain wave pattern, or electroencephalogram, was of "confirmatory value" in establishing brain death. It outlined the procedure for performing such tests for lack of brain activity.

## Repeated Observations

All tests and observations should be repeated at least 24 hours later to confirm that there has been no change, the report stipulated. But it noted that the criteria could not be used if the body had been chilled below 90 degrees or if the central nervous system were affected by depressants, such as barbiturates. Patients have been known to exhibit flat electroencephalogram waves under such conditions yet revive later.

Once brain death is established, the report said, the family and all medical personnel involved should be informed; then the respirator supporting the patient should be turned off.

"The decision to do this and the responsibility for it are to be taken by the physician-in-charge," the committee said. "It is unsound and undesirable to force the family to make the decision."

The recent proliferation of transplant operations has underscored the problem of definition of death because organs must be kept viable after death. A controversy arose in Houston recently when the heart of Clarence Nicks, a murder victim, was kept beating mechanically for three hours after death had been declared. Such controversies would be obviated, Dr. Beecher said, if the Harvard criteria were accepted.

The report recommended that the decision to turn off the respirator be made by physicians not involved later in transplant of the patient's organs—"to avoid any appearance of self-interest."

An increasing number of medical men and others concerned with medical ethics and law have been urging that death be determined by brain damage. The question was discussed at the meeting last month of heart transplant specialists in Capetown. It also is to be the subject of a conference to be held by the American College of Cardiology next month in Bethesda, Md.

*August 5, 1968*

# Transplant Frontiers: A Special Report: Healthy Give Organs to Dying, Raising Issue of Risk and Ethics

By DENISE GRADY

On a gray morning in Minneapolis, Tammy Hoff and Dormae Gebhardt sat in adjacent hospital beds making brave jokes with their husbands while waiting to be wheeled off to the operating room. It was a typical hospital scene, except for one detail: the two women, both in their early 30s, were perfectly healthy, and about to have major surgery that they did not need.

In another bed across the room was 31-year-old Kimberly Miles, Ms. Hoff's sister and Ms. Gebhardt's friend. Thin and pale, with oxygen tubing looped about her face, Ms. Miles, too, put up a bold front, kidding with her 8-year-old son and his father.

Unlike the others, Ms. Miles did need surgery, desperately. Her lungs were so damaged by the genetic disease cystic fibrosis that she had barely enough breath to walk across the room. She needed a lung transplant. But most transplants come from cadavers, and the waiting period for lungs is two years or more. Ms. Miles was not expected to live that long.

And so the three women cast their fates together. Ms. Hoff and Ms. Gebhardt each offered to donate half of one lung to Ms. Miles, whose own diseased lungs would be removed. The two donated halves would become her new lungs, smaller than normal but still large enough to let her live a normal life.

"She will walk and probably even run," predicted Dr. Soon Park, her surgeon at Fairview-University Hospital and an assistant professor at the University of Minnesota Medical School.

Once unthinkable, using healthy people as organ donors to provide kidneys and portions of livers and lungs is gaining wide acceptance.

Ethically, emotionally and medically, this is uncharted territory. There is no doubt that living donors can save the lives of people who are languishing on transplant lists. But no matter how well the operations go, performing major surgery on someone who does not need it still violates the historical admonition that doctors must "do no harm."

One live donor has died in the United States and others have suffered complications.

481

"The donors worry me a lot," Dr. Park said. "Perfectly healthy people, having major operations. They are good people with a kind heart. Some donate and feel wonderful. Others may donate, go through a big operation and the recipient dies. We are creating questions I don't have answers for."

Dr. Park himself donated a kidney to his ailing sister while he was a college student.

The very existence of these operations forces patients and their relatives to look within and confront their fears, values and feelings about themselves and each other. Patients must decide whether they can bear to ask a relative or friend to endure the pain and risk of major surgery on their behalf. An organ is a gift that they will never be able to repay. And the friends and relatives must decide whether they are willing to put their own health on the line. Some learn things about themselves that they might have preferred not to know.

"Whether you say yes or no, it will affect you for a lifetime," Dr. Park said.

Increasingly, surgeons are telling people who need transplants that their relatives, spouses and friends are potential organ donors. In most cases, the recipients' insurance pays the medical expenses of donors. Hospitals are setting up education programs and support groups for potential donors and recipients. The existence of the surgery has created a pressure on families that did not exist before. In some cases people as young as 19 are being asked to act as liver donors for their parents.

Fueled by the severe shortage of organs from cadavers, the number of living donors in the United States rose by 16 percent in 2000, to 5,500, the largest increase in any one year. Most donors gave a kidney, an operation that has become routine and provides 40 to 50 percent of kidney transplants.

Although ethical objections were raised about living kidney donors when the practice began, the operations have become so safe and are so successful that they are not questioned today.

But liver transplants from live donors require a far more complicated and risky operation, removing part of the organ. Nonetheless, these transplants have increased sharply, to 347 in 2000 from 86 in 1998. In New York State last year, a third of all liver transplants came from live donors. And the number of live donors for lung transplants—also riskier than kidney donation—has slowly grown in the last decade, though each recipient requires two donors.

The vast majority of the operations have been successful. But no surgery is without risk. Aside from the liver donor who died in the United States, several others are reported to have died in Europe. But none of the deaths have been written about in medical journals, and no one is certain of the number. Doctors estimate the risk of death to liver donors to be 10 to 20 in 10,000 compared with 3 in 10,000 for kidney donors.

The shift to living donors is a major change in the history of transplants, and it is happening quietly, on its own, with no centralized control. Unlike drugs, new operations do not have to be approved or regulated by any government agency or medical group, so individual hospitals make their own decisions about whether to go ahead with live donor programs. In a sense, the expanding use of live donors is a vast scientific and social experiment.

"There is no Food and Drug Administration for surgeons," said Dr. Jay Hoofnagle, director of the division of digestive diseases and nutrition at the National Institutes of Health. "So procedures just get adopted."

Given the rapid growth of the field, some doctors are troubled by the lack of formal control over the operations and the lack of long-term follow-up and reporting on the donors. Different doctors use different surgical techniques, and there have been no major comparative studies to determine which work best. There are no mandatory registries to keep track of donors or complication rates and no means of certifying transplant programs.

## Pressure of Donating: Facing a Relative Who Is Facing Death

Wendy Marx, a 34-year-old woman in San Francisco who has had two liver transplants, both from cadavers, said her doctor suggested that she consider asking a relative to donate if she ever needed a third transplant. Ms. Marx said she found the idea very disturbing.

"It's not right," Ms. Marx said. "You have to think of the worst-case scenario. If I woke up and found out that my mother or brother had died so that I could have a transplant, I wouldn't want to be alive."

Her husband strongly disagrees, Ms. Marx said, and she conceded that if she were facing death she might feel differently.

Transplant teams say that they never ask anyone to donate and that donors must come forward on their own. But of course, they cannot know what was said at home before the donor came forward.

Some doctors are reluctant as a matter of principle to take organs from live donors. Some doctors worry, too, that even though donors and recipients are screened by psychiatrists and social workers and evaluated by different medical teams to avoid conflict of interest, donors may not truly be acting freely. They may be caving in to pressure from the recipient and other family members, and blinded to the risks by their own guilt and distress over seeing a loved one suffer.

Those who have never had major surgery may have no idea how difficult and painful it can be. In any case, a relative's fatal illness itself can be coercive, evoking a powerful sense of obligation and the feeling that to say no is to let the patient die without trying to help.

Dr. Myron Schwartz, a liver transplant surgeon at Mount Sinai Hospital in Manhattan, said, "I often wonder how well prospective donors hear the risks we tell them about."

Dr. Richard J. Battafarano, a lung transplant surgeon at Washington University in St. Louis, said: "You can imagine, you have a sick child that's been told if they don't have a transplant they're going to die, and all of a sudden all the family members are looking at one another to see who's a match. Even if it's not spoken, there's a lot of pressure."

But if doctors disagree with someone's decision to be a donor, do they have the right to refuse to operate? The answer is not always clear. At one hospital, when a young man offered to be a liver donor for his mother, surgeons rejected him because he had a baby. At another hospital, a similar donor was accepted. Surgeons say they are sometimes torn between their needs to protect donors and to respect the donors' rights as adults to make their own decisions.

## Liver Transplants: Few Children Now Die on Waiting Lists

The first live donor liver transplants were from adults to children, and the procedure, which grew rapidly in the 1990s, has unquestionably been a great boon. Before it came into use, 20 percent to 30 percent of children who needed livers died on the waiting list. Now, hardly any do. Many receive livers from their parents or other relatives. Around the world, more than 1,500 pediatric operations with live donors have been done.

To provide a transplant for a child, doctors remove all or part of the left lobe of the donor's liver, the smaller of its two lobes, making up about 30 percent of the organ. Because the liver has an extraordinary ability to regenerate, the donor's liver grows back to its normal size within a few weeks, and the transplanted piece also grows with the child.

Initially, surgeons took a cautious approach to liver transplants for children using live donors, and they did not begin performing them until the operations had been studied and proved to work by doctors at the University of Chicago, in 1991. But that wariness did not extend to adult-to-adult transplants, even though they require a much riskier procedure, removing the right lobe of the donor's liver, 50 to 70 percent of the organ. Instead, the surgery caught on quickly, before anyone had a chance to do a detailed study. Although no one questions the use of live donors for children, using them for adults is controversial.

Dr. Hoofnagle said: "The adult operation is different from the pediatric one. It's a big step. Ethically, you're no longer talking about parents and child, the image of a child in a burning building. This is not a child anymore. Sometimes it's a parent who's 60 years old. It's a very different level of ethical decision. The operation is much bigger. You are right at the edge of putting someone into liver failure. In fact, in the immediate post-op period the donor is suffering from borderline liver failure. It's tenuous."

In May, Dr. Mark Siegler, a medical ethicist who was involved in planning the pediatric clinical trial of liver transplants in Chicago, joined two liver surgeons in writing an article in the *New England Journal of Medicine* that criticized the rapid expansion of live donor programs for adult liver transplants and called for government control. They said that although the operations were extremely valuable, too many hospitals in the United States were doing them or planning to start, including some centers that might lack the experience needed to perform the operations safely. And they suggested that some surgeons and medical centers that were starting to do the operation might have been motivated in part by the desire for prestige and money.

Dr. Siegler and his coauthors also questioned whether all serious complications and deaths among donors were being reported.

"I suspect that if we had full reporting of the complications and mortality of the operation from the U.S. and Europe, we would discover that there are more complications and additional deaths that have been thus far unreported," Dr. Siegler said in an interview.

The one donor death known in the United States occurred in July 1999, at the University of North Carolina. The donor was a 41-year-old man, Danny Lee Boone, who suffered complications and died three weeks after donating a portion of his liver to his half brother, who survived.

Other problems have occurred. At a meeting last fall of medical social workers specializing in liver transplants, one participant described a case in which the recipient died and the donor, his brother, began drinking shortly after the surgery. His liver did not regenerate fully, and he refused treatment and broke off contact with the doctors.

In a similar case, described by doctors at New York Presbyterian Hospital in Manhattan, the recipient was a woman with fulminant liver failure, a type that comes on suddenly and is fatal in 48 hours without a transplant. A much younger relative became the donor, but had far less time than most donors to think over her decision. The recipient died. The young relative became depressed, not only because of the death, but because she herself had gone through a painful operation and felt disfigured by the big abdominal scar it had left, while nothing had been gained. She, too, stopped seeing the doctors, and the hospital team decided not to use any more live donors for patients with fulminant liver failure.

Doctors said they had encountered cases in which desperate, frightened parents tried to pressure their own adult children into acting as donors for them. Dr. Silvia Hafliger, a psychiatrist at New York Presbyterian Hospital, said one woman called her daughter every day, begging her to be a donor, even though the daughter had just had a baby. The young woman did not want the surgery, and Dr. Hafliger said she urged the mother to let her daughter alone.

"I yelled at her," Dr. Hafliger said. "I said, 'How could you even think of that?'"

Children donating livers to parents are surprisingly common, and the process brings up difficult issues for some families. This is particularly true if the cause of the failure has been hepatitis C, the leading reason for liver transplants in the United States. Many people with the disease contracted it long ago through drug abuse, which they never revealed to their children. During transplant discussions, the secret inevitably comes out, and both donor and recipient must decide whether it is fair to ask someone else to give up an organ in those circumstances.

Similar questions come up when the recipient's liver disease resulted from alcoholism, particularly if there are doubts about the recipient's ability to stay sober.

Every transplant group has encountered people who volunteer to be donors but who, away from their families and alone with a doctor or social worker, reveal that they actually do not want to go through with the surgery. Some do not fully realize it themselves until they begin discussing it, and most are ashamed to admit it to their families. Most medical teams help cover for them by telling relatives that they were medically unsuitable but not specifying why.

At the social workers' meeting last fall, one participant said he felt he had really done his job when potential donors declined, not because he had talked them out of it, but because he had helped them decide what they really wanted to do.

Another participant, Carol Holzer, from New York Presbyterian, said there was a constant tension between social workers and surgeons because the surgeons were eager to operate and the social workers were eager to pick up signs of ambivalence and rule out reluctant donors.

## The Rewards: Painful Recoveries Don't Dim Elation

For people with cystic fibrosis, the age of 31 can be close to the end of life, and Kimberly Miles's past two years had been a constant struggle. She spent more and more time in the hospital with lung infections and could no longer breathe without supplemental oxygen. In April 2000, at her mother's urging, the family began considering a live-donor lung transplant. Family members volunteered, but Ms. Miles's parents, her cousin and one sister were ruled out for medical reasons.

The sister, Debra Bloczynski, 38, said: "You have mixed feelings. You love her and you want to help. But you think about yourself. You want to do it and you don't."

The idea that anyone could have mixed feelings about being a donor angered Ms. Miles's mother, and Ms. Bloczynski said she felt guilty that she had not qualified. So did the cousin, who referred to herself as "the big reject."

Ms. Miles's friend, Dormae Gebhardt, meanwhile, said she decided instantly to volunteer. But Ms. Miles's other sister, Tammy Hoff, hesitated, all the while feeling considerable pressure from her mother.

"It was not easy," Ms. Hoff said. "I had mixed emotions."

Members of the transplant team sensed her ambivalence and rejected her. She grappled with her feelings for a month, then decided to go ahead. She met with the team again and was accepted.

"You have to decide, and when you do you feel a lot better about yourself," Ms. Hoff said. "What actually got me was when I went to a checkup with Kim. There were these people that had had cadaver transplants, and this one lady had this look in her eye that said, 'Just do it.' It was like she was some kind of guardian angel, like a sign from above that said, 'Do it. It's going to work.'"

Lungs for transplant are difficult to obtain, because they can be harvested from only 10 percent to 15 percent of cadaveric organ donors. Often, infection or other conditions make them unusable, and the scarcity has led surgeons to turn to live donors.

Surgeons say that donors recover fully and rarely feel different than they did before the surgery.

A report last year on 62 lung donors at Barnes-Jewish Hospital in St. Louis showed no deaths, but many had complications after surgery. The authors of the study concluded that the operation should be done only on patients who could not wait for cadaver transplants, and that donors must be warned about the high rate of complication.

The St. Louis doctors found that 38 of the 62 donors, or 61 percent, had complications, including 12 major problems and 55 minor ones. The major complications included a hemorrhage that required transfusions and a nerve injury that partly paralyzed a patient's diaphragm, though it did not cause symptoms or other problems. In another case, the surgery caused an abnormal heart rhythm and the patient needed a procedure to destroy damaged nerve fibers that were disrupting his heartbeat. Another patient had two lobes removed from his right lung instead of one, because of a surgical problem.

The minor complications included pneumonia, temporary problems with heart rhythm and infections of the pericardium, the sac around the heart.

"Our feeling was that we wouldn't expand the use of the procedure," said Dr. Battafarano, the lung transplant surgeon who was an author of the paper. "This review confirmed our view that we should reserve it for recipients who have no alternative. And that has to do not only with the donor operation but also that if the recipient can survive on the list, they'll get two full lungs."

The extra tissue from a cadaver, he said, could lengthen survival.

Dr. Park said that the chance of death for donors was very small, and that he had not heard of any deaths in lung donors. "But that's biased," he said. "If it happened, people would not be likely to brag about it."

For people with cystic fibrosis, a lung transplant offers a 75 percent chance of living one year and a 65 percent chance of living five. To Ms. Miles, who had been hospitalized for four months before the surgery, those odds sounded pretty good.

"Her ability to survive outside the hospital is nonexistent," said Jackie Zirbes, a transplant coordinator.

On the morning of the surgery, three operating rooms and three surgical teams, about 25 people in all, were ready. And as the surgeons required, a backup donor, another friend of Ms. Miles, stood by, ready to be taken into surgery in case doctors found that they could not remove a lung section from one of the primary donors.

Ms. Hoff's operation, a three-hour procedure to remove the lower lobe of her right lung, began first. After about an hour, when it was clear that the lobe could be taken out, doctors began to remove Ms. Miles's right lung. Replacing both her lungs was expected to take about six hours.

While Ms. Hoff's lobe was being sewn into Ms. Miles, doctors began to remove Ms. Gebhardt's. By late afternoon, Ms. Hoff and Ms. Gebhardt were in recovery. And Ms. Miles's new lungs were in place. They puffed up like balloons to fill her small chest, to the delight of the surgical team.

Ms. Miles recovered slowly but surely, despite a bout with pneumonia shortly after the surgery. Her new lungs worked well, she was freed from her tether to an oxygen tank and she was able to return briefly to her home in Black River Falls, Wis. But other problems set in, possibly related to her cystic fibrosis, which affects the digestive system as well as the lungs. Since the transplant, Ms. Miles has suffered from such severe nausea and vomiting that she has been unable to eat and has required a feeding tube. She was back in the hospital for gallbladder surgery by early June and remained there yesterday.

Ms. Hoff and Ms. Gebhardt recovered quickly, though with far more pain and fatigue than either of them had expected. Two months after surgery, both were back at work full time. Six months after the surgery, both were reported fully recovered by their surgeons.

Ms. Gebhardt said that giving up a few weeks of her life seemed a small price to pay for the chance to add years to Ms. Miles's life.

"Even with the pain I had to go through, I would do it all over again if I had to," she said.

In the weeks after the surgery, Ms. Hoff was delighted to see the changes in her sister. "Her cheeks are rosy, her eyes have a little glitter, her fingertips aren't purple anymore," Ms. Hoff said. But, she added, "She's got a heck of a road to go."

As for herself, Ms. Hoff said: "I have no regrets at all. It's a scar you're proud of."

*June 24, 2001*

# French, in First, Use a Transplant to Repair a Face

By LAWRENCE K. ALTMAN; with reporting from CRAIG S. SMITH

Surgeons in France have for the first time performed a partial face transplant, a surgeon who led one of the two teams that performed the operation said yesterday.

The recipient of the transplant was a 38-year-old woman who had been severely disfigured in an attack by a dog, said the surgeon, Dr. Jean-Michel Dubernard of Lyon. The operation was carried out in Amiens on Sunday.

In a brief telephone interview, Dr. Dubernard said the two surgical teams had grafted a nose, lips and chin from a donor who had been declared brain dead onto the woman's face.

Hospital officials said the woman who received the transplant did not wish to be identified. They gave no details about what measures, if any, had been taken to reconstruct her face short of a transplant. "The patient is well and fine, and the graft is O.K.," Dr. Dubernard said. He said a news conference would be held tomorrow in Lyon to discuss the case.

The surgery represents the first foray into a much-debated realm of medicine. A number of other surgical teams in the United States, France and the Netherlands have announced plans to perform various types of face transplants. But none are known to have performed the procedure. Face transplants are among the most disputed frontiers in transplantation science because they are so risky and no one can say what a patient will look like afterward.

Ethics committees in France and England have rejected proposals to perform full face transplants until more research is done. The committees were concerned about the unknown risks of the long-term use of large doses of immunosuppressive drugs for a procedure that does not save lives. The aim of face transplants is to improve the quality of life for patients who have suffered severe injuries from burns, accidents and shootings, for example.

The French committee did approve partial face transplants of the type performed on the woman in Amiens. But the committee cautioned in a report last year that even a partial transplant—the mouth and the nose, for example—was "high-risk experimentation."

In the United States, an institutional review board that oversees the safety of human experiments at the Cleveland Clinic last year became the first such body to approve a full face transplant. Full and partial face transplants can involve the transfer of attached muscles, blood vessels, nerves and other tissues. The tissues are needed to help restore an acceptable appearance for the recipient.

Among the risks of either type are the chance that the graft will be rejected, leaving a patient in a worse condition than before the operation, the development of cancer from the immunity suppressing drugs given to prevent organ rejection, and the chance that a patient will suffer psychological problems in adjusting to a new identity and appearance.

The woman who received the transplant on Sunday had been attacked by a dog last May. Dr. Dubernard said she was transferred on Tuesday from Amiens to the Edouard-Herriot Hospital in Lyon, where Dr. Dubernard works, for long-term monitoring of the immunosuppressive therapy that she will need. The transfer was according to a scientific blueprint that Dr. Dubernard said he and Dr. Bernard Devauchelle of Amiens had agreed on before the operation. He said Dr. Devauchelle's team was "very well trained for this type of surgery."

In 1998, Dr. Dubernard headed the team that performed the first hand-forearm transplant. He is also a politician and member of the French Parliament.

Outside experts said it was difficult to know whether the partial transplant was as difficult to perform as a full face transplant. For example, it is not known how badly injured the woman was, or how much of the donor's face and underlying muscle, blood vessels and tissue were transplanted Sunday. Also, the experts said they could not determine how well the French team had informed and prepared the woman psychologically for the transplant.

The relatively short interval of about six months between the dog bite and the surgery raised questions among some experts about what, if any, efforts had been made to perform reconstructive surgery first. "The major question is: what were the indications" for the transplant, said Dr. Maria Siemionow, a surgeon at the Cleveland Clinic who plans to perform a full face transplant.

Questions about the timing of the French surgery are relevant because the first patient to receive a hand transplant, Clint Hallam, did not comply in taking his prescribed antirejection therapy. He had his transplanted hand amputated in 2001, three years after receiving it.

Dr. Laurent Lantieri, a surgeon who was not directly connected with the French woman's surgery but who has reviewed some of her records, said he was puzzled about why she was put on the list for a face transplant in June or July, so soon after she received her injuries. Dr. Lantieri has published articles about his intention to perform partial face transplants, and was a consultant to the ethics committee in France that approves such procedures.

Face transplants, the committee said, should not be performed on an emergency basis. One reason, it said, is because "the very notion of informed consent is an illusion," even if all standard techniques have been exhausted, a candidate patient insists on receiving the transplant and a donor is available. "The surgeon cannot make any promises regarding the results of his restorative efforts, which are always dubious," the committee said. The report continued, "Authentic consent, therefore, will never exist."

The national committee was intended only to give advice and not to approve individual cases, Dr. Lantieri said in a telephone interview. French surgeons are supposed to have their experimental protocol reviewed by an independent committee of experts before carrying out a partial face transplant, he said.

Dr. Lantieri said he had reviewed a summary of the woman's medical record and examined a photograph of her damaged face. The woman's type of injury seemed consistent with proposals to do a partial facial transplant, he said. "She had very strong psychological problems," Dr. Lantieri said. "I said I would not go further if I did not have more examinations by additional psychiatrists to know that she would be able to pursue lifelong immunosuppression therapy." Dr. Lantieri said he believed that Dr. Dubernard "wanted to be first" to do a face transplant, as he had done a hand transplant.

Dr. Dubernard said his team planned to do another transplant—of bone marrow—on the woman while she was in the hospital in Lyon. Although bone-marrow transplants are a standard treatment for some conditions, in this case the hope would be that it would increase the patient's tolerance to a graft.

Dr. Lantieri said if a bone-marrow transplant was carried out on the patient it would mean that she would be undergoing two experiments at the same time. The extra experiment would be unethical, Dr. Lantieri said, because "every ethical committee says that only one experiment should be carried out at a time. That is a basic rule of clinical research."

But, he added, "I really hope the partial face transplant will work."

*December 1, 2005*

**CHAPTER 21**

# Ulcers

# Say Gastric Ulcers May Be Infectious

Two important announcements were made to the members of the International Surgical Association at yesterday morning's session of the fourth congress, which is meeting at the Hotel Astor, during a discussion of ulcers of the stomach and duodenum. The first tended to show that these ulcers, which are comparatively common in persons of middle age, belong to the category of infectious diseases, while the second positively indicates the evolutionary character of bacterial life.

The second announcement substantiates in a measure the report cabled from Europe the other day to the effect that a new infectious agent, producing a new disease, had been produced by the simple process of subjecting a known and well-defined bacterium to the action of ultra-violet rays. The morphological characteristics of the germ underwent an immediate change.

Dr. Arthur D. Bevan, Professor of Surgery at the University of Chicago, made the announcement relative to the origin of gastric and duodenal ulcers. He said that his colleague, Dr. Edward C. Rosenau, who occupies the Chair of Pathology at the Chicago University and has a wide reputation as a research worker, had demonstrated that these ulcers could be caused by the injection of bacteria taken from other ulcers. The injections were made intravenously, that is, directly into the blood, whereupon the disease made its appearance at the usual sites of ulceration, both in the stomach and intestines of animals. The duodenum is that portion of the small intestine immediately contiguous to the stomach and is about twelve inches long. The stomach empties directly into it through the pyloric orifice. Ulcers of the stomach and duodenum are annoying, painful, and sometimes fatal. Their treatment offers at best a perplexing problem to both physician and surgeon.

## Dr. Rosenau's Experiments

It developed in the course of Dr. Bevan's remarks that Dr. Rosenau's experiments in creating ulcers by bacterial injection were based on logical deductions following an earlier and equally fascinating—to the scientific mind—series of experiments. He had taken certain strains of bacteria, that is, bacteria cultivated in a certain medium, and injected the germs into animals by the intravenous method. He found that endocarditis, or inflammation of the lining of the heart, followed. Invariably this strain of bacteria produced endocarditis.

Next, the investigator took the same variety of bacteria and cultivated them in a different medium. Some subtle change in product resulted, producing another strain, which, when injected into animals by the same method as before, produced inflammatory infectious lesions in the joints. The joint lesions also invariably followed the injection of this second strain.

Dr. Rosenau concluded that each strain produced possessed a selective or affinitive action for some distinctive type of tissue in the body. Proceeding on this theory, he isolated bacteria from the exudate of gastric and duodenal ulcers, cultivated them in suitable media, and set up diseased processes similar to those from which they were taken by the injection of a solution of the bacteria which he had isolated and cultivated. That is, he produced the pathological lesions by the injection of one particular strain of the bacteria taken from the ulcers, as will be shown later. "Dr. Rosenau would say," Dr. Bevan remarked in conclusion, "that a particular strain of bacteria has a particular selective action for some particular tissue."

Dr. John B. Murphy of Chicago, who followed Dr. Bevan, corroborated the latter's statement and added enough information to indicate the evolutionary processes going on in bacterial life under the comparatively slight stimulus afforded by a change in environment.

## Produces Different Lesions

"Dr. Bevan," said Dr. Murphy, "took a single strain of streptococcus, cultivated it in different media, and produced different lesions by injecting the resulting strains. For instance, the streptococci when cultivated in a certain medium changed to diplococci, and when these were injected into an animal they produced pneumonia, and the original strain of streptococci was then cultivated in another medium. The resulting products were injected into other animals and produced ulcers of the stomach and duodenum."

Several papers were read on ulcers of the digestive tract, and the only session of the day was devoted to reading and discussing them.

Dr. P. de Quervain of Basel set forth in his paper the actual condition of the clinical and radiological diagnostic features of gastric and duodenal ulcer and the problems concerned therein. He asserted that apart from certain well-established facts there existed a great number of open and controversial questions. He discussed several of these, which were of a technical nature.

Dr. H. Hartmann and Dr. P. Lecene of Paris presented a joint paper in which they asserted that duodenal ulcer is more frequent than was supposed several years ago. In their opinion, however, its frequency has been exaggerated. They have found one ulcer of the duodenum to eight or ten of the stomach.

## Cancer Possible Outcome

They also found that about one-fifth of the cases of the callous ulcers of the stomach degenerate into cancer. "The importance of radioscopy and radiography in the diagnosis of gastric ulcers is to-day universally recognized," they asserted.

"The surgical treatment of gastric or duodenal ulcer," they continued, "must therefore not be opposed to the medical treatment. The first is only the frequently necessary complement of the second. The real results, observed at a lapse of time, of the medical treatment are far from being as good as was formerly supposed. Without speaking of serious complications, such as hemorrhage, perforation and stenosis, which are indisputably urgent surgical indications, we consider that all ulcers (gastric or duodenal) showing resistance to medical treatment belong to the surgeon."

They described in detail several of the operative procedures which are depended upon nowadays for the relief and cure of these ulcers.

Dr. William T. Mayo gave a historic review of the diagnosis and treatment of chronic ulcers of the stomach and duodenum, as observed and carried on in St. Mary's Hospital at Rochester, Minn., since 1893.

Dr. E. Payr of Leipsic reviewed the origin and pathology of the ulcers, so far as known, but none of these theories, he acknowledged, was sufficient to explain every case. He did not mention the theory which Dr. Rosenau has brought forward, which may explain these obscure cases.

Those who took part in the discussion of these papers were: Dr. Block of Copenhagen; Dr. Sonnenburg of Berlin; Dr. Kummell of Hamburg; Dr. Lambotte of Brussels; Dr. Ullmann of Vienna; Dr. Manninger of Budapest; Dr. Gautitano of Naples; Dr. Brunning of Giessen; Dr. Zahradmicky of Nemeky-Brod; Dr. Krynski of Warsaw; and Dr. Howard Lilienthal of New York.

Prof. Charles Willems of Ghent, President of the Association, and twenty-five noted Dutch and Russian surgeons, arrived yesterday on the Rotterdam. Among the new arrivals was Dr. Jan Schoemaker, head of the hospital at The Hague, who is one of the best-known surgeons in Europe. Dr. Schoemaker before he returns home will visit clinics in the chief cities between New York and Chicago.

Instead of holding the usual afternoon session, an adjournment was taken at noon until this morning, to give the visitors an opportunity to visit Mt. Sinai Hospital, where the system of management was explained to them by Dr. A. C. Gerster. Some of the foreign surgeons attended clinics at St. Luke's, Roosevelt, and the New York Hospitals.

Mrs. William T. Mayo entertained the wives of the visitors at luncheon at the Biltmore, and later they attended a matinée performance of *Peter Pan*. All the members and their wives were the guests of the American Medical Association at a special performance at the Metropolitan Opera in the evening.

*April 15, 1914*

# New Bacterium Linked to Painful Stomach Ills

By LAWRENCE K. ALTMAN

Two Australian researchers have discovered what seems to be a new spiral-shaped bacterium living in the human stomach. The finding of one more microorganism among the thousands known might have been no more than a curiosity if the Australian bacterium were not now being tentatively linked to some of the most painful ailments known: gastritis, peptic ulcers in the stomach and duodenum, and perhaps other problems as well. Several million Americans have these ailments whose origins are often unknown.

The story of how the finding was made and how the research is being conducted on several continents has much to say about how science really works, not so much as a matter of breakthroughs but rather in fits and starts, with optimism, pessimism and rivalries that sometimes impede potentially important advances. Thus, while there is a great deal of skepticism about the importance of this finding, there is a great deal of excitement, too, as the potential implications begin to emerge.

It is possible, for instance, that if bacteria contribute to or lie at the root of stomach and intestinal pains, these now intractable problems may be helped, even cured, by antibiotics. Such drugs might be used in place of or in addition to the medications now prescribed.

Another possibility is that some day a blood test may be developed to help doctors diagnose and treat stomach conditions without patients' having to swallow chalky barium while standing behind X-ray machines and without going to examining rooms for the insertion of tubes called gastroscopes that enable doctors to look directly at the stomach. Underscoring the potential importance of the Australian finding is the fact that in recent years previously undetected bacteria were discovered to be the cause of Legionnaire's disease and other disorders, including some that affect the intestines. In a few such cases where the findings were first made outside of the United States, American researchers were slow to confirm and accept them.

The excitement this time centers on a spiral-shaped bacterium that Dr. Barry J. Marshall and Dr. J. Robin Warren in Perth have detected in a study of 100 patients suffering from an inflammatory stomach condition known as gastritis and from stomach ulcers. The researchers detected the bacterium in 58 of the patients. It was identified in 27 of 31, or 87 percent, of patients who had a gastric or duodenal

498

ulcer, and in 38 of 40, or 95 percent of patients with pathological evidence of active gastritis. The bacteria were detected on biopsies of stomach obtained through a gastroscope. When such biopsies were studied under a microscope, the bacterium were mostly seen beneath the mucus, which apparently protects it against the hydrochloric acid produced by the stomach.

The new bacteria resemble the S-shaped ones that belong to the genus *Campylobacter*. But an important difference is that whereas *Campylobacter* have at most one slender projection known as a flagellum emerging from one end of the S, the newly discovered organisms have up to four flagella. The resemblance to *Campylobacter* is a reminder of how with time and new knowledge doctors change their minds about the importance of certain microorganisms. About half a century passed from 1909 when *Campylobacter* were discovered in animals until doctors linked them to human disease. In the past decade, however, *Cambylobacter* have been recognized increasingly as a cause of such disease. There are two main types, *C. jejuni* and *C. intestinalis,* that cause distinctly different human conditions. *C. jejuni* is one of the most commonly recognized causes of diarrhea throughout the world; *C. intestinalis* generally affects only debilitated adults with serious chronic diseases.

Speaking of the Australian bacterium, Dr. George Buck, a microbiologist at the University of Texas at Galveston, said, "It definitely is a new organism." He also said that he believed "it is a new genus, but it is hard to say that without definitive genetic studies, and they have not been done yet." Dr. Buck said his opinion was based on comparisons of samples he and the Australians have sent each other. Dr. Buck's findings add to the reports that have come from several research teams in England, the Netherlands, Scotland and West Germany confirming the existence of the spiral stomach bacterium.

The editors of the *Lancet,* which is published in London and in which most of the reports have appeared, said that proof of the theory would make the Australian work "very important indeed." Such proof might come from attempts to infect animals. However, researchers have been hindered by the lack of a good animal model for chronic ulcers so that if animals fed the organism do not develop ulcers or gastritis, the negative findings may not be significant.

Researchers may have to seek proof from various long-term epidemiologic, pathologic and other studies on humans, according to one researcher, Dr. Robert M. Donaldson Jr., a Yale medical professor. "It would take a long time—my guess is a decade—to provide really convincing evidence" of the infectious cause, he said. Even then, Dr. Donaldson added, he seriously doubts the infectious theory "would pan out." One test is the response of patients to antibiotic therapy. Dr. Marshall contended that by adding a bismuth containing drug and antibiotics to the standard treatment regimen for ulcers and gastritis, and then documenting the disappearance of the bacteria, he had prevented relapses of the ailments.

But before such therapy is applied on a wider basis, Dr. Sherwood L. Gorbach, who heads the division of infectious diseases at Tufts Medical School in Boston, urged a careful, scientifically controlled study. The aim would be to determine how well, if at all, patients with gastritis and ulcers who harbor the bacterium respond to therapy with different antibiotics. "If I were to bet now," Dr. Gorbach said, "I would say that antibiotics are not going to reverse this condition. But I would not want to let my bet prevent a legitimate therapeutic trial because I think there is enough evidence now to allow an ethical trial, and it should be the No. 1 priority."

## Dismissed as Curious Contaminants

The availability of antibiotics is just one of the many scientific changes that have occurred since the beginning of the modern microbiological era. At the turn of this century, many doctors saw spiral-shaped bacteria in human stomachs and thought they were linked to gastric ailments. But largely because the bacterial identification techniques were then too crude to permit the crucial further studies, the spiral bacteria became curiosities and were dismissed as contaminants. Doctors then considered the stomach a sterile organ and abandoned the infectious theory of gastric ailments.

In 1979, while working at Royal Perth Hospital, Dr. Warren noticed the bacteria as he looked through a microscope at the biopsy specimens taken through gastroscopes. Dr. Warren had used a special silver stain to easily spot what was difficult to see in specimens prepared with more conventional chemical stains.

In 1981, Dr. Marshall was looking for a research project and soon after joining Dr. Warren, he found a picture of similar organisms in a physiology book. Later, he consulted librarians and the computerized listings of medical references gathered by the National Library of Medicine in Bethesda, Md., and found articles dating to late in the last century that described spiral-shaped bacteria in the stomachs of humans and animals. "Much of the work supporting our hypothesis had already been done, and it was only a matter of pulling it out of the literature and making sense of it," he said.

Still, the Australians had the advantages of modern technology that were not available to many of earlier researchers. Flexible fiberoptic gastroscopes allowed the Australians to take more biopsy samples from a larger area of the stomach than their predecessors could. The Australians availed themselves of newer microbiologic techniques that permitted the spiral bacteria to grow in the laboratory for the first time. They also had access to electron microscopes that allowed clearer definition and other techniques that, in turn, permitted better biochemical and molecular biological analyses.

It remains to be seen whether the Australian bacterium is the same as one of those described in past decades. Also, no one has determined how humans acquire the Australian bacterium.

The Australians and one British group have developed blood tests to detect evidence of the presence of the bacteria, a tool that may help in further studies. Dr. Marshall contended such tests might show that the organism accounts for some intestinal symptoms that many patients suffer but that doctors cannot now diagnose and treat effectively.

## Reasons for Skepticism

At this point, European interest in the research has exceeded that in the United States. At a recent national meeting of the American Gastroenterology Association, Dr. Donaldson, the Yale researcher, said, "There was no talk about this and no fire."

Dr. Donaldson also said that one reason for his skepticism was that reports in the *Lancet* "are so preliminary."

"An awful lot of things have appeared in that journal that have not panned out," he said.

Researchers are well aware of a history in this field in which enthusiastic claims for bacterial answers to intestinal ailments have led down blind avenues or proved false. The fact that an organism is present in the body of an ill person does not necessarily mean it is a cause of the problem. The intestines are cluttered with bacteria; more than 500 species of bacteria are present in what is known as the intestinal flora, though few have been studied in the stomach.

It takes extensive studies to determine whether the presence of the bacteria is a primary, or causative, event, or whether the organisms are present merely as secondary invaders. The current controversies focus on that very point—the meaning of the presence of the Australia bacteria.

However, one American researcher, who asked not to be named, said that too many of his colleagues had the attitude that "if we don't describe it first, our first reaction is always negative. We are very chauvinistic and have the attitude that if we haven't found something, it's probably wrong," he said. "But we have been wrong in that line of thinking."

Still another American researcher, Dr. Charles E. Pope 2d, a gastroenterologist at the University of Washington in Seattle, said that at first he had been skeptical about the Australian findings. But after a visit, he said he had "come away thinking it was a really new and intriguing observation." The bacteria may not be the cause, Dr. Pope said. "It may be that something else like drugs or alcohol starts it, and then these organisms grow there, making it worse and difficult to reverse." Dr. Pope urged more American doctors to carry on the research because "there really might be something there" and because treatment for gastritis is mostly ineffective.

*July 31, 1984*

# New Study Backs Ulcer-Cure Theory

By GINA KOLATA

New research has lent more support to the belief that a common bacterium lies behind most ulcers. The researchers, from Baylor College of Medicine in Houston, said almost all ulcer patients could be completely cured by taking a combination of drugs to eradicate the bacteria.

The idea that the bacteria, *Helicobacter pylori*, could be linked to ulcers has long been the subject of debate. Gastroenterologists say the new study is the most convincing one to be conducted in this country, and the researchers said they hoped it, along with previous research in Europe and Australia, would promote general acceptance of the idea that killing bacteria could cure ulcers.

About 10 million Americans suffer from ulcers, sores in the stomach or intestine. Ulcers heal after patients take drugs that suppress stomach acid production but they often recur again and again.

## Convincing Doctors of Cure

In their study, Dr. David Graham and his colleagues studied 109 ulcer patients who had been randomly assigned to receive the ulcer drug Zantac, a standard treatment that inhibits production of stomach acid, or a two-week regimen of four drugs: two antibiotics to kill the ulcer-causing bacteria, Zantac and an over-the-counter drug for an upset stomach.

The study found that 95 percent of patients with gastric ulcers who were treated with the new therapy had no recurrence in the next two years. But just 12 percent of those who received the standard treatment were ulcer-free in that period. Among patients with duodenal ulcers, 74 percent had no recurrence, as against 13 percent with the standard therapy.

The results of the study are described in the current issue of *Annals of Internal Medicine*.

"Most physicians are not yet aware that ulcers are curable," said Dr. Graham, the principal author of the new study. He said his findings "tell us what is possible."

Dr. Daniel Hollander, a professor of gastroenterology at the University of California at Irvine, said the findings "show you can prevent recurrence of ulcers if you eradicate *H. pylori*," and added, "That's truly important."

## Similar Findings

Dr. Hollander said the new therapy was neither difficult nor expensive. The two antibiotics, tetracycline and metronidazole, are available as generic drugs and the treatment lasts just two weeks.

Dr. Graham's study comes on the heels of similar studies in Europe and Australia that gradually convinced some gastroenterologists to revise their view of ulcers. Dr. Barry Marshall, a gastroenterologist at the University of Virginia Medical Center, described the new data as "the most convincing so far."

But some gastroenterologists said the four-drug approach to eradicate *Helicobacter* is not ideal and advised reserving it for patients with the most intransigent ulcers.

In an editorial in the *Annals*, Dr. John H. Walsh of the University of California in Los Angeles said the bacteria could become resistant to the antibiotics if they were used too widely, antibiotics could cause side effects, and patients could become reinfected and develop ulcers again. And he said there were not sufficient data on the long-term effectiveness of the treatment.

Dr. James H. Lewis, a gastroenterologist who is vice president of medical development at Glaxo Pharmaceuticals, also urged caution in interpreting the results. "No one in the gastroenterology community is saying this isn't relevant in some way," he said. "But it is still too early to say that this is the best approach to treating ulcers."

He said that "nobody really knows" whether *Helicobacter* was the cause of ulcers, adding that although most people with an ulcer had the bacterial infection, so did many who did not have an ulcer.

Ulcers, he said, are "multifactorial," and their occurrence can be influenced by a variety of factors, including a genetic predisposition, the amount of acid in the stomach and intestine, whether the person is taking aspirin or ibuprofen, and whether they smoke cigarettes.

## Origin of Theory

The *Helicobacter* hypothesis dates to 1984, when Dr. Marshall, then working in Australia, proposed it; the organism has also been called *Campylobacter*. Since then, he and others have found that as many as 90 percent of patients with duodenal ulcers were infected with *Helicobacter* and 70 percent of gastric ulcer patients had the bacterial infection. Most of the remaining patients had developed ulcers because they overused aspirin or ibuprofen. Their ulcers could be cured if they stopped taking the analgesics.

But acceptance of the *Helicobacter* theory has been hard to achieve in the United States, in part because many people infected with the bacteria do not develop ulcers. Dr. Hollander said that a group of 20 gastroenterologists at his university recently polled themselves. "A third are convinced and two-thirds are still skeptical," he said.

Drugs like Zantac, made by Glaxo, and Tagamet, made by Smithkline Beecham Inc., are among the best-selling drugs in medicine.

Dr. Marshall said many doctors stay with the standard drug treatment. If patients ask about the antibiotic approach, he said, "their doctor will say 'it's only experimental.'" He predicted that with the increasing body of evidence, more and more gastroenterologists and ulcer patients will start using antibiotics.

"Over the next year or so, I think many will change over," he said.

*May 6, 1992*

## CHAPTER 22

# Vaccines

# Measles Vaccine Reported at U. of P.

By WILLIAM L. LAURENCE

A vaccine for immunizing children and adults against measles, a disease which often leads to serious complications when it occurs during Winter months, was announced today at the bicentennial conference of the University of Pennsylvania.

Measles is one of the numerous diseases caused by a virus, the general name given to a wide group of micro-organisms too small to be seen by the most powerful microscopes or to be caught in a porcelain filter that prevents ordinary bacteria from passing through.

In recent researches by Dr. Wendell M. Stanley at the Rockefeller Institute of Medical Research it was established that viruses, instead of being living organisms like bacteria, are protein molecules, large chemical aggregates of atoms, neither living nor non-living, but existing in the twilight borderland between the animate and the inanimate.

The new vaccine was hailed by authorities attending the conference as "an important development toward active immunization against this common contagious ailment."

It was announced at a symposium on "Problems and Trends in Virus Research" by Professor Joseph Stokes Jr. of the University of Pennsylvania Medical School and Dr. Geoffrey Rake of the Squibb Institute for Medical Research, New Brunswick, N.J.

While most people think of measles as a rather harmless childhood sickness, the fact is, it was pointed out, that Wintertime cases are often followed by middle-ear infections, mastoiditis or bronchopneumonia. Furthermore, it was added, measles frequently attacks adults, particularly those who escaped childhood exposure to it.

## Measles a World War Hazard

During the World War, it was recalled, measles struck heavily at thousands of country lads who, because of their relative degree of isolation during childhood, had not contracted it then. Measles became one of the commonest causes of death, it was pointed out, by producing severe cases of pneumonia.

In view of this potential danger in the ranks of peacetime Army trainees, it was stated, the new measles vaccine might become a valuable national defense as well as public health measure.

The vaccine is grown on chick embryos in the shell. While this technique has been successfully used in the culture of many other viruses, previous efforts by other scientists to cultivate the measles virus have been inconclusive.

Apparently the virus becomes weakened or attenuated while growing in this strange environment, the chorio-allantoic membrane surrounding the chick membrane, and when injected under the skin or placed within the nose produces a modified measles of a very mild type in some children and no symptoms at all in others. Subsequent tests upon thirteen vaccinated children, made two to eight months later with nasal washings or blood from typical cases of measles, indicated that the vaccination might afford protection against the disease.

The first children to receive the measles vaccine were in three large New Jersey institutions. Later permission was obtained from the Philadelphia Department of Health to inoculate children who had been followed every two weeks since birth in a special well-baby clinic at Children's Hospital and who were known not to have contracted measles up to that time.

Dr. Stokes and Dr. Rake pointed out that 98 per cent of children were susceptible to measles, and since control over the time, place and manner of infection is apt to insure greater safety for the child, it was not difficult to obtain parental permission for these tests.

## Influenza Virus Resisted

Studies showing that the nasal membranes possess two mechanisms for resisting the virus of influenza, one of which may also act as a defense against infantile paralysis, were reported by Dr. Thomas Francis Jr., Professor of Bacteriology at the New York University College of Medicine, formerly on the staff of the international health division of the Rockefeller Foundation.

One defensive mechanism, revealed in ferrets, one of the few animals susceptible to influenza, a change in the character of the epithelial cells in the mucous membrane of the upper respiratory tract. The other, studied in human beings, is an antibody or germ-neutralizer in the nasal secretion which is capable of inactivating the influenza virus.

"These two manifestations of local immunity, one cellular, one serological, may conceivably complement one another," Professor Francis suggested. "Each represents a method by which an injurious agent reaching the tissue of predilection may be combated."

Most evidence to date, Dr. Francis stated, indicates that the influenza virus enters the body by way of the nose and that the nasal and upper respiratory membranes therefore constitute the "tissue of predilection."

The importance of these local mechanisms of resistance, Dr. Francis said, becomes apparent in the light of certain heretofore puzzling features of immunity and non-immunity to the disease. At the onset of the attack of epidemic influenza the blood of a majority of the patients, he pointed out, contains sufficient antibodies to protect experimental animals against many lethal doses of influenza virus. Yet the antibodies apparently do not check the progress of disease in the patients themselves.

"On the other hand," Dr. Francis continued, "it is not uncommon to find individuals who possess little or no demonstrable antibody but who escape infection although intimately exposed."

Thus the amount of antibody circulating in the blood does not always bear a direct relationship to the extent of the patient's immunity to the disease. This situation, paralleled by experiments in ferrets, suggests that other factors than circulating antibodies play a role in resistance and immunity. The local mechanisms in the nasal membranes seem to offer an explanation.

Extensive serological and biological tests led Dr. Francis to conclude that the substances in the nasal secretions have the properties of antibodies, and that they are possibly derived from the blood. He doubted that they were formed as the result of a specific infection, however, but said they probably represented a physiological product or "natural antibodies."

Dr. Francis observed that the protective effect of nasal secretions was not limited to influenza virus, that the capacity of nasal secretions to inactivate infantile paralysis virus, for example, had been demonstrated by other workers.

## Ferrets Develop Immunity

In the studies of the mucous membranes of the respiratory tract of the ferret Dr. Francis found that infection with the influenza virus destroyed the ciliated epithelial cells, leaving only a thin basement membrane covering the respiratory area. The mucous membrane over the olfactory area, however, was unharmed.

By the fourth day after the beginning of the infection the damaged membranes had begun to repair themselves.

The regenerating tissue was composed of abnormal, primitive cells which appeared to be highly resistant to subsequent injury by either influenza virus or zinc sulfate solution applied in the presence of an ionizing electric current. But by the fifteenth day of convalescence the abnormal repair cells had been replaced by normal cells, which were vulnerable to the ionized chemical but not to the virus. Subjected to a second inoculation of virus at a later date, the membranes were again damaged, even though circulating antibodies were present in the ferret's blood.

When ferrets were subjected to three or four inoculations with influenza virus, at suitable intervals, however, all but one were completely immune to the virus, nor was there any evidence of cellular injury in the respiratory membranes.

"These results," commented Dr. Francis, "suggest that following repeated exposures to influenza virus the nasal epithelium has developed a capacity to resist injury, a property which after a single infection was exhibited in incomplete form."

Long-standing cases of schizophrenia (dementia praecox), the commonest form of "split-personality" insanity, have responded in encouraging manner to a new operation in which fibers of the frontal lobe of the brain, seat of the intelligence, are severed, it was reported at a symposium on "Therapeutic Advances in Psychiatry" by Dr. Edward A. Strecker, Professor of Psychiatry and chairman of that department at the University of Pennsylvania Medical School.

This new form of "surgery of the psyche," it was stated, promises to become an important addition in the treatment of hopeless cases of insanity for which the other new methods of treatment, such as induced sleep, insulin shock and modified convulsive therapy, have not resulted in improvement. Insulin shock and convulsive therapy were discovered by Dr. Manfred Sakel, formerly of the University of Vienna and now in New York, who was among the distinguished psychiatrists attending the symposium.

The surgical procedure described by Dr. Strecker is known technically as pre-frontal leucotomy (referring to the cutting of white matter in the pre-frontal lobes of the brain). It was devised by Dr. Egas Moniz of Spain and was introduced into this country a few years ago by Dr. Walter Freeman and Dr. James W. Watts of the George Washington University School of Medicine, Washington, who have modified the technique.

## Brain Tissue Is Cut

A narrow spatula-shaped instrument is inserted through a hole drilled in the region of the temple and a fan-shaped cut is made in the brain tissue. On the basis of the symptoms which it seemed to control in the agitated melancholia cases of late middle life, for which Dr. Freeman and Dr. Watts employed it, Dr. Strecker proposed the operation for schizophrenia.

He selected only patients who had been insane for a long time, who had not been helped by any other methods of treatment and whose symptoms made life difficult for themselves and those caring for them. All of the eight cases operated upon to date have been insane for more than ten years. The surgery was done by Dr. Francis Grant, Professor of Neurosurgery at the U. of P.

"The results were interesting and sometimes truly amazing," Dr. Stecker reported. "The aggressiveness, in some instances homicidal in degree, disappeared; mental material which one would have believed irretrievably lost was apparently salvaged by the operation and was utilized by the patient in establishing realignments with life; panic reactions due to hallucinosis were terminated. The hallucinosis continued but a recall of the patient to reality in some of the cases was very easy, a few simple questions sufficing."

Dr. Louis I. Dublin, third vice president of the Metropolitan Life Insurance Company, reported that studies indicated that by 1980 14.4 per cent of the population of the United States would be sixty-five years old or over, as contrasted with 6.3 per cent today and 4.1 per cent in 1900.

This means, he declared, that one of medicine's major problems would become that of treating the "over sixty-five" group, while the whole economic and political life of the nation might be expressed in a new pattern because of the growing old-age group.

*September 18, 1940*

# Vaccine for Polio Successful;
# Use in 1 to 3 Years Is Likely

By WILLIAM L. LAURENCE

A vaccine against polio that has been used safely and successfully in preliminary trials on ninety children and adults, producing protective immunity bodies against all the three viruses causing the disease, was announced last night at a special meeting at the Waldorf-Astoria Hotel under the auspices of the National Foundation for Infantile Paralysis.

The vaccine was described by Dr. Jonas E. Salk, Professor of Research Bacteriology at the University of Pittsburgh, who headed the team of scientists in developing it with the aid of March of Dimes funds. A technical report by Dr. Salk and his associates appears in the issue of the *Journal of the American Medical Association* out today.

There are three types of polio virus, known as Brunhilde, Lansing and Leon. The vaccine has been found to provide protection against all three. In many cases, Dr. Salk reported, the quantity of antibodies (immunity factors) produced by the vaccine was greater than the number produced naturally in persons who had been exposed to one or more of the viruses.

Dr. Salk warned, however, that further experimentation would be required before the vaccine could be safely given to the general public.

## Precise Effectiveness Sought

"Although the results obtained in these studies can be regarded as encouraging," Dr. Salk said, "they should not be interpreted to indicate that a practical vaccine is now at hand.

"However, it does appear that at least one course of further investigation is clear. It will now be necessary to establish precisely the limits within which the effects here described can be reproduced with certainty."

In the medical journal he wrote:

"Because of the great importance of safety factors in studies of this kind, it must be remembered that considerable time is required for the preparation and study of each new batch of experimental vaccine before human inoculations can be considered.

"It is this consideration, above all else, that imposes a limitation on the speed with which this work can be extended. Within these intractable limits every effort is being made to acquire the necessary information that will permit the logical progression of these studies into larger numbers of individuals in specially selected groups."

## Discoveries Are Cumulative

These considerations indicate that it may take at least another year, and more likely two to three years, before the vaccine can be made available with safety for general use. There are about 46,000,000 in the United States, 1 to 19 years old, who may require vaccination.

The vaccine is the culmination of one of the greatest concentrated efforts in history. It was made possible by several important discoveries in recent years which, in turn, were made possible by the response of the public to the annual March of Dimes appeal.

One of these discoveries was the recognition that polio could be produced by three species of virus, instead of only one as had been believed, and that protection against one type would not provide protection against the other two.

Another major discovery was that the viruses could be grown on non-nervous tissue, either human or simian.

Another discovery was the fact that the polio viruses might be killed by formaldehyde so that they no longer could produce the disease while they still retained their ability to produce protective antibodies (immunity).

Finally, it was found that emulsification of the killed viruses with mineral oil greatly increased the powers of the vaccine to produce immunity agents.

## Process of Preparation

The vaccine is prepared by first growing the viruses of the three types separately in testicular or kidney tissue of the monkey. These are harvested by centrifugation, in which the viruses are separated from the monkey tissues and then killed with formalin.

After tests on animals to make certain that the viruses no longer can produce polio, they are prepared in the form of a mineral oil emulsion for experimental testing on carefully selected human subjects.

The first persons to participate in these studies were patients paralyzed in recent years by a polio infection, who were at D. T. Watson Home for Crippled Children at Leetsdale, Pa. Additional studies were undertaken at the Polk State School, Polk, Pa.

In all, ninety subjects were tested with the multiple emulsified vaccine for all three types while seventy-one others received a single-virus aqueous vaccine.

## Success with Emulsion

The tests disclosed that the emulsified vaccine produced antibodies within six weeks and that they were still present after four and a half months, with indications that they would last much longer. The aqueous vaccine was described as spotty, some developing antibodies, while others failed to do so.

Associated with Dr. Salk were Maj. Byron L. Bennett, retired, L. James Lewis, Elsie N. Ward, and J. S. Youngner.

Disease-forming organisms such as bacteria or viruses are known as antigens, that is, they stimulate the body's defensive mechanisms to produce agents to counteract them. These agents are known as antibodies. The immunity agents may last an individual for years, if not a lifetime, depending on the type of organism.

The presence of these immunity bodies in the blood of an individual is determined by taking a sample of the blood and testing it against any organism desired.

For example, a person's serum containing immunity bodies against contracting polio, either by having been exposed to the disease or as, the result of vaccination, would inactivate polio viruses in a test tube. Such inactivation could be determined by injecting the virus into a monkey and observing whether or not the animal contracted the disease.

*March 27, 1953*

# Smallpox Wiped Out in Its Worst Form

By LAWRENCE K. ALTMAN

The worst form of smallpox, the kind that kills, blinds and maims, has been eradicated, but a much milder form remains in Somalia on the horn of Africa, Dr. Halfdan Mahler, the head of the World Health Organization, said here today.

The last case of the most virulent form of smallpox, called variola major, occurred in Bangladesh in October 1975 in a 3-year-old girl, Rahima Banu. She survived her attack of the viral infection.

For the last two years, 12,000 Bangladesh health workers, aided by 100 W.H.O. and international staff workers, have made repeated house-to-house searches for additional, hidden cases. None were found.

And tomorrow a nine-member international commission of physicians will formally declare smallpox eradicated from Bangladesh.

"We have signed the death certificate of smallpox in Asia," Dr. Mahler said. That act leaves just the milder form in the horn of Africa.

## "A Day of Victory"

"Make no mistake about it, this is a day of victory," Dr. Mahler said from Dacca, Bangladesh, to reporters here. "It is here, on these densely populated plains, so often ravaged by flood, famine and war, that smallpox had its most ancient and tenacious roots."

Victory was accomplished by applying modern management and technological methods to the discovery of smallpox vaccination, which was made in the 18th century by the English physician Edward Jenner. The Geneva-based World Health Organization began its drive to eradicate smallpox from the world 10 years ago.

"To do within that remarkably short time what had not been done in more than a century is nothing short of a public health miracle," Dr. Mahler said.

The health organization has still not achieved total victory over smallpox because the African horn is still considered infected. More than 3,200 cases occurred in Somalia this year, but there have been none in the last seven weeks, Dr. Mahler said.

Dr. Donald A. Henderson, who formerly directed the smallpox program from Geneva and is now dean of the School of Public Health at Johns Hopkins University in Baltimore, said: "If anyone put up $1 million and asked to be shown a case of smallpox now, we would not be able to accept the $1 million."

## Too Early to Know

But Dr. Henderson and Dr. Mahler stressed that it was too early to know if the last case had been detected in the horn of Africa. Flooding and conditions in the war-affected area have added to the difficulties of searching for smallpox cases there now.

After the last case is detected, African health workers will spend two more years searching the area, as was done in Bangladesh and the dozens of other countries from which the disease was eradicated in the last decade, before an international commission declares the infection eradicated from the world.

Dr. Mahler said that before eradication of all forms of smallpox was declared the organization would require documentation from all member states, including those like China where the health organization did not conduct a program to eradicate smallpox.

"From all the signals we have, I have not the slightest doubt that we will be able to satisfy the most inquisitive kind of tribunal of scientists and public health administrators," he said.

## Huge Saving Foreseen

Dr. Henderson said that when total eradication was attained, there would be no need for smallpox vaccinations for anyone. That will save the world $2 billion each year, he added.

The United States and 15 other countries have already stopped routine vaccinations, and others are expected to follow shortly. Most smallpox vaccinations given to Americans now are given only to those who plan to travel.

Although World Health Organization member countries passed a resolution stating that requirements for smallpox vaccination certificates should be limited to people coming from countries where smallpox existed, such documents have been demanded of many people traveling between areas not affected by smallpox.

Dr. Henderson said that, according to international health regulations, the absence of smallpox cases in Somalia for the last seven weeks meant that "no country should request a smallpox vaccination certificate of any traveler coming from anyplace in the world."

He added, "This is the way it should be, but the wheels of bureaucracy move slowly, and it will take a little time for all travelers to travel freely without any worry about" smallpox vaccination certificates.

## Aid to Family Planning Seen

Dr. Mahler said that people in developing countries that have been freed from smallpox would gain confidence that their children would survive and that the quality of their lives would improve. As a result, he said, parents would be more accepting of family planning programs.

Dr. Henderson said that with the virulent form of smallpox now eradicated, the causative virus, variola major, was probably extinct in nature. It exists in test tubes in a few laboratories where scientists are tightening security to prevent accidental infections such as occurred in England a few years ago.

*December 14, 1977*

•

# Vaccine for Hepatitis B, Judged Highly Effective, Is Approved by F.D.A.

By HAROLD M. SCHMECK JR.

The Food and Drug Administration yesterday announced approval of the first vaccine against hepatitis to be licensed for use in the United States.

The vaccine required about 13 years of research and development. It has been judged highly effective in protecting against hepatitis B virus, a major cause of liver disease throughout the world.

Of the 200,000 to 300,000 new infections with the virus in the United States every year, an estimated 56,000 cases are serious enough to involve jaundice and other effects, such as nausea, fatigue and substantial liver damage. Roughly 10,000 hospitalizations and 200 deaths a year result.

Hepatitis B virus is considered a major public health problem in Africa and Asia and is believed to be a significant factor in liver cancer in those regions. Liver cancer accounts for 20 to 40 percent of all cancers in some regions of Africa and Asia.

In some Asian populations as many as 20 or even 50 percent of the population are carriers of the virus, according to Dr. Maurice R. Hilleman, vice president for virus and cell biology research of Merck Sharp & Dohme Research Laboratories, where the new vaccine was developed.

Because liver cancers in Asia seem closely linked to prior infection with the virus, some public health experts have speculated that widespread use of a vaccine against it would eventually bring about major reductions in the toll of liver cancer there. Liver cancer is relatively uncommon in the United States.

For the time being the new vaccine is expected to be too expensive for large-scale use anywhere. Dr. Hilleman said the vaccine's price was currently estimated at $75 to $120 for three injections given over six months. It is expected that the three doses will give protection for at least five years. Supplies of the vaccine will be available for general use by mid-1982, according to Merck Sharp & Dohme, which will market it as Heptavax-B.

Expense of the vaccine is said to be partly related to the complexity and length of time required for the production process. "This is the first completely new viral vaccine in 10 years and the first vaccine ever licensed in the United States that is made directly from human blood," said Dr. Arthur Hull Hayes Jr., Commissioner of Food and Drugs, in announcing the approval.

Dr. Hilleman said it takes about six months to isolate, purify and otherwise prepare the material for the vaccine from blood serum that contains the virus. After concentration and purification, six to seven months are required for testing in monkeys to demonstrate the product's safety and efficacy. Thus, a batch of the vaccine takes more than a year to prepare, the longest for any vaccine.

A different hepatitis B vaccine has been marketed in France since May. Experimental vaccines against the virus are reported in use in Japan and the Netherlands.

The illness produced by the hepatitis B virus was once called serum hepatitis because it was known to be passed through blood transfusions. Because of blood screening programs, hepatitis B virus is no longer a leading cause of serum hepatitis. Persons considered at high risk of infection today are medical workers, kidney dialysis patients and others who need frequent blood transfusions, as well as people in close contact with infected persons. It has been especially troublesome among drug addicts and persons with numerous sexual contacts.

At least two other kinds of virus-caused hepatitis are known. Hepatitis A, which used to be called infectious hepatitis, is caused by a virus that is passed through the human digestive tract and can be transmitted from person to person through the contamination of food, shellfish or utensils by human wastes. An experimental vaccine for that virus is under development, according to Dr. Hilleman. A third category of viral hepatitis is simply called "non-A, non-B," signifying that it is caused by one or more still unidentified viruses distinct from the first two. Hepatitis, which means inflammation of the liver, can also have causes other than virus infection.

The drug concern cited Dr. Hilleman and three associates, Dr. William J. McAleer, Dr. Arlene A. McLean and Dr. Eugene B. Buynak as leaders in the vaccine development project, which began in 1968.

Recent major trials of the vaccine have been done in about 6,000 persons and showed it to be about 95 percent effective, according to published reports.

*November 17, 1981*

# Medicine Timeline

**1858:** public health officials rail against "swill milk" that they say is poisoning children

**1865:** germ warfare terrorism in American cities—a doctor tries to spread yellow fever with infected bedding and clothing

**1866:** new code of health in New York requires reporting of infectious diseases, including smallpox

**1882:** Robert Koch finds the tuberculosis bacterium

**1893:** Caesarean operation performed

**1896:** X-rays discovered

**1897:** yellow fever epidemic in southern cities leads to quarantines

**1904:** X-rays said to cure a woman of breast cancer

**1908:** doctor claims to cure patients with a mix of toxins that act to stimulate immunity

**1912:** first cornea transplant

**1914:** surgery said to be the only cancer cure

**1914:** doctors say stomach ulcers may be infectious

**1915:** scientists treat diabetes by starving patients

**1916:** polio in New York said to have infected 10,000 and killed 2,500

**1918:** world's worst flu epidemic reaches United States

**1922:** insulin is discovered, used to treat diabetes

**1922:** laughing gas used as anesthesia during labor and delivery

**1937:** lobotomies said to cure mental illness

**1938:** Typhoid Mary dies of a stroke

**1940:** electroshock used to treat depression

**1940:** first measles vaccine

**1941:** penicillin discovered to be powerful antibiotic

**1942:** first blood pressure drug, chlorothiazide, found to be effective

**1943:** life insurance company issues tables of ideal heights and weights for men and women and says that as people go above those weights they are less healthy and their lives are shortened

**1945:** spinal block anesthesia used in labor and delivery

**1945:** new antibiotic, streptomycin, cures typhoid for the first time

**1947:** Nazi trials reveal medical experiments that horrify the world

**1950:** first kidney transplant

**1952:** first use of a heart-lung machine

**1952:** birth control pills found to prevent pregnancy

**1953:** Salk vaccine for polio can prevent the disease

**1953:** Watson and Crick announce structure of DNA, a double helix

**1955:** first schizophrenia drugs found effective

**1959:** drug for depression, Nardil, being tested

**1959:** U.S. Surgeon General says smoking and cancer are linked

**1962:** dialysis machine used to save lives of patients with kidney failure

**1962:** thalidomide's effects reported—babies being born with stumps for arms and legs

**1965:** first report of mammography finding cancers

**1965:** bariatric surgery helps obese people lose weight

**1965:** report on unethical medical studies in the United States shakes medical establishment

**1966:** obesity deemed a major health problem

**1968:** new category, brain death, proposed to enable organ donation for transplants

**1969:** first bypass surgery

**1971:** surgeons question mainstay of breast cancer treatment—radical mastectomy

**1972:** revelation that U.S. government left poor black men with syphilis untreated as part of a medical experiment in Tuskegee

**1974:** U.S. government issues rules for protection of human subjects

**1974:** colonoscopy used to view colon and remove polyps, which can be precursors of colon cancer

**1975:** CT scanner developed

**1977:** smallpox eradicated from the earth

**1978:** doctors in England report birth of first IVF baby

**1981:** first report of an unusual cancer in gay men; it will eventually become known as a symptom of AIDS

**1981:** discovery of cause of a cholesterol disorder—finding will lead to development of statins

**1981:** hepatitis B vaccine is approved by the F.D.A.

**1982:** a dentist, Barney Clark, receives first artificial heart

**1984:** AIDS virus isolated

**1984:** Australian researchers link bacterium to stomach ulcers

**1986:** first evidence that a drug, AZT, can help treat HIV

**1987:** first statin approved

**1990:** three years after it was introduced, Prozac becomes the most widely prescribed antidepressant

**1991:** gene mutation that causes Alzheimer's found—first opening to understand the disease

**1992:** a four-drug combination can kill bacteria causing stomach ulcers and cure almost all patients

**1993:** mammograms questioned for women under age 50

**1995:** mice genetically engineered to develop Alzheimer's—will allow testing of drugs and ideas of the disease's genesis

**1997:** first cloned mammal, the sheep named Dolly

**1997:** the 1918 flu virus is reconstructed from shards found in preserved tissue

**1998:** human embryonic stem cells isolated

**2000:** completion of mapping of human genome

**2001:** routine cancer screening tests questioned, issues of whether they are saving lives

**2004:** opening arteries with angioplasty and stents is found not to protect against heart attacks

**2005:** National Cancer Institute plans to sequence the genomes of the most common cancers

**2005:** lowest death rates among the overweight, not those of normal weight

**2005:** first face transplant

**2007:** scientists find a way to generate embryonic stem cells without using embryos

**2011:** Institute of Medicine says there is no link between vaccines and autism

**2012:** one in 88 American children said to have an autism spectrum disorder

**2012:** Human Microbiome project announces first results of study of the 100 trillion bacteria that live in people

**2014:** first Ebola cases treated in United States

# CONTRIBUTORS' BIOGRAPHIES

**Lawrence K. Altman, M.D.** is a longtime medical reporter for *The New York Times* who regularly writes The Doctor's Life column.

**Natalie Angier** is a Pulitzer Prize-winning science writer for *The New York Times* and author of several books, mostly recently *Woman: An Intimate Geography*.

**Homer Bigart** (1907–1991) was a two-time Pulitzer Prize-winning reporter and war correspondent for *The New York Times* and *The New York Herald Tribune*.

**Sandra Blakeslee**, a science writer who frequently contributes to *The New York Times*, is the author, most recently, of *Missing Microbes*.

**Jane E. Brody** writes the Personal Health column for *The New York Times* and is the author of numerous books on health and nutrition.

**Alan Cowell** is a senior *New York Times* foreign correspondent based in London.

**Leonard Engel** (1916–1964) was a contributor to many national magazines, including *The New York Times Magazine*, and author of several books on science.

**Lucy Freeman** (1916–2004) was a reporter and author whose early coverage of psychiatry and mental health for *The New York Times* led to wider coverage of the subjects.

**Erica Goode** is a national correspondent for *The New York Times*.

**Denise Grady** is a science reporter for *The New York Times* and the author of *Deadly Invaders*, a book about emerging viruses.

**Amy Harmon** is a domestic correspondent for *The New York Times* who won a Pulitzer Prize for her 2008 series, The DNA Age. She is also the author of the ebook *Asperger Love: Searching for Romance When You're Not Wired to Connect*.

**Gardiner Harris**, who has been a science reporter for *The New York Times*, is currently a foreign correspondent for the paper based in New Delhi.

**Emma Harrison** (1921–1970) was a *New York Times* reporter whose coverage of mental health news won several awards.

**Waldemar Kaempffert** (1877–1956) was a science writer and museum director who worked for *The New York Times* from 1922 to 1953.

**Gina Kolata** reports on science and medicine for *The New York Times*. A two-time Pulitzer Prize finalist, she is the author of several books, including *Flu: The Story of the Great Influenza Pandemic of 1918* and the *Search for the Search for the Virus That Caused It*.

**William L. Laurence** (1888–1977) was a science writer for *The New York Times* and winner of two Pulitzer Prizes.

**Steve Lohr**, a technology reporter for *The New York Times*, is the co-author of *U.S. vs. Microsoft* and author of *Digital Revolutionaries*.

**Richard D. Lyons** (1928–2013) was a reporter who covered science and medicine, as well as Congress and the United Nations, for *The New York Times*.

**Donald G. McNeil Jr.** is a reporter in the science department of *The New York Times*.

**Adam Nossiter** is the Dakar bureau chief of *The New York Times*.

**Norimitsu Onishi** is the Johannesburg bureau chief of *The New York Times*.

**John A. Osmundsen** is a former science reporter for *The New York Times* and the author of a number of books, including *Sweet Reason: On Life, Love and War in the Nuclear Age*.

**Robert K. Plumb** (1922–1972) was a reporter for *The New York Times* for 18 years and later wrote for *Medical World News*.

**Robert Reinhold** (1941–1996) was a science writer and national correspondent for *The New York Times*.

**Howard A. Rusk, M.D.** (1901–1989), whose specialized in the rehabilitation of the physically disabled, wrote a weekly column for *The New York Times* from 1946 to 1969.

**Emanie N. Sachs** (1894–1981), a novelist and biographer, also wrote for *The New York Times* and for a number of magazines.

**Harold M. Schmeck Jr.** (1923–2013) was a science writer for *The New York Times* who specialized in covering medical research.

**Dana Adams Schmidt** (1915–1994) was a *New York Times* foreign correspondent who covered Europe, North Africa and the Middle East.

**Craig S. Smith**, a former *New York Times* foreign correspondent and Shanghai bureau chief, is now managing director of *The Times*'s business operations in China.

**Michael Specter**, a former reporter for *The Washington Post* and *The New York Times*, is a staff writer for *The New Yorker.*

**Walter Sullivan** (1918–1996) was an award-winning science reporter and editor for *The New York Times.*

**M.A. Taft** (1861–1944) was a reporter for *The New York Times* for more than a quarter of a century who covered the early years of the women's suffrage movement, among other subjects.

**Van Buren Thorne, M.D.** (1870–1935) was on the staff of *The New York Times* for 30 years.

**Abraham Verghese** is the author of the novel *Cutting for Stone* and other books. He is a the Linda R. Meir and Joan F. Lane Provostial Professor at Stanford University and Vice Chair of the Department of Medicine.

**Nicholas Wade** is a former editorial writer, science reporter and editor for *The New York Times* and author, most recently, of *A Troublesome Inheritance: Genes, Race and Human History.*

# INDEX

Also available:

*The New York Times Book of Wine*
edited by Howard G. Goldberg, foreword by Eric Asimov

*The New York Times Book of Physics and Astronomy*
edited by Cornelia Dean, foreword by Neil deGrasse Tyson

*The New York Times Book of Mathematics*
edited by Gina Kolata, foreword by Paul Hoffman